Serono Symposia Publications from Raven Press
*Volume 46*

# HERPES AND PAPILLOMA VIRUSES

Their Role in the Carcinogenesis of the Lower Genital Tract - II

# Serono Symposia Publications from Raven Press

Serono Symposia Publications from Raven Press
*Volume 46*

# Herpes and Papilloma Viruses

Their Role in the Carcinogenesis of the Lower Genital Tract
Vol. II

Editors

### G. De Palo, M.D.
*Division of Diagnostic
Oncology and Out-patient Clinic
Istituto Nazionale Tumori
Milan, Italy*

### F. Rilke, M.D.
*Division of Pathology
Istituto Nazionale Tumori
Milan, Italy*

### H. zur Hausen, M.D.
*Deutsches Krebsforschungszentrum
Heidelberg, F.R.G.*

Raven Press ■ New York

**Raven Press, 1185 Avenue of the Americas, New York, New York 10036**

HERPES AND PAPILLOMA VIRUSES, vol. II
(Serono Symposia Publications from Raven Press; v. 46)

International Standard Book Number 0-88167-322-6
Library of Congress Catalog Number 87-043071

*Printed in Rome, Italy
by Christengraf*

# Preface

This volume contains the contributions of speakers invited to the Symposium held in Milan early in 1987, the second of a series on Herpes and Papilloma Viruses and their possible role in the carcinogenesis of the lower genital tract, in addition to other aspects of their pathogenicity.

Two years have passed since the first Symposium held in 1985, nevertheless a great deal of new information has become available in the meantime and, interestingly enough, many of the investigators who reported at the first meeting were now able to present either follow-up data or new observations on the same topic within a framework of conceptual continuity.

Two presentations, which are at same time position papers and state-of-the-art contributions, open the proceedings and come respectively from M.A. Epstein (UK) and H. zur Hausen (FRG). The first clarifies the present problems related to the anti EB-virus vaccination to prevent EB-virus-induced infectious mononucleosis and, perhaps, in the long run, nasopharyngeal carcinoma. The second paper reviews a timely topic of viral oncology which is the role of the some fifty plus types of papillomavirus in human cancer, not only of the lower genital tract, but also of other sites, including the skin and the respiratory tract.

The lack of tissue culture systems for the in vitro propagation of papillomaviruses has not inhibited major advances being achieved in molecular biology of these agents, particularly following the advent of recombinant DNA technology which has permitted the molecular cloning of a number of papillomavirus genomes. Three contributions, from the NCI (USA) by P.M. Howley, from the Istituto Nazionale Tumori (Italy) by G. Della Torre et al., and from the University of Ferrara (Italy) by D. Di Luca et al., actually deal with the molecular biology of papillomaviruses. These data have a counterpart in the elegant experiments of J.W. Kreider (USA) and associates, who describe further studies on the development of a model to test potential co-factors in cervical carcinogenesis.

A substantial number of the presentations deal with one of the most modern aspects of oncology, the application of molecular biologic investigations to clinical material by both extra-situm and in situ techniques. There are observations on head and neck tumors, tumors of the digestive tract and skin tumors reported by E.-M. de Villiers (FRG), on benign and malignant ano-genital tumors by R.S. Ostrow (USA) and co-workers, on the diagnostic applicability of in situ hybridization by K.V. Shah (USA) and associates, on the molecular mechanisms underlying the development of cervical cancer, including adenocarcinoma, by HPV 16 and 18 by Y. Tsunokawa (Japan) and her group, on the role of several HPV types in vulvar warty and neoplastic lesion by S. Pilotti (Italy), and on neoplasia of the male and female lower genital tract by K. Syrjanen (Finland), who also reported on the progression rates to real neoplasia of HPV-induced lesions. Progression, persistence and regression rates, as well as recurrences following eradication, were extensively related to the type of virus involved. Follow-up studies on an Italian population by G. De Palo at al. (Italy) showed a less pronounced tendency to progression of this type of lesion in the cervix uteri.

The feared outbreak of a dangerous increase of cancer of the uterine cervix in relation to the higher prevalence of sexually transmitted diseases, including HPV infections, is not supported by the body of information available to the Nordic Cancer Registries as reported by M. Hakama et al. (Finland). Nonetheless, to support adequately the epidemiologic hypothesis of there being an association between HPV infection and anogenital cancer, well designed studies seem to be essential and some of these are outlined by N. Munoz et al. from IARC.

Laryngeal papillomatosis is a well defined clinico-pathologic entity with viral etiology which may arise before or after puberty. It runs a benign course, with a few exceptions, and benefits nowadays from interferon therapy adjuvant to surgical treatment, as outlined by A. Bomholt (Denmark).

Four papers deal more specifically with herpes simplex virus. One, by B. Roizman et al. (USA) describes the HSV-1 transacting factors that operate early in infection, the second by C.A. Benson et al. (USA) gives a detailed account of the clinical manifestations and longterm sequelae of herpes virus infections, as well as of HPV infections. The third and fourth papers discuss present-day views on the therapeutic approaches, including an historical review of the topic, with a special reference to vaccines by G.D. Wilbanks et al. (USA) and topical interferon-beta treatment by M. Glezerman et al., respectively.

Finally a different point of view on pathogenesis of cervical carcinoma was discussed by B. Reid (Australia).

In conclusion, the wide spectrum of contributors working in the different areas of viral oncology provides a remarkably well documented insight into this rapidly moving area. The continuously changing scenario is best expressed by the considerable amount of data obtained over the last two years and presented in this publication. Particularly impressive is the progressive closing of the gap that used to exist between basic science and investigation in clinical medicine, epidemiology, pathology and allied applicative fields.

The Editors

# Acknowledgements

We wish to express our appreciation to the Members of the Scientific Committee who contributed in achieving the high scientific standard of the Symposium, to the distinguished Chairmen and Moderators (Prof. L. Carenza, Prof. G. Della Porta, Prof. G. De Thè, Prof. F. Dianzani, Prof. M. Ghione, Prof. G. Remotti) who ensured a smooth running of the Sessions and finally to Ares-Serono Symposia, for the cooperation and efficiency in publishing within a period of a few months the Proceedings of this International Symposium.

The Editors

# Contents

# Contributors

**C.A. Benson**
*Section of Infectious Disease*
*Department of Medicine*
*Rush Medical College*
*Rush-Presbyterian-St. Luke's*
*Medical Center*
*1753 West Congress Parkway*
*Chicago, Illinois 60612*
*USA*

**A. Bomholt**
*Ear, Nose and Throat Department*
*Roskilde Hospital*
*DK-4000 Roskilde*
*Denmark*

**F.X. Bosch**
*Unit of Field and Intervention Studies*
*International Agency for Research*
*on Cancer*
*150 cours Albert Thomas*
*69372 Lyon Cedex 08*
*France*

**L.F. Carson**
*Department of Obstetrics*
*and Gynecology*
*University of Minnesota*
*Minneapolis, Minnesota 55455*
*USA*

**E. Cassai**
*Institute of Microbiology*
*University of Ferrara*
*Via Borsari, 46*
*44100 Ferrara*
*Italy*

**B.A. Clark**
*Department of Obstetrics*
*and Gynecology*
*University of Minnesota*
*Minneapolis, Minnesota 55455*
*USA*

**P.O. De Campos Lima**
*Division of Experimental Oncology A*
*Istituto Nazionale Tumori*
*Via Venezian, 1*
*20133 Milan*
*Italy*

**G. Della Porta**
*Division of Experimental Oncology A*
*Istituto Nazionale Tumori*
*Via Venezian, 1*
*20133 Milan*
*Italy*

**G. Della Torre**
*Division of Experimental Oncology A*
*Istituto Nazionale Tumori*
*Via Venezian, 1*
*20133 Milan*
*Italy*

**M. Del Vecchio**
*Division of Medical Statistic*
*Istituto Nazionale Tumori*
*Via Venezian, 1*
*20133 Milan*
*Italy*

**G. De Palo**
*Division of Diagnostic Oncology*
*and Out-patient Clinic*
*Istituto Nazionale Tumori*
*Via Venezian, 1*
*20133 Milan*
*Italy*

**E-M. de Villiers**
*Referenzzentrum fur humanpathogene*
*Papillomviren*
*Deutsches Krebsforschungszentrum*
*Im Neuenheimer Feld 280*
*6900 Heidelberg*
*F.R.G.*

**D. Di Luca**
*Institute of Microbiology*
*University of Ferrara*
*Via Borsari, 46*
*44100 Ferrara*
*Italy*

**T. Doerner**
*InterYeda Ltd*
*Ness-Ziona*
*Israel*

**R. Donghi**
*Division of Experimental Oncology A*
*Istituto Nazionale Tumori*
*Via Venezian, 1*
*20133 Milan*
*Italy*

**M.A. Epstein**
*Nuffield Department of*
*Clinical Medicine*
*University of Oxford*
*John Radcliffe Hospital*
*Headington*
*Oxford OX3 9DU*
*U.K.*

**F. Falcetta**
*Division of Medical Statistic*
*Istituto Nazionale Tumori*
*Via Venezian, 1*
*20133 Milan*
*Italy*

**A.J. Faras**
*Department of Microbiology and*
*Institute of Human Genetics*
*University of Minnesota*
*Minneapolis*
*Minnesota 55455*
*USA*

**M. Glezerman**
*Soroka Medical Center*
*Beer-Sheva*
*Israel*

**J.W. Gupta**
*Department of Immunology*
*and Infectious Diseases*
*The Johns Hopkins School*
*of Hygiene and Public Health*
*615 N. Wolfe Street*
*Baltimore, MD 21205*
*USA*

**S.J. Gustafson**
*Department of Microbiology and*
*Institute of Human Genetics*
*University of Minnesota*
*Minneapolis, Minnesota 55455*
*USA*

**M. Hakama**
*Department of Public Health*
*University of Tampere*
*P.B. 607, SF-33101*
*Tampere*
*Finland*

**M.K. Howett**
*Departments of Pathology*
*and Microbiology*
*College of Medicine*
*The Milton S. Hershey Medical Center*
*The Pennsylvania State University*
*Hershey, Pennsylvania 17033*
*USA*

**P.M. Howley**
*Laboratory of Tumor Virus Biology*
*National Cancer Institute*
*Bethesda, Maryland 20892*
*USA*

**Y. Inagaki**
*Genetics Division*
*National Cancer Center*
*Research Institute*
*1-1, Tsukiji 5-chome,*
*Chuo-ku*
*Tokyo 104*
*Japan*

**B.E. Kloster**
*Institute of Human Genetics*
*University of Minnesota*
*Minneapolis, Minnesota 55455*
*USA*

**J.W. Kreider**
*Departments of Pathology*
*and Microbiology*
*College of Medicine*
*The Milton S. Hershey Medical Center*
*The Pennsylvania State University*
*Hershey, Pennsylvania 17033*
*USA*

**T.M. Kristie**
*Marjorie B. Kovler Viral*
*Oncology Laboratories*
*University of Chicago*
*910 East 58th Street*
*Chicago, Illinois 60637*
*USA*

**K. Louhivuori**
*Finland and Finnish Cancer*
*Registry Helsinki*
*Liisankatu 21*
*SF-00170 Helsinki*
*Finland*

**D.A. Manias**
*Department of Microbioloy and*
*Institute of Human Genetics*
*University of Minnesota*
*Minneapolis, Minnesota 55455*
*USA*

**J.L.C. McKnight**
*Marjorie B. Kovler Viral*
*Oncology Laboratories*
*University of Chicago*
*910 East 58th Street*
*Chicago, Illinois 60637*
*USA*

**N. Michael**
*Marjorie B. Kovler Viral*
*Oncology Laboratories*
*University of Chicago*
*910 East 58th Street*
*Chicago, Illinois 60637*
*USA*

**P. Monini**
*Institute of Microbiology*
*University of Ferrara*
*Via Borsari,46*
*44100 Ferrara*
*Italy*

**M. Movshovitz**
*Sheba Medical Center*
*Tel-Aviv*
*Israel*

**N. Munoz**
*Unit of Field and Intervention Studies*
*International Agency for Research on*
*Cancer*
*150 cours Albert Thomas*
*69372 Lyon Cedex 08*
*France*

**M. Muttini**
*Division of Experimental Oncology A*
*Istituto Nazionale Tumori*
*Via Venezian, 1*
*20133 Milan*
*Italy*

**S. Nozawa**
*Department of Obstetrics and*
*Gynecology*
*School of Medicine*
*Keio University*
*35 Shinanomachi*
*Shinjuku-ku*
*Tokyo 160*
*Japan*

**T. Okagaki**
*Department of Laboratory*
*Medicine and Pathology and*
*Department of Obstetrics and*
*Gynecology*
*University of Minnesota*
*Minneapolis, Minnesota 55455*
*USA*

**R.S. Ostrow**
*Department of Microbiology and*
*Institute of Human Genetics*
*University of Minnesota*
*Minneapolis, Minnesota 55455*
*USA*

**M.A. Pierotti**
*Division of Experimental Oncology A*
*Istituto Nazionale Tumori*
*Via Venezian, 1*
*20133 Milan*
*Italy*

**S. Pilotti**
*Division of Pathology and Cytology*
*Istituto Nazionale Tumori*
*Via Venezian, 1*
*20133 Milan*
*Italy*

**B.L. Reid**
*Queen Elizabeth II*
*Research Institute*
*for Mothers and Infants*
*The University of Sydney*
*Sydney 2006*
*Australia*

# Epstein-Barr Virus. Infection and Tumour Induction: Progress Towards Vaccine Control

## M.A. Epstein

*Nuffield Department of Clinical Medicine*
*University of Oxford, John Radcliffe Hospital,*
*Headington, Oxford, U.K.*

The Epstein–Barr (EB) virus was discovered in 1964 (16) in the course of sustained investigations designed to reveal an infectious agent aetiologically related to endemic Burkitt's lymphoma (BL)(5). Since that time an immense body of information has been accumulated on every aspect of EB virus from the epidemiological at one end of the spectrum to the molecular biological at the other (14,15), and constantly growing evidence indicates that the virus is an important link in a chain of events which ultimately leads to some forms of human cancer. Thus, many authorities now believe that EB virus is aetiologically related to BL, to undifferentiated nasopharyngeal carcinoma (NPC)(46), and to the malignant lymphomas seen with unusual frequency in immunodepressed individuals. Theories and counter-theories regarding the mode of action of the virus in the induction of these cancers have not yet finally been resolved (10,25,26) but it does seem generally agreed that the virus plays some essential causative role.

For many years considerable efforts have been devoted to the search for human cancer viruses (2) but it must not be forgotten that apart from the scientific interest of discovering such agents, there has also been the profoundly important longterm goal of cancer control by anti-viral vaccination. For, if a virus could be shown to cause a particular tumour, then the vaccine prevention of infection by the virus would theoretically lead to a decrease in the incidence of that cancer.

Against this background it was evident already by 1976 that the links between EB virus and both BL and NPC were so strong as to make it essential that an

anti-viral vaccine programme should be considered (12).
Although BL is not of great importance in world  cancer
terms NPC has long  been recognized as the most  common
tumour of men and the  second most common of women  for
very large  population  groups  including  all those  of
Southern Chinese  origin,  and  there  are  substantial
peoples amongst  whom the  tumour has a  less high  but
nevertheless significant incidence (46). When the  proposals for a vaccine against EB virus were put  forward
(12) attention was drawn  to the precedent provided  by
the anti-viral  vaccine control  of Marek's  lymphomas.
Marek's herpesvirus-induced disease of chickens (30,41)
became a serious  economic problem  with the advent  of
broiler-house and  battery poultry  farming because  of
huge losses from the  malignant lymphomas which  follow
infection, yet  these lymphomas  were virtually  eliminated when vaccines against Marek's disease herpesvirus
became available  (6,40).  Furthermore,  the  proposals
suggested the EB virus-determined membrane antigen (MA)
as immunogen since  antibodies to it  were known to  be
virus-neutralizing, and  pointed out  that supplies  of
the rare cotton-top tamarin (Saguinus oedipus  oedipus)
should be  secured because  this  small Columbian  non-
human primate was the only animal which regularly  gave
lesions after  experimental  infection with  the  virus
(32) and was then about to be placed on the  endangered
species list.

## DEVELOPMENT OF A PROTOTYPE SUBUNIT VACCINE
## AGAINST EB VIRUS

Work towards the elaboration of a vaccine against EB
virus gathered pace in the following years and culmina-
ted in  the recent  successful testing  of a  prototype
subunit preparation.  The aim  from the  outset was  to
base this on MA and experiments in several laboratories
demonstrated that this antigen complex consists of  two
immunologically related  large glycoprotein  components
with molecular weights of  340,000 and 270,000  daltons
(MA gp340 and gp270)  (reviewed in 13). The largest  of
these molecules was  selected for  work in the  present
programme, but the development  of an MA-based  vaccine
calls for  five essential  requirements,  and as  shown
below, each of these had to be provided.

### Test Animals: the Cotton-Top Tamarin

A colony of  tamarins was set  up and the  necessary
dietary, management,  and husbandry  conditions  for
breeding were worked  out (22-24).  But to ensure  that
the successful  breeding  led to  the build-up of  the
colony, only small numbers of animals could be used for
experiments in the early stages, the constraints  being

similar to those operating with hepatitis B virus where biological tests can only be done in chimpanzees (31). Because of the small numbers available it was essential that any dose of virus to be given as a challenge after vaccination would be capable of causing lesions in all unprotected animals. Such a dose was therefore devised and shown in numerous experiments to be 100% lymphoma-genic (17).

## Suitable MA gp340 Immunogens

To purify MA gp340 efficiently a sensitive test was needed for the antigen in order to monitor production methods, and a quantitative radioimmunoassay (RIA) (38) was elaborated. This RIA was used to perfect a separa-tion procedure based on molecular weight using sodium dodecyl sulphate polyacrylamide gel electrophoresis (SDS-PAGE) (34) and another dependent upon monoclonal antibody immunoaffinity chromatography (44). Although the RIA indicated that the latter readily yielded high amounts of gp340 it also made clear that the method collected less than half of the go340 epitopes.

Purified gp340 was found to have only a feeble capa-city to induce neutralizing antibodies when injected into animals, and immunogenicity had therefore to be enhanced. This was achieved by incorporating gp340 in artificial liposomes (39) in which the siting of the antigen resembles, at least to some extent, the natural arrangement in cell membranes.

## A Sensitive Assay for Antibodies to MA gp340

In order to exploit immunogenicity studies with various types of gp340 to the full, a highly sensitive test to quantitate antibody responses was required. Accordingly, a rapid enzyme-linked immunosorbent assay (ELISA) was developed based on the monoclonal antibody immunoaffinity chromatography-purified gp340 (43). This ELISA proved 1000 times more sensitive than conven-tional tests and enabled the sequential production of specific antibodies to gp340 to be followed accurately and quickly during the immunization of animals.

## VACCINE PROTECTION OF COTTON-TOP TAMARINS

As already explained, the present vaccine programme was guided by the assumption that procedures that worked with the herpesvirus of Marek's disease and its lymphomas would be applicable to EB virus (12), a seemingly oncogenic herpesvirus of man. Current Marek's disease vaccines make use of live apathogenic viruses (6,40) but earlier laboratory studies had shown that antigen-containing membranes from infected cells markedly reduced lymphoma incidence when used as an experimental vaccine (21) and that even soluble antigens from such cells also protected (27). The first and simplest step in the present experiments was to determine whether plasma membranes from EB virus-infected cells expressing MA could be used in a comparable manner.

## Protection with MA-Positive Cell Membranes

Plasma membranes were collected from cells showing maximum MA expression by sucrose density gradient centrifugation. Tamarins were immunized with the resulting material and serological responses were measured by indirect immunofluorescence, by the highly sensitive ELISA, and by virus neutralization tests (9,36). Satisfactory immunization was considered to have been achieved when the levels of neutralizing antibody equalled or exceeded the highest titres found in sera from naturally infected human subjects.

When the immunized tamarins were challenged with the 100% lymphomagenic dose of EB virus they remained entirely free of clinically detectable lesions in contrast to control animals inoculated at the same time.

## Protection with SDS-PAGE-Purified MA gp340

In both a first pilot experiment and in a confirmatory experiment, animals immunized with liposomal gp340 prepared by the molecular weight-based method were found to be protected against the 100% tumour-inducing dose of EB virus when their levels of neutralizing antibody were equal to or higher than those in the sera of naturally infected human subjects.

These experiments demonstrate that gp340 prepared by the SDS-PAGE method and incorporated in liposomes can be used as an efficient prototype subunit vaccine to protect experimental animals against tumour induction by a massive challenge dose by EB virus.

## Failure of Protection with
## Monoclonal Antibody-Purified MA gp340

gp340 from the immuno-affinity chromatography purification procedure also gave high titre antibodies in the tamarins. The neutralizing capacity of sera from these animals was the same as that of the tamarins successfully protected by vaccination with SDS-PAGE-purified material. Yet when challenge virus was administered in the usual dose all the immunized animals rapidly developed gross, multiple tumours (17).

It was known from the outset that the monoclonal antibody used only bound and collected about 50% of the MA epitopes (44) and this failure of the inoculated

product to induce full protection was not wholly un-
expected. What does surprise is the finding that powerful neutralizing antibodies elicited although not protective, were indistinguishable in the neutralization
tests from those which were. It is clear that the SDS-
PAGE purification method must isolate a component
important for protection which is not selected by the
monoclonal antibody. Current investigations of differences in the repertoire of immunological responses of
tamarins depending on which of the two types of immunogen they received seem likely to shed light on the
nature of the epitope(s) crucial for protection.

### DEVELOPMENT OF A VACCINE SUITABLE FOR MAN

In order to plan the development of subunit vaccines
against EB virus for human use the general structure of
the MA gp340 molecule was investigateed. gp340 was
analysed after treatment with various glucosidases and
V8 protease, with and without preliminary exposure to
tunicamycin during synthesis. The results showed that
carbohydrate represents more than 50% of the total mass
of the molecule, that gp340 is both 0- and N-linked,
that V8 protease fragments are antigenic, and that
specific antibody appears to bind the protein not the
sugar moiety (11,35). The major importance of the protein in the immunogenicity of gp340 makes it likely
that new and sophisticated procedures can be exploited
for vaccine development. In this connection it is also
important that the region of the EB virus genome coding
for MA has already been identified (20) and that the
nucleotide sequence is known (4).

### MA-Based Vaccines

Using the foregoing information and exploiting the
latest tools of biotechnology, the main directions in
which progress is being made, or might be made, are set
out in Table 1.
For subunit production in genetically engineered
cells the MA gene has been cloned and expressed in
cultures of E.coli (3), yeast, and three types of
mammalian cell, and efforts have been directed to the
extraction and purification of gp340 subunits from some
of the systems (Table 1 - 1).
As regards the use of genetically engineered viral
vectors (Table 1 - 2), the MA gp340 gene has been
inserted into a recombinant WR strain vaccinia virus
and has been expressed under the control of a vaccinia
virus promotor during replication of the recombinant
(29). Furthermore, antibodies induced in rabbits by the
recombinant vaccinia virus included some directed
against MA gp340 which neutralized EB virus in the

standard test (9,36). This vaccinia construct has been
shown significantly to protect cotton-top tamarins
against challenge with the standard 100% lymphomagenic
dose of EB virus, but the skin lesions induced by the

**TABLE 1.** Prospective Vaccines against EB Virus

---

1. Subunit production in genetically engineered cells

         bacterial
         yeast
         mammalian

2. Use of recombinant viral vectors

         vaccinia
         varicella

3. Synthetic subunit peptides

4. Attenuation of virulence by genetic manipulation

5. Use of novel adjuvants

         immunostimulating compounds (ISCOMS)
         muramyl dipeptide analogues

---

recombinant during intra-dermal vaccination of the
animals were extensive and severe. The WR strain of
vaccinia virus is a neurotropic laboratory strain
considerably more virulent than accepted vaccine
strains. When the experiments were repeated using a
recombinant based on the Wyeth vaccine strain of vaccinia virus, skin lesions in the tamarins were minimal
and no protection was induced. It would appear that
much further work will be required to develop an effective recombinant based on vaccinia virus suitable for
human use.
    In an analogous way the gp340 gene has quite re-
cently been incorporated into a varicella virus vector
(28) using from the outset the acceptable Oka vaccine
strain (47) to construct the recombinant (Table 1 - 2).
It will be of considerable interest to see how well
this novel engineered agent protects against EB virus
in vivo.
    Since the nucleotide sequence of the MA gene is
known (4) it should be feasible to prepare the relevant
peptides synthetically and use these as immunogens
(Table 1 - 3). However, success with this approach has
proved difficult to achieve with some other comparable

systems and many problems remain to be overcome.

A different type of genetic manipulation involves the induction of site-specific mutations to attenuate viral virulence (Table 1 - 4), but although some progress has been reported in this direction with small RNA viruses work with large DNA viruses is only just beginning (45).

Quite recently, MA gp340 has become available in considerable amounts and in a form sufficiently pure for use in man as a result of the application of fast protein liquid chromatography (7). This advance has provided material which can now be used in conjection with exciting new adjuvants designed to enhance immunogenicity (Table 1 - 5).

Immunostimulating compounds (ISCOMS) based on Quil A micelles (33) have already been shown to be capable of incorporating gp340 and newly introduced muramyl dipeptide analogues (1) are likewise being exploited.

## Strategies for Human Trials

An EB virus vaccine for use in man will be tested in three stages as soon as its efficacy has been fully established experimentally in tamarins. In the first phase, a small number of informed volunteers will receive the preparation to demonstrate its safety and capacity to induce neutralizing antibodies in those who have not been infected by the virus or to augment such antibodies in those who have been.

For second phase, studies will be undertaken in the context of EB virus-induced infectious mononucleosis (IM). Young adults who have escaped the usual silent primary EB virus infection of childhood can be readily detected and it is well-known that such individuals are at risk for delayed primary infection which is accompanied by the clinical manifestations of IM in 50% of cases (37). There are thus good grounds for applying such a screening programme to a group of university or college students and then undertaking a double-blind vaccine trial amongst volunteers who are sero-negative and hence have never been infected by the virus. The efficacy of the vaccine in preventing primary infection should be evident in a rather short time and there would be the added advantage that those who were successfully vaccinated would not have to face a possible attack of IM. Already at this stage, there are strong ethical reasons for administering even an unproven vaccine to the rare individuals at risk for developing the genetically determined X-linked lymphoproliferative (XLP) syndrome following primary EB virus infection, since this condition is invariably a very serious, often life-threatening, disease in affected males (42).

Once vaccine prevention of primary EB virus infection has been demonstrated with co-incidental protection against IM and the grave manifestations of XLP syndrome, the way would be open for the final phase of trials. For this, the vaccine would have to be deployed in an appropriate area where endemic BL has a high incidence. By definition, this will need to be in some developing country (5) and special considerations will thus arise. Primary EB virus infection occurs at a very early age in the social conditions and standards of hygiene of the third world (19) and vaccination would have to be carried out during the first months of life. Such a schedule is exactly comparable to that required for hepatitis B vaccination (8) and the logistics for an EB virus vaccine control against BL in the tropics are in no way more complicated. Since the peak age incidence for endemic BL is at about age 7 (5) the influence of EB virus vaccination should be apparent within ten years.

Anti-EB virus vaccination to prevent NPC, a tumour of later life (46), will be more difficult. Immunity will have to be maintained for many decades but even so, progress with a vaccine against EB virus is continuing so fast that what may appear daunting now is likely to prove possible sooner rather than later.

## REFERENCES

1. Allison, A.C., and Byars, N.E. (1986): J. Immunol. Methods, 95: 157-168.
2. Baker, C.G., Carrese, L.M., and Rauscher, F. (1966): In: Some recent developments in comparative medicine, edited by R.N.T-W-Fiennes, pp. 259-278. Academic Press Inc., London and New York.
3. Beisel, C., Tanner, J., Matsuo, T., Thorley-Lawson, D., Kezdy, F., amd Kieff, E. (1985): J. Virol., 54: 665-674.
4. Biggin, M., Farrel, P.J., and Barrell, B.G. (1984): EMBO J., 3: 1083-1090.
5. Burkitt, D. (1958): Br. J. Surg., 46: 218-223.
6. Churchill, A.E., Payne, L.N., and Chubb, R.C. (1969): Nature, 221: 744-747.
7. David, E.M., and Morgan, A.J. (1987): Rapid and efficient purification of Epstein-Barr virus membrane antigen gp340 by fast protein liquid chromatography (FPLC). Submitted to press.
8. Deinhardt, F., and Jilg, W. (1986): Ann. Inst. Pasteur Virol., 137E: 79-95.
9. De Schryver, A., Klein, G., Hewetson, J., Rocchi, G., Henle, W., Henle, G., Moss, D.J., and Pope, J.H. (1974): Int. J. Cancer, 13: 353-362.
10. Duesberg, P.H. (1985): Science, 228: 669-677.

11. Edson, C.M., and Thorley-Lawson, D.A. (1983): J. Virol., 46: 547-556.
12. Epstein, M.A. (1976): JNCI, 56: 697-700.
13. Epstein, M.A. (1984); Proc. R. Soc. Lond., 221: 1-20.
14. Epstein, M.A., and Achong, B.G., editors (1979): The Epstein-Barr virus. Springer, Berlin, Heidelberg and New York.
15. Epstein, M.A., and Achong, B.G., editors (1986): The Epstein-Barr virus: recent advances. Heinemann, London.
16. Epstein, M.A., Achong, B.G., and Barr, Y.M. (1964): Lancet, i: 702-703.
17. Epstein, M.A., Morgan, A.J., Finerty, S., Randle, B.J., and Kirkwood, J.K. (1985): Nature, 318: 287-289.
18. Epstein, M.A., Randle, B.J., Finerty, S., and Kirkwood, J.K. (1986): Clin. Exp. Immunol., 63: 485-490.
19. Henle, W., and Henle, G. (1969): East Afr. Med. J., 46: 402-406.
20. Hummel, M., Thorley-Lawson, D.A., and Kieff, E. (1984): J. Virol., 49: 413-417.
21. Kaaden, O.R., and Dietzschold, B. (1974): J. Gen. Virol., 25: 1-10.
22. Kirkwood, J.K. (1983): Primates, 24: 515-520.
23. Kirkwood, J.K., Epstein, M.A., and Terlecki, A.J. (1983): Lab. Animals, 17: 35-41.
24. Kirkwood, J.K., Epstein, M.A., Terlecki, A.J., and Underwood, S.J. (1985): Lab. Animals, 19: 269-272.
25. Klein, G. (1983): Cell, 32: 311-315.
26. Lenoir, G.M., and Bornkamm, G.W. (1987): In: Advances in Viral Oncology Series Vol. 7, edited by G. Klein, pp. 173-206. Raven Press, New York.
27. Lesnick, F., and Ross, S.J.N. (1975): Int. J. Cancer, 16: 153-163.
28. Lowe, R.S., Keller, P.M., Keech, B.J., Danison, A.G., Whang, Y., Morgan, A.J., Kieff, E., and Ellis, R.W. (1987): Varicella-zoster virus as a live vector for expression of foreign genes. Submitted to press.
29. Mackett, M., and Arrand, J.R. (1985): EMBO J., 4: 3229-3234.
30. Marek, J. (1907): Beutsch Tierarztl. Wschr., 15: 417-421.
31. Maynard, J.E., Berquist, K.R., Krushak, D.H., and Purcell, R.H. (1972): Nature, 237: 514-515.
32. Miller, G., Shope, T., Coope, D., Waters, L., Pagano, J., Bornkamm, G.W., and Henle, W. (1977): J. Exp., Med., 145: 948-967.
33. Morein, B., Sundquist, B., Hoglund, S., Dalsgaard K., and Osterhaus, A. (1984): Nature, 308: 457-

460.

34. Morgan, A.J., North, J.R., and Epstein, M.A. (1983): J. Gen. Virol., 64: 455-460.

35. Morgan, A.J., Smith, A.R., Barker, R.N., and Epstein, M.A., (1984): J. Gen. Virol., 65: 397-404.

36. Moss, D.J., and Pope, J.H. (1972): J. Gen. Virol., 17: 233-236.

37. Niederman, J.C., Evans, A.S., Subrahmanyan, L., and McCollum, R.W. (1970): N. Engl. J. Med., 282: 361-365.

38. North, J.R., Morgan, A.J., Thompson, J.L., and Epstein, M.A. (1982): J. Virol. Methods, 5: 55-65.

39. North, J.R., Morgan, A.J., Thompson, J.L., and Epstein, M.A. (1982): Proc. Natl. Acad. Sci. USA, 79: 7504-7508.

40. Okazaki, W., Purchase, H.G., and Burmester, B.R. (1970): Avian Dis., 14: 413-429.

41. Payne, L.N., Frazier, J.A., and Powell, P.C. (1976): In: International Review of Experimental Pathology, edited by G.W. Richter, and M.A. Epstein, pp. 59-154. Academic Press, New York, San Francisco, London.

42. Purtilo, D.T., editor (1984): Immune deficiency and cancer. Epstein-Barr virus and lymphoproliferative malignancies. Plenum Medical Book Co., New York and London.

43. Randle, B.J., and Epstein, M.A. (1984): J. Virol. Methods, 9: 201-208.

44. Randle, B.J., Morgan, A.J., Stripp, S.A., and Epstein, M.A. (1985): J. Immunol. Methods, 77: 25-36.

45. Roizman, B., and Jenkins, F.J. (1984): Science, 229: 1208-1214.

46. Shanmugaratnam, K. (1971): In: International Review of Experimental Pathology, edited by G.W. Richter, and M.A. Epstein, pp. 361-413. Academic Press, New York and London.

47. Takahashi, M., Otsuka, T., Okuno, Y., Asano, Y., Yazaki, T., and Isomura, S. (1974): Lancet, ii: 1288-1290.

# Papillomaviruses in Human Genital Cancer

## H. zur Hausen

*Deutsches Krebsforschungszentrum*
*Heidelberg, F.R.G.*

Human papillomaviruses represent a heterogeneous group (43). At present more than 50 distinct types of human papillomaviruses (HPV) have been analyzed. Probably this number will increase in the future.

Papillomaviruses reveal a very characteristic pattern in their infectious cycle: they appear to require the availability of cells still capable of dividing for successful infection. The uptake of viral DNA by such cells, usually exposed to the surface in micro-lesions of epiderm is or mucosa or at specific sites (e.g. the transition zone of the cervix) results in its episomal persistence. The persisting DNA stimulates enhanced proliferation. Its own independence replication appears to be blocked by host cell factors. During steps in differentiation and keratinization this cell-mediated block obviously is released, resulting in viral DNA replication, synthesis of structural proteins and the maturation of viral particles. Thus, the keratinized superficial layer of a wart containing infectious particles points to an underlying proliferating layer of cells haboring viral DNA which stimulates cell proliferation.

The dependence of particle maturation on specific stages of cell differentiation is probably the main reason for the present inability to propagate papillomaviruses in tissue colture. The analysis of their biological functions is further restricted by a remarkable host specifity with a pronounced preference of individual types for specific types of tissue. Thus, human papillomaviruses do not produce recognizable changes in animal hosts.

The DNA of several papillomavirus types has been sequenced. In contrast to polyoma-type viruses, transcripts are read from one strand only, revealing the same polarity. Several open reading frames (ORF) exist, 2 of them (L1 and L2) appear to code for structural proteins, a varying number of additional ORFs (E1 to

E8) contain information responsible for early functions
(25). E6 and E5 of bovine papillomaviruses apparently
code for transforming functions (27,35), E2 reveals
transactivating for the E6, E7 region (31) and E1, and
possibly also E7 somehow regulate the episomal state of
persisting papillomavirus DNA (20). Very little is
known of the proteins coded for by early ORFs. Their
expression in bacterial vector systems is presently
being explored.

## PAPILLOMAVIRUS INFECTIONS OF THE GENITAL TRACT

More than twelve types of papillomaviruses have been
isolated from the human genital tract (41). The majority of these types has only rarely been found in
genital tumors. The most prevalent types clearly are
HPV 6, 11, 16 and to a lesser extent 18 and HPV 33.

HPV 6 and 11 are closely related, 82% of their nucleotides are identical (6). These viruses are found in
typical genital warts (condylomata acuminata). In these
tumors HPV 6 is found in about 60%, HPV 11 in about
30%. Invasively growing, non-metastasizing giant condylomata have been described, frequently labelled as
Buschke-Lowenstein tumors. HPV 6 DNA was found in
almost all of such tumors so far analyzed, the only
exceptional one contained HPV 11 (4).

The histology of genital warts is characterized by
the exophytic papillary growth and the typical appearance of koilocytotic cells. The latter represent the
sites of viral DNA replication, protein synthesis and
particle maturation, thus being an expression of cytopathogenic changes induced by events leading to the
synthesis of infectious virus.

Although condylomatous changes are also noted upon
infections of the vaginal wall, most notably HPV 11
infections of cervical sites reveal a different pattern
(43). Colposcopically they are observed as flat dysplastic lesions which histologically show features of mild
dysplasias (cervical intraepithelial neoplasia, CIN-1),
usually with extensive koilocytosis.

HPV 6 and 11 infections are very rare at non-genital
epidermal sites. They occur, however, at low frequency,
at oral sites or within the respiratory tract (7). The
most frequent non-genital predilection site is infection of the vocal cords, resulting in laryngeal papillomatosis (13,22). This represents a serious clinical
condition, sometimes spreading into the bronchial
tract. Laryngeal papillomatosis occurs at higher frequency as a perinatal infection, most likely occurring
during delivery due to maternal genital warts. HPV 11
is found in this condition more often than HPV 6.

HPV 6 or 11 containing condylomatous proliferations
are occasionally found in the buccal mucosa, the lips,

or located directly on the tongue. The histology shows less koilocytotic changes, probably reflecting a substantially reduced virus production at these sites.

Recently a technique has been developed which permits the direct study of the causative role of papillomavirus infection in the induction of condylomatous proliferations (17). Inoculation of normal cervical tissue beneath the renal capsule of nude mice results in the development of cysts outlined at their inner surface by cervical epithelium. These cysts persist for several months. Infection of the cells with HPV 11 prior to inoculation results in dysplastic proliferations revealing extensive koilocytosis and, within the koilocytes, virus-specific antigens and particles.

In addition, tissue culture studies indicate the transforming potential of HPV 16 infections. Yasumoto et al. (36) were able to malignantly transform NIH 3T3 cells after HPV 16 DNA transfection. Genomic DNA obtained from an HPV 16 positive cervical cancer biopsy also transformed NIH 3T3 cells (34). The transformed cells contained HPV 16 DNA which was transcribed. More recently, Durst et al. (10) showed that transfection with HPV 16 DNA leads to immortalization of human foreskin epithelial cells. The immortalized cells revealed an aneuploid karyotype, contained integrated HPV 16 DNA and transcripts from the early region. The cells were non-tumorigenic in nude mice.

In HPV 16 and 18 infections, the macroscopic and microscopic pattern of the induced lesions differs markedly from that described for HPV 6 and 11. Most available data result from HPV 16-containing proliferations. This virus type is by far the most frequently HPV found in Bowenoid papulosis or genital Bowen's disease, which represent rather discrete and incospicuous looking white or redish plaques found at vulvar, penile and perianal sites (15). Their histology, however, reveals marked atypia and usually all characteristics of a carcinoma in situ. Spontaneous regression of these tumors does occur, although the majority of these lesions seem to persist for long periods of time, in many instances for years, and possibly for decades.

HPV 16 infections of the cervix are associated with marked atypia, changes characteristic for CIN II or CIN III and carcinoma in situ (5). Usually, little or no koilocytosis is noted in these proliferations, although in some biopsies an extensive koilocytosis may originate from simultaneous infections with additional HPV types.

Simultaneous infections with either HPV 6/11 or HPV 16 and 18 appear to be relatively frequent. A recent survey of smears analyzed from more than 10,000 women indicated the presence of both groups of viruses in about 12% of this population (8). More than 5% of these women revealed evidence of infections by more than one of these agents.

## PAPILLOMAVIRUSES IN ANOGENITAL CANCER

The original isolations of HPV 16 and HPV 18 DNA were both obtained from cervical cancer samples (3,11). Thus, it was of interest to analyze other tumor samples for the presence of HPV DNA. Up to now a large number (< 200) of cervical cancer biopsies and a limited number of penile and vulvar cancers have been analyzed (3,11,29). HPV 16 DNA is found in close to 50% of biopsies tested from various parts of the world. Individual results differ in the range between 30 and 80%. HPV 18 DNA is less frequently found. In our own studies the percentage of positive biopsies (including penile and vulvar cancer) comes close to 20%. In additional tumors, other types of papillomaviruses have been detected. In a few samples, HPV 11 DNA was detected (14); in others, more recently, HPV 31 (19), HPV 33 (1) and HPV 35 (Lorincz and Temple, personal communication) DNAs have been found. Approximately 80% of all of these biopsies contain specific types of HPV DNA. In the majority of the remaining tumors hybridization under conditions of low stringency discloses the presence of HPV-related, yet unidentified sequences, most likely due to the presence of new types of papillomaviruses. Thus, we encounter the regular presence of DNA from specific HPV types in cervical, vulvar and penile cancer.

Perianal and anal cancer have also been found to frequently contain HPV 16 DNA (2).

Metastatic tissue derived from cervical cancer usually contains HPV DNA in quantities similar to the primary tumor tissue.

A number of cell lines have been derived from cervical cancer, including HeLa cells. Southern blot analysis of these cells revealed the presence of HPV DNA in the majority of lines thus far tested (3,24,30,37). Interestingly, the otherwise rare HPV 18 DNA is present in most lines analyzed up to now, including HeLa cells. The copy number of HPV genomes in these cells differs considerably from about 1 genome copy in C4-1 cells (30) to up to 600 or more copies in the Caski line.

The availability of HPV-positive cell lines permitted a convenient testing for the state of the persisting HPV DNA. At least the vast majority of HPV DNA in these lines, but also HPV DNA in fresh biopsy samples from cervical cancer, contains integrated sequences. The integrated viral DNA is frequently amplified, usually involving the flanking host cell DNA. Some primary tumors contain, in addition to the integrated sequences, episomal viral DNA.

It is interesting to note that HPV 16-positive precursor lesions (cervical dysplasias and Bowenoid papulosis) seem to contain only episomal DNA (12). It therefore appears that malignant conversion is associated with a shift in the state of persisting viral DNA.

The persistence and chromosomal localization of viral DNA can be visualized by in situ hybridizations, most easily in the Caski line with a large number of viral genome copies. Several integration sites are evident from these studies, revealing high copy numbers for individual sites (21).

The integration pattern reveals some specifity (30). In most primary tumors, metastases - and in all positive cell lines tested so far, at least some of the viral DNA molecules - integrate within the E1-E2 open reading frames. This obviously disrupts an intragenomic regulation which has recently been reported by Spalholz and her associated (31) for bovine papillomavirus genomes.

The integrated viral DNA is transcribed in cell lines exclusively involving the E6-E7 open reading frames (30). In addition, fusion transcripts between E6-E7 and adjacent host cell sequences are formed. Their biological significance is at present unknown. Transcriptions from the same regions also appear to be a regular feature of primary tumors, although in some of them the transcriptional pattern appears to be more complicated.

The transcripts have been analyzed by c-DNA cloning, revealing exclusive transcription of the E6-E7 region with a peculiar splicing pattern within the E6 open reading frame (28). Since similar splicing sites do not exist in genital papillomaviruses infections with types not commonly associated with malignant tumors (HPV 6 or 11), this may point to a specific role of these events in the process of malignant conversion.

Sequencing of cDNA clones of HPV 18 transcripts in 3 cervical cancer lines revealed the existence of a small intron within the E6 open reading frame (28). The second E6 exon is read in a different reading frame resulting in a putative protein which shows some distant relationship to epidermal growth factor. It is interesting to note that the same splice donor and acceptor sites also exist in HPV 16 and 33 DNA, but are absent in HPV 6 and 11 DNA. It remains to be seen whether this has any functional significance.

The regularity of transcription in HPV positive cervical cancer cells and the consistent expression of the E6-E7 open reading frames suggest a role of this genetic activity in the maintenance of the transformed state. Integration of viral DNA within E1-E2 with a likely disruption of an intragenomic regulation may represent another event important for malignant conversion.

Recently some still somewhat preliminary studies further emphasize the role of HPV expression in the maintenance of the malignant phenotype.

Stanbridge and his co-workers (32) demonstrated that fusion of HeLa cells to normal human fibroblast or keratinocytes results in a suppression of the malignant phenotype. Loss of chromosomes from the non-transformed donor, apparently in particular of chromosome No. 11, leads to a reacquisition of malignant growth upon heterotransplantation into nude mice. Since HeLa cells express HPV 18 RNA, it was of obvious interest to analyze HPV 18 expression in the non-malignant HeLa hybrids as well as in their malignant revertants.

The data obtained thus far indicate that no remarkable differences exist in HPV 18 expression in HeLa cells, their hybrids with normal cells or in malignant revertants upon cultivation of these cells in tissue culture. Under these conditions also no differences are noted in clonability and growth in soft agar. Implantation of the cells in diffusable chambers into nude mice however significantly changes the pattern. Whereas HeLa cells and malignant revertants continue to express HPV 18 DNA under these conditions, a virtually complete block of HPV 18 expression became apparent in the non-malignant hybrid lines.

These initial experiments were obscured by the fact that mouse macrophages selectively invaded chambers containing the non-tumorigenic hybrid cells. Therefore attempts have been made to mimic the in vivo situation in vitro by adding a variety of factors to the tissue culture medium. Upon addition of retinoic acid or 5-azacytidin it has indeed been possible to selectively suppress HPV transcription in nontumorigenic hybrid cells without affecting c-myc, β-actin or ribosomal RNA transcription. In contrast, in parental HeLa cells or tumorigenic segregants obtained from non-tumorigenic hybrids no selective suppression of HPV transcription has been observed. Concomitantly, growth suppression was noted in the non-tumorigenic hybrids, whereas the tumorigenic segregants as well as the parental HeLa-cells were not influenced.

In vitro HPV 16-immortalized keratinocytes showed a similar pattern of suppression of HPV-transcription as non-tumorigenic hybrids. The repression of transcription can be inhibited by cycloheximide addition.

The interpretation of these data points to an intracellular control of HPV expression by cellular genes. These genes most likely are modified and functionally inactive in HeLa cells but are contributed to the hybrids by the normal donor. Obviously, they are not expressed in tissue culture but require their activation by a putative humoral factor. This occurs upon heterotransplantation to the nude mouse.

These data, if confirmed for other human tumor cell lines, support a concept viewing the development of human cancer as a failing host cell control of persisting viral genes (38,39). The model derived therefrom can readily explain the frequently observed synergism between papillomavirus infections and initiating events (40). Initiators should interact by modifying cellular control functions or the binding sites recognized by the cellular suppressing factor within the viral genome.

Factors modifying cellular genes in the development of genital cancer are presently poorly defined. Smoking, viral inections with initiating properties (e.g. herpes simplex virus and cytomegalovirus), potentially mutagenic metabolites in chronic inflammations should be of particular risk for cervical sites and are probably much less active at external genital sites. This could account for the much higher risk of cervical cancer in comparison to vulvar and penile cancer and for a different age distribution of the latter in comparison to cancer of the cervix.

The data suggest the existence of an intracellular surveillance mechanism which controls papillomavirus infections. It may have far reaching implications for other human tumor virus infections as well, possibly controlled by a similar mechanism. This could represent an ancestral defense mechanism, preceding immunological control functions, protecting the host at the cellular level against potentially lethal functions of co-evolving viruses. The expression of these viral functions in differentiating cells which are unable to proliferate permitting now replication and maturation of the respective papillomaviruses, points to a fine tuning of host-virus and virus-host adaptions.

Cancer as a result of a failing host cell control of persisting viral genes could readily explain long latency periods between primary infections of cancer-linked viruses and tumor appearance. It also provides a convenient explanation why only a small number of infected individuals develops the respective cancer type. Since besides a persisting viral genome modifications in both alleles of suppressing genes are required, monoclonality of the arising tumor can be predicted.

## PAPILLOMAVIRUS DNA IN NON-GENITAL CANCER

Specific types of papillomaviruses, most notably HPV 5, have been detected in squamous cell carcinomas of patients with a rare condition, epidermodysplasia verruciformis (23).

Our own group became interested in the presence of papillomavirus DNA in carcinoma of the human respiratory tract and the oral mucosa. Since papillomavirus infections seem to interact synergistically with chemical or physical carcinogens in carcinoma development (38,40), human tumors clearly linked etiologically to chemical factors (smoking) like laryngeal and lung cancers were the primary target for this investigation. The analysis of more than 100 individual cancer biopsies indeed led to the identification of HPV-positive carcinomas which are listed in Table 1. It is interesting to note that 5 of these tumors contained HPV-16 sequence, demonstrating that this type of infection also occurs at extragenital sites, leading again to a remarkable association with malignant growth.

**TABLE 1.** HPV DNA in Cancer of the Oral Mucosa
and the Respiratory Tract

| HPV-Type | Site of Cancer | References |
|----------|----------------|-----------|
| HPV - 11 | Buccal mucosa | 18 |
| HPV - 16 | Buccal mucosa | 18 |
| HPV - 2 | Tongue | 9 |
| HPV - 16 | Tongue | 9 |
| HPV - 16 | Tongue | 9 |
| HPV - 16 | Larynx | 26 |
| HPV - 30 | Larynx | 16 |
| HPV - 16 | Lung | 33 |

Some rather preliminary data point to the existence of additional, yet not fully characterized HPV types in other laryngeal and lung carcinomas. The availability of some HPV-containing carcinomas derived from this region provides an encouraging baseline for the concept that carcinomas of the oral mucosa and the respiratory tract may originate from an interaction of cells persistently infected by specific HPV types and environmental chemical factors. This, in addition, would open a new pathway for strategies in preventing very common types of human cancers.

## REFERENCES

1. Beaudenon, S., Kremsdorf, D., Croissant, O., Jablonska, S., Wain-Hobson, S., and Orth, G. (1986): Nature, 321: 246-249.
2. Beckmann, A.M., Daling, J.R., and McDougall, J.K. (1985): J. Cell Biochem. Suppl., 9c: 68.
3. Boshart, M., Gissmann, L., Ikenberg, H.,

Kleinheinz, A., Scheurlen, W., and zur Hausen, H. (1984): EMBO J., 3: 1151–1157.

4. Boshart, M., and zur Hausen H. (1986): J. Virol., 58: 963–966.
5. Crum, C.P., Mitao, M., Levine, R.U., and Silverstein, S. (1985): J. Virol., 54: 675–681.
6. Dartmann, K., Schwarz, E., Gissmann, L., and zur Hausen, H. (1986): Virology, 151: 124–130.
7. de Villiers, E.M., Neumann, C., Le, J.Y., Weidauer, H., and zur Hausen, H. (1986): Med. Microbiol. Immunol., 174: 287–294.
8. de Villiers, E.M., Wagner, D., Schneider, A., Wesch, H., Miklaw, H., Wahrendorf, J., Papendick, U., and zur Hausen, H. (1987): Lancet (in press).
9. de Villiers, E.M., Weidauer, H., Otto, H., and zur Hausen, H. (1985): Int. J. Cancer, 36: 575–579.
10. Durst, M., Dzarlieva-Petrusevzka, R.T., Boukamp, P., Fusenig, N., and Gissmann, L. (1987): Oncogene (in press).
11. Durst, M., Gissmann, L., Ikenberg, H., and zur Hausen, H. (1983): Proc. Natl. Acad. Sci. USA, 80: 3812–3815.
12. Durst, M., Kleinheinz, A., Hotz, M., and Gissmann, L. (1985): J. Gen. Virol., 66: 1515–1522.
13. Gissmann, L., Diehl, V., Schultz-Coulon, H.J., and zur Hausen H. (1982): J. Virol., 44: 393–400.
14. Gissmann, L., Wolnik, H., Ikenberg, H., Koldovsky, U., Schnurch, H.G., and zur Hausen, H. (1983): Proc. Natl. Acad. Sci. USA, 80: 560–563.
15. Ikenberg, H., Gissmann, L., Gross, G., Grussendorf, E.I., and zur Hausen, H. (1983): Int. J. Cancer, 32: 563–565.
16. Kahn, T., Schwarz, E., and zur Hausen, H. (1986): Int. J. Cancer, 37: 61–65.
17. Kreider, J.W., Howett, M.K., Wolfe, S.A., Bartlett, G.L., Zaino, R.J., Sedlacek, T.V., and Mortel, R. (1985): Nature, 317: 639–641.
18. Loning, T., Ikenberg, H., Becker, J., Gissmann, L., Hoepfer, I., and zur Hausen, H. (1985): J. Invest. Dermatol., 84: 417–420.
19. Lorincz, A.T., Lancaster, W.D., and Temple, G.F. (1985): J. Cell Biochem., Suppl. 9c: 75.
20. Lusky, M., and Botchan, M.R. (1984): Cell, 36: 391–401.
21. Mincheva, A., Gissmann, L., and zur Hausen, H. (1986): Med. Microbiol. Immunol. (in press).
22. Mounts, P., Shah, K.V., and Kashima, H. (1982): Proc. Natl. Acad. Sci. USA, 79: 5425–5429.
23. Orth, G., Favre, M., Breitburd, F., Croissant, O., Jablonska, S., Obalek, M., Jarzabek-Chrozelska, M., and Rzesa, G. (1980): In: Viruses in Naturally Occurring Cancers, edited by Essex, M., Todaro, G., and zur Hausen, H., pp. 259–282. Cold

Spring Harbor Lab. Press, Cold Spring Harbor, N.Y.

24. Peter, M.M., and Pater, A. (1985): Virology, 145: 313-318.
25. Pfister, H. (1984): Rev. Physiol. Biochem. Pharmacol., 99: 111-181.
26. Scheurlen, W., Stremlau, A., Gissmann, L., Hohn, D., Zehner, H.P., and zur Hausen, H. (1986): Int. J. Cancer (in press).
27. Schiller, J.T., Vaas W.C., and Lowry, D.R. (1984): Proc. Natl. Acad. Sci. USA, 82: 7880-7884.
28. Schneider-Gaedicke, A., and Schwarz, E. (1986): EMBO J., 5: 2285-2292.
29. Scholl, S.M., Pillers, E.M., Robinson, R.E., and Farrell, P.J. (1985): Int. J. Cancer, 35: 215-218.
30. Schwarz, E., Freese, U.K., Gissmann, L., Mayer, W., Roggenbuck, B., Stremlau, A., and zur Hausen, H. (1985): Nature, 314: 111-114.
31. Spalholz, B.A., Yang, Y.C., and Howley, P.M. (1985): Cell, 42: 183-191.
32. Stanbridge, E.J., Der, C.J., Doersen, C.J., Nishimi, R.Y., Peehl, D.M., Weissman, B.E., and Wilkinson, J.E. (1982): Science, 215: 252-259.
33. Stremlau, A., Gissmann, L., Ikenberg, H., Stark, M., Bannasch, P., and zur Hausen, H. (1985): Cancer, 55: 737-740.
34. Tsunokawa, Y., Takebe, N., Kasamatsu, T., Terada, M., and Sugimura, T. (1986): Proc. Natl. Acad. Sci. USA, 83: 2200-2203.
35. Yang, Y.C., Okayama, H., and Howley, P.M. (1985): Proc. Natl. Acad. Sci. USA, 82: 1030-1034.
36. Yasumoto, S., Burkhardt, A.L., Doniger, J., and DiPaolo, J.A. (1986): J. Virol., 57: 572-577.
37. Yee, C., Krishnan-Howlett, I., Baker, C.C., Schlegel, R., and Howley, P.M. (1985): Am. J. Pathol., 119: 361-366.
38. zur Hausen, H. (1977): Curr. Top. Microbiol. Immunol., 78: 1-30.
39. zur Hausen, H. (1980): In: Adv. Cancer Res., edited by Klein, G., and Weinhouse, S., Vol. 33, pp. 77-107.
40. zur Hausen, H. (1982): Lancet, ii: 1370-1372.
41. zur Hausen, H. (1986): Int. Med., 7: 66-79.
42. zur Hausen, H. (1986): Lancet, ii: 489-491.
43. zur Hausen, H., and Schneider, A. (1986): In: The Papillomaviruses, edited by Howley, P.M., and Salzmann, N.P. (in press).

# The Trans-Activation of Viral Gene Expression in Herpes Simplex Virus Infected Cells

B. Roizman, T.M. Kristie, N. Michael, J.L.C. McKnight, P. Mavromara-Nazos and D. Spector

*Marjorie B. Kovler Viral Oncology Laboratories,*
*University of Chicago, Chicago, Illinois, USA*

The herpes simplex virus (HSV) gene expression is tightly regulated at the transcriptional and post transcriptional levels. The genes identified and studied to date form 5 groups designated as $\alpha$, $\beta 1$, $\beta 2$, $\gamma 1$ and $\gamma 2$ whose expression is coordinately regulated and sequentially ordered in a cascade fashion (17). At least 3 viral trans-inducing regulatory proteins have been identified. These are the $\alpha$ gene trans-inducing factor ($\alpha$TIF), a virion protein which induces $\alpha$ genes after infection (3), the major regulatory protein $\alpha 4$ which appears to regulate all viral genes, either or both positively and negatively (18), and the $\alpha 0$ gene whose function as a promiscuous viral trans-acting factor has been demonstrated in transient expression systems only (11,14,31,38).

Interest in HSV trans-acting regulatory proteins stems from three considerations. Foremost, understanding of the mechanisms by which HSV regulates its gene expression is key to the understanding of viral pathogenesis in humans. HSV gene regulation is also an important model of eukaryotic gene regulation inasmuch as for at least two of the three trans-acting factors both the sequence of the gene and of the cis site required to effect the trans-activation are known (6, 12,23,25,32, 40). Equally important, the ecological niche of human HSV infections, i.e., the oral and genital tracts, is also the site of latent infections with the members of the human papillomavirus group found in association with certain cancers. In this instance, the key question is whether HSV trans-acting factors are responsible for the trans-activation of transforming papillomavirus genes that might be responsible for the genesis of the cancers with which they are associated. This paper shall address itself to the two best known HSV trans-acting factors, αTIF and α4, and the cis sites required for their function.

## αTIF AND ITS CIS SITE

### αTIF

The operational definition of α TIF is that it is capable of inducing the transcription of the α genes in the absence of de novo viral or host cell protein synthesis (3,44). The protein, approximately 64,000 in apparent molecular weight (6,40), is packaged in the tegument, i.e. between the capsid and the envelope, in approximately 500 to 1,000 copies per virion (15). The αTIF gene has been mapped and sequenced (6,40); the gene is not spliced and its coding domain does not appear to overlap with that of other genes (Fig. 1). Attempts to delete the gene have not been successful and the data suggest that it might be essential (unpublished observations). The function of αTIF in transient expression systems appears to be affected by the products of two genes mapping 3' to αTIF (35); their role in the induction by αTIF in natural infections is not known. Although α genes are expressed in eukaryotic cultured cells in the absence of αTIF, the level of expression is significantly lower than that in its presence (21,44).

### αTIC Sequence

Activation of α genes by αTIF requires that the promoter regulatory domain contain one or more homologs of a sequence designated as the α trans-induction cis (αTIC) site (24,25,30,47). αTIC is present in the domains of all α genes in one (α27) to three (α0) copies per gene (19, 30). DNA fragments containing the consensus sequence 5'-GyATGnTAATGArATTCyTTGnGGG-3' (Table 1) are capable of conferring αTIF-dependent regulation upon a chimeric α promoter-thymidine kinase gene (21, 29,33,44). αTIC is partially homologous to some viral enhancer elements (19,26).

### Host Proteins Bind to the α-TIC Sites of HSV-1 α Genes

αTIF does not bind to its cis site. In DNA bandshift assays, DNA fragments containing the αTIC sites of α0, α4 and α27 genes form several major DNA - protein complexes with nuclear extracts from either HSV-1 infected or mock infected cells (20,24,25). The major complexes formed by mock-infected nuclear extracts were not significantly different from those formed by infected cell extracts.

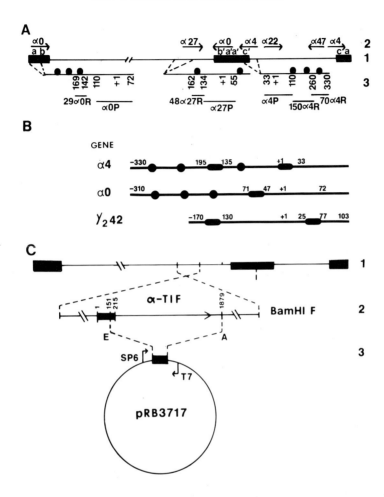

**FIG. 1.** Panel A, line 1: schematic diagram of the HSV-1 genome. The thin lines represent unique sequences. The filled rectangles represent the terminal sequences **ab** and **ca** repeated internally in an inverted orientation as **b'a'a'c'** (50); line 2: the arrows indicate the location and direction of transcription of the 5 α genes, 4, 0, 27, 22, and 47 (51); line 3: the promoter domains of the α4, α0, and α27 genes are expanded to show the location of the DNA fragments used in these studies (19–25, 34,35). Circles indicate the locations of the αTIC site homologs. Panel B. The mapped locations of the α4 (ovals) and αH1, αH2–αH3 (circles) binding sites in α4, α0, and $\gamma_2$42 gene (19, 20,22–25, 55 and work in progress). The nucleotides are numbered relative to the transcription initiation site (+1). Panel C, line 1: the location of the BamH1 F fragment containing the αTIF coding sequences; line 2: expanded map of the BamH1 F

fragment. The ATG codon is at nucleotide +215 (40); line 3: structure of the pGEM-1 derived plasmid, pRB3717, used for in vitro transcription of αTIF RNA under the control of the bacteriophage SP6 promoter (34).

**TABLE 1.** Summary of the Results of Analyses of the αH1, αH2-αH3 Binding Sites in the Promoter Domains of the α0, α27, and α4 Genes[a]

α - T I C  C o n s e n s u s:        GyATGnTAATGArATTCyTTGnGGG        NC

T e s t   h o m o l o g s :

                48α27R            ATATGCTAATTAAATACATGCCACG
              150α4R-1           CGTGCATAATGGAATTCCGTTCGGG
              150α4R-2           GGGCGGTAATGAGATGCCATGCGGG
                70α4R            GCATGCTAACGAGGAACGGGCAGGG
                29α0R            GCATGCTAATGATATTCTTTGGGGG

B i n d i n g   s i t e s:

                                                    *  * **
48α27R-αH1      cggaagcggaacggtgtatgtGATATGCTAATTAAATACATGccacgtgg      NC

               gccttcgccttgccacATACACTATACGATTAATTTAtgtacggtgcacc      C
                                 * **  *

                                                        *  *  *  *
48α27R-αH2/3   cggaagc●●●●●●●●●●●●●●atgtgatatgctaattAAATACATGCCACGTGG      NC
                       gggaacggtgt

               gccttcgccttgccacatacactatacgattaATTTATGTACGGTGCACC      C
                                                          ** * *
29α0R-αH1                       * * *  **
               ccgtGCATGCTAATGATATTCTTtggggg      NC

               ggcACGTACGATTACTATAAGaaacccccc      C
               * **  *

[a] The top line shows the consensus sequence of the αTIC sites of the HSV-1 α genes. The list below the consensus sequence includes the nucleotide sequence of the αTIC homologs of the α4, α0 and α27 genes. The large letters identify the purines whose methylation interferes with the binding of the respective proteins. The intermediate size letters show the domains protected from DNase 1 digestion. The circles indicate a sequence motif that is homologous to the immunoglobulin gene enhancer element. NC - non coding strand; C - coding strand; Y - pyrimidine; R - purine; N - any nucleotide (20,24,25).

The major complexes designated as αH1 and αH2-αH3 were formed by all fragments tested that contain complete αTIC sites. αH1 can be readily differentiated from αH2-αH3 complexes by their electrophoretic mobility, and by competition with synthetic polymers (24,25). The syntheti polymers poly(dA)·poly(dT) or poly(dAdT)· poly(dAdT), readily compete with the probe DNA for αH1 whereas poly(dI)·poly(dC) or poly(dIdC)·poly(dIdC) compete with the probe DNA for the αH2-αH3 proteins (Fig. 2). The host proteins forming the αH1 complex were readily separated from those forming the αH2-αH3 complex by chromatographic fractionation on a variety of substrates including DNA cellulose (Fig. 3), heparin agarose, an DEAE-sepharose suggesting that they are common components of the host repertoire of DNA binding proteins (25). We have not been able to separate the αH2 from the αH3 proteins by any of the procedures tested. Competition studies indicated that an αH1 protein binding site is present in the SV40 72bp enhancer element whereas in an αH2-αH3 protein binding site is present in the metallothionein promoter (-152 to +64) domain (20,24).

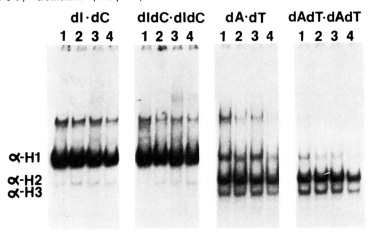

**FIG. 2.** Autoradiographic image of DNA protein complexes formed by labeled 48α27R DNA fragments reacted with HeLa cell nuclear protein extract in the presence of increasing amounts of synthetic DNA polymers and them electrophoretically separated in non denaturing polyacrylamide gels. The polymers (dI.dC, dIdC.dIdC, dA.dT, or dAdT.dAdT) were present in the following concentrations in the reaction mixtures: lane 1, 1.3 µg; lane 2, 2.6 µg; lane 3, 3.9 µg; lane 4, 5.2 µg. The position of the DNA-protein complexes are indicated as αH1, αH2, and αH3. The experimental protocol is described in detail elsewhere (22-24).

## The Binding Sites of αH1 and αH2-αH3 Proteins

DNase 1 protection studies on a 29 bp fragment from the α0 gene containing an αTIC site (29α0R) and on a 48 bp fragment containing the single αTIC sequence of the α27 gene (48α27R) showed that αH1 protected most of the sequence of the αTIC sites. The αH2-αH3 protected the 3' domain of the 48α27R fragment. The DNase protection footprints of the αH1 and αH2-αH3 proteins overlapped by approximately 8 to 9 nucleotides (24,25). Examples of the methylation interference and DNase protection studies are shown in Fig. 4.

The methylation interference studies indicated that

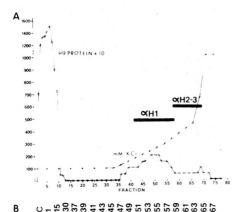

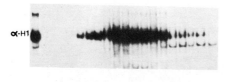

p(dI)·p(dC)

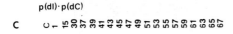

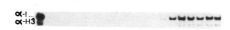

p(dAdT)·p(dAdT)

FIG. 3. Separation of αH1 and αH2-3 proteins by chromatography on DNA-cellulose. Panel A: the elution profile of the proteins. The fractions containing the peak activities of the αH1 and αH2-3 proteins are indicated by the filled bars. Panel B: autoradiographic images of the electrophoretically separated complexes formed in the presence of poly(dI).poly(dC) between labeled 48α27R DNA probe and αH1 proteins from selected DNA cellulose chromatographic fractions. Panel C: electrophoretically separated complexes formed in the presence of poly(dAdT).poly(dAdT) between the labeled DNA probe and the αH2-αH3 proteins in the chromatographic fractions (24,25). The lanes designated as C contain the complex formed by labeled probe with proteins in crude HeLa cell nuclear extract in the presence of the respective synthetic polymer.

the purines whose methylation interfered with the binding of αH1 are located at the 5′ end of the αTIC sequence and are adenine rich (Table 1 and Fig.4). Conversely, the purines whose methylation interfered with the binding of the αH2-αH3 are mostly guanines located at the 3′ terminus of the αTIC homolog. The dominant motif of the αH1 binding sites in the several αTIC sites tested is the sequence **GCATGCTAAT** whereas that of the αH2-αH3 protein in the αTIC sequence of the α27 gene is **ACGTGGCATGC** (24,25). As illustrated in Fig. 4, consistent with the failure to separate αH2 and αH3, their DNase 1 protection and methylation interference footprints determined from the individual DNA - protein complexes excised from non denaturing polyacrylamide

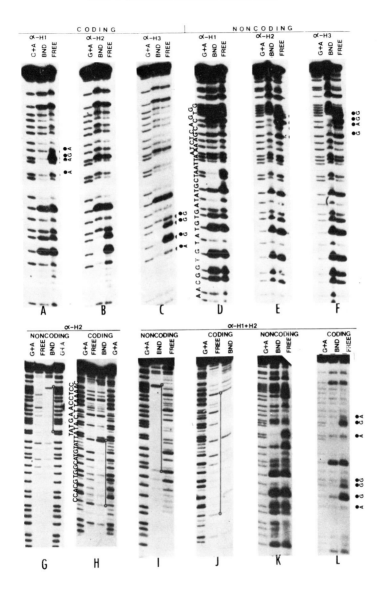

**FIG. 4.** Analyses of the αH1 and αH2-αH3 binding sites in the 48 α27R DNA fragment by methylation interference and DNase 1 protection assays. Panels A and D, B and E, C and F: the positions of the methylated purines which preclude the binding of αH1, αH2, and αH3 respectively on the coding and noncoding strands. Panels G and H: DNA sequences protected from DNase 1 digestion by αH2 on the coding and non coding strands. Panels I and J: the position of DNA sequences protected from DNase 1 digestion by a reconstituted mixture of αH1 and αH2-αH3

proteins. Panels K and L: the positions of the methylated
purines which precluded the binding of a reconstituted mixture
of αH1 and αH2-αH3. The position of interfering methylated
purines is shown by solid circles. The domains protected from
DNase 1 digestion are indicated by the vertical lines (25).

gels appeared to be identical (25). Therefore, these
proteins may differ only with respect to post transla-
tional modifications.

In addition to the αH1 and αH2-αH3 binding sites,
the 48α27R fragment also contains a sequence element,
the GA tract, which bears a strong homology to the
immunoglobulin enhancer element characterized in vivo
by Church et al. (7) and in vitro by Sen and Baltimore
(53). Homologs of this sequence are also present within
the promoter domains of the α4 and α0 genes and have
been implicated in the basal level expression of these
genes (5).

### The Molecular Properties of αH1 and αH2-αH3 Proteins

UV light crosslinking of [$^{32}$P]-labeled probe DNAs to
αH1 and αH2-αH3 proteins fractionated by chromatography
(Fig. 5) revealed that the maximum apparent molecular
weights of the bound proteins were 110,000 and 64,000,
respectively (25).

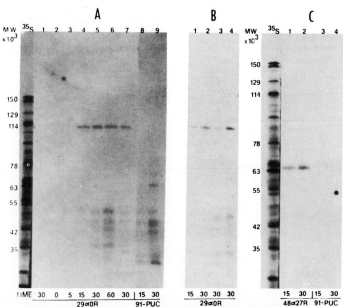

**FIG. 5.** Autoradiographic images of the proteins labeled by
crosslinking to internally labeled DNA probes containing the
αTIC sites and electrophoretically separated in non denaturing

gels. Panel A: the electrophoretic mobility of the proteins crosslinked to the 29αOR fragment (25). Lane 1, plus additional bovine serum albumen (BSA) only; lane 2-6, plus partially purified αH1 and BSA; lane 7, plus partially purified αH1 only; lanes 8-9 show the electrophoretic mobility of the proteins present in the partially purified αH1 fraction crosslinked to the control 91 bp fragment from pUC9. Panel B: the electrophoretic mobility of proteins crosslinked to the labeled 29αOR fragment in the presence of synthetic polymer and additional competitor DNA; lane 1 and 2, no additional competitor DNA; lane 3, 60 fold excess unlabeled 29αOR DNA fragment; lane 4, 60 fold excess unlabeled 91 bp DNA fragment from pUC9. Panel C: electrophoretic mobility of the proteins crosslinked to the labeled DNA. Lanes 1 and 2: proteins crosslinked to 48α27R DNA fragment. Lanes 3 and 4: proteins crosslinked to the 91 bp pUC9 fragment. The duration of UV light irradiation in minutes is shown at the bottom of each lane. The arrows in panels A, B and in Panel C indicate the position of the labeled αH1 and αH2-αH3 proteins, respectively (25).

## αTIF Binding to DNA Fragments Containing the αTIC Site Requires the Participation of Host Proteins

To determine whether αTIF binds to DNA, the αTIF gene was cloned into the pGEM-1 transcriptional vector under the control of the bacteriophage SP6 promoter. The mRNA synthesized in vitro was translated in vitro to yield a 64,000 molecular weight protein that comigrated with the infected cell polypeptide No. 25 (ICP25), the ICP designation for αTIF (Fig. 6). In addition, a polyvalent antibody to αTIF was made by immunizing rabbits with a synthetic 12 mer peptide whose amino acid sequence was predicted from the nucleotide sequence of the αTIF gene. This antibody reacted with a protein band which comigrated with αTIF (34). Studies utilizing these reagents (FIG. 7,8) indicated the following:
(i) The DNA - protein complexes formed by mock infected cell extracts in the presence of the αTIF made in vitro formed a new band which comigrated with that formed by the labeled probe DNA in the presence of extracts of nuclei of infected cells. Substitution of unlabeled αTIF with that labeled with [$^{35}$S]-methionine and of [$^{32}$P]-labeled probe DNA with unlabeled probe DNA yielded a single band which comigrated with the new band described above. The presence of the αTIF in the new DNA - protein complex was verified by the observation that antibody to αTIF decreased the electrophoretic mobility of this complex. Preimmune serum failed to react with the DNA-protein complexes. The in vitro synthesized αTIF did not form a complex with the DNA in the absence of extracts of nuclei of mock infected cells (34).

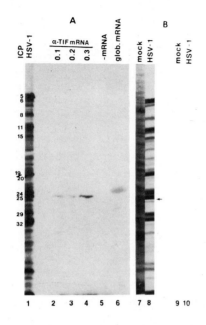

**FIG. 6.** Autoradiographic and photographic images of infected (HSV-1) or mock-infected (mock) cell extracts, and in vitro translated αTIF electrophoretically separated in denaturing polyacrylamide gels and transferred to nitrocellulose. Lanes 1, 7, and 8: Vero cell extracts labeled 20 to 24 hours post infection with [$^{35}$S]-methionine (51). Lanes 2 – 6: [$^{35}$S]-methionine labeled protein translated in vitro from the in vitro synthesized αTIF mRNA (Fig. 1C) or rabbit globin mRNA. Lanes 9 – 10: mock and infected cell extracts, as in lanes 7 and 8, reacted with rabbit serum containing a polyvalent antibody to αTIF and then with anti rabbit antibody coupled to peroxidase (34). The arrow indicates the position of ICP25, the numerical designation of αTIF.

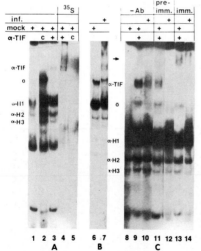

**FIG. 7.** Autoradiographic images of DNA-protein complexes with, or without αTIF, separated in a polyacrylamide gel. Panel A. Mock-infected HeLa cell nuclear extract was reacted with 48α27R DNA. In addition, 5 μg of control (c) or reticulocyte extract containing the in vitro translated αTIF were included where indicated (+). Lanes 1-3: The DNA fragment was labeled with [$^{32}$P], the reticulocyte extract was unlabeled. Lanes 4-5: The DNA fragment was unlabeled, the reticulocyte extract was labeled with [$^{35}$S]-methionine. Panel B: 3 μg of mock-infected (mock) or 12 hour infected (inf.) nuclear extracts were reacted with 2 ng [$^{32}$P]-labeled 48α27R DNA. Panel C: 1 μg of mock-infected (mock) or 12 hour infected (inf.) extract was reacted with labeled 48α27R DNA. The reactions were done in the absence of antibody (-Ab) or in the presence of preimmune (pre-imm.) or immune (imm.) rabbit serum containing polyvalent antibody to αTIF. The open circles mark the location of the αH1 + αH2-αH3 complex.

(ii) The evidence that αTIF requires the participation of αH1 in the formation of these complexes is suggested by three series of experiments. First, the αTIF – DNA complex was formed in the presence of poly(dI).poly(dC) but not in the presence of poly(dAdT).poly(dAdT)polymers. Second, while the probe DNA fragment 29α0R competes for αH2–αH3 proteins, it does not bind them. The 29α0R probe DNA readily formed complexes with αTIF in the presence of chromatographic fractions containing αH1. Lastly, chromatographic fractions containing αH2–αH3 failed to support the formation of DNA protein complexes containing αTIF (24,25,34).

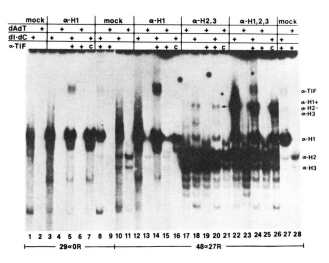

**FIG. 8.** Autoradiographic images of protein–DNA complexes formed by 48α27R and the 29α0R DNA fragments in the presence of different competitor DNAs (34). The DNA fragments were labeled with [$^{32}$P]. The competitor DNAs were either poly(dI)·poly(dC) [dI·dC] or poly·(dAdT)·poly(dadT) [dAdT]. The source of protein was unfractionated mock–infected HeLa cell nuclear extract (mock), DEAE Sepharose fraction 4 (αH1), or fraction 22 (αH2–αH3) (23). 10 µg of control (c) or reticulocyte extract containing the in vitro translated αTIF (+) was added as indicated.

## α4 PROTEIN AND ITS CIS SITES

Biochemical and genetic studies indicate that the transition from α to β and γ protein synthesis requires the expression of functional α proteins, and particularly of the products of the α4 gene. Moreover, the expression of the α genes is negatively regulated by the α4 proteins (51). The α4 polypeptide is found in at least three electrophoretically distinct forms due to

post-translational modifications which include poly-
(ADP) – ribosylation and phosphorylation (41,48,58).

## Binding of the HSV-1 α4 Protein to the
## Promoter-Regulatory Domains of HSV-1 Genes

In contrast to the apparent indirect regulation of α
gene expression by αTIF, the α4 protein has been detected in protein – DNA complexes with the promoter-
regulatory domains of several HSV-1 genes (4,12,22,23,
36). The evidence that the α4 protein binds to DNA
rests on two observations. First, several independently
derived monoclonal antibodies to the α4 protein decreased the electrophoretic mobility of infected cell protein – DNA complexes. A few of the monoclonal antibodies block the formation of the complex (22). Second,
electrophoretically separated infected cell lysates
electrically transferred to a nitrocellulose sheet and
renaturated formed bands which bound labeled DNA fragments known to contain α4 protein binding sites but not
control DNA fragments (Fig. 9). Electrophoretically
separated lysates of mock infected cells failed to form
these bands. The identity of these bands as the three
forms of the α4 protein was determined by their reactivity with monoclonal antibodies to the α4 protein (20).

## The Location of the α4 Protein Binding Sites in
## HSV-1 Genes

The binding sites for the α4 protein in the α and $\gamma_2$
gene DNA fragments used in these studies have been
mapped by a variety of techniques including deletion
analysis, protection from DNase 1 or exonuclease III
and methylation interference analyses illustrated in
part in Fig. 10 (20,23). In the initial studies, the α4
protein was found to bind to DNA fragments containing
sequences from its own gene's promoter and regulatory
domains as well as those derived from the promoter
domains of the α0, α27, and $\gamma_2$42 genes. The binding of
the α4 protein to the promoter of the thymidine kinase,
a β gene was weaker and was seen only in the presence
of the monoclonal antibody (22,23). The two sites
identified in the α4 gene sequences are located at in
the promoter domain and across the transcription initiation site of the gene (22,23,30,36). The α0 gene
contains a single binding site positioned directly 3'
to the CCAAT sequence within the promoter domain (22,
30). Binding studies on several DNA fragments from the
5' regulatory sequences of this gene have not yet
identified additional binding sites for the α4 protein.
It is likely, therefore, that this cis element represents the target for the negative regulation of the α0
gene expression. Binding sites have also been detected

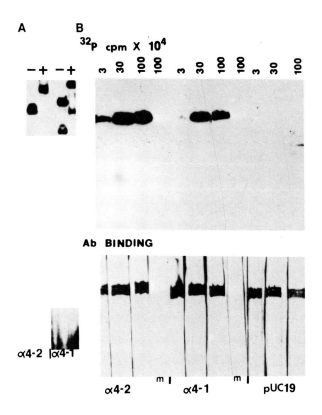

**FIG. 9.** Autoradiographic image of labeled HSV-1 DNA fragments reacted with α4 proteins. Panel A: autoradiographic image of labeled DNA fragments containing α4 gene promoter (α4-2; -44 to +33) or regulatory (α4-1; -134 to -195) domains reacted with infected cell proteins in the presence (+) or absence (-) of antibody against α4 protein (22). Panel B top: autoradiographic image of the labeled DNA fragments reacted with lysates of HeLa cells mock infected (m) or harvested 14 hrs post infection with HSV-1, electrophoretically separated in denaturing gels, transferred to nitrocellulose and renatured. Individual strips were cut and hybridized with increasing amounts of 5'end-labeled DNA fragments. The control (pUC19) DNA probe was the PuvII to HindIII fragments of pUC19. Panel B bottom: photograph of the strips in the top panel after reaction with monoclonal antibody to α4 proteins and staining with rabbit anti mouse IgG coupled to peroxidase (20).

in the transcribed non coding domains of $\gamma_1$ (αTIF) and $\gamma_2$ ($\gamma_2$42 and glycoprotein C) genes (unpublished observations). Thus, the $\gamma_2$42 gene contains at least two binding sites, one mapped in the promoter domains and one in the 5' transcribed non coding domains. Faber and

Wilcox (12) have identified three additional α4 binding sites; one is within the promoter domain of the glycoprotein D, a $\gamma_1$ gene, and two are in the pBR322 plasmid DNA sequences.

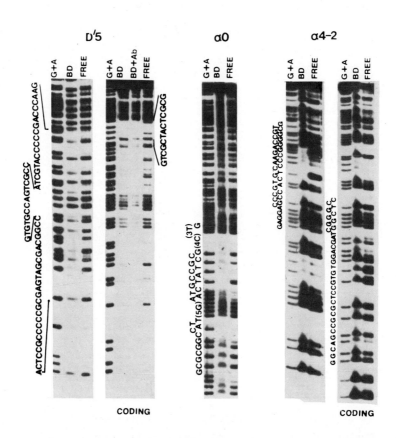

CODING          CODING

**FIG. 10.** Mapping of the α4 protein binding sites in three HSV-1 DNA fragments by methylation interference. The DNA fragments were from the α4 promoter domain (α4-2; -44 to +33), the α0 gene (-110 to +72) and the transcribed non coding domain of the $\gamma_2 42$ gene (D'5; +15 to +98). The DNA fragments were labeled at the 5' terminus of the coding or the non coding strand, partially methylated with dimethyl sulfate, and reacted with proteins from HSV-1 infected HeLa cell nuclei. The bound (BD) and free (FREE) DNA were separated on a non denaturing gel, extracted, cleaved to reveal modified G residues, and electrophoretically separated on a standard 8% sequencing gel as described (23-25). G+A, purine specific sequencing reaction. The nucleotide sequence of the relevant region is shown adjacent to each reaction set.

## The Nature of the α4 Protein Binding Site in HSV-1 DNA

The initial consensus sequences published by Faber and Wilcox (12) was based on one HSV-1 and two pBR322 binding sites. Subsequent analyses of binding sites have generally upheld this consensus, but there exist binding sites which do not conform (manuscript in preparation). The summary of sequences of DNA fragments shown to bind to the α4 protein shown in Table 2, together with available methylation interference and DNase protection studies (Fig. 10) suggest a possible second consensus sequence, but much remains to be done to define the motif of the binding site.

**TABLE 2.** The Nucleotide Sequence of the HSV-1 and Non Viral DNA Binding Sites of the α4 Protein[a]

| GENE | NUCLEOTIDE No. | SEQUENCE |
|------|----------------|----------|
| CONSENSUS 1 | | ATCGTCNNNNCNGNN |
| **α4 BINDING SITES IN PROMOTER DOMAINS OF HSV-1 GENES:** | | |
| GD | -115 | TGTGACACTATCGTCCATACCGACCACACCGACGAATCCCCTAAGGGG |
| α0 | -75 | ATTGGGGGAATCGTCACTGCCGCCCCTTTGGGGAGGGGAAAGGCGTGG |
| α4-2 | -12 | GACGCCCCGATCGTCCACACGGAGCGCGGCTGCCGACACGGATCCACG |
| **α4 BINDING SITES IN 5' TRANSCRIBED NON CODING DOMAINS OF HSV-1 GENES:** | | |
| D'L2 | +55 | CCAGTCGCCATCGTACCCCCGACCCAAGCTGTCCGGCTGGACAAGGA |
| αTIF | +145 | AAGCCCGATATCGTCTTTCCCGTATCAACCCCACCCAATGGACCTCTT |
| **α4 BINDING SITES IN NON HSV-1 DNA SEQUENCES:** | | |
| PBR322 | | AATGCGCTCATCGTCATCCTCGGCACCGTCACCCTGGATGCTGTAGGC |
| PBR322 | | TTGCGGGATATCGTCCATTCCGACAGCATCGCCAGTCACTATGGCGTG |
| **α4 BINDING SITES THAT DO NOT FIT CONSENSUS 1:** | | |
| CONSENSUS 2 | | YYNRGTRNYR |
| α4 | -172 | TCGACCAACGGGCCGCGGCCACGGGCCCCCGGCGTGCCG<br>AGCTGGTTGCCCGGCGCCGGTGCCCGGGGGCCGCACGGC |
| D'P1 | -151 | GTGGTGCCCTGGGCTGGATAGCGCGGGGGCGTGAATAATCGCA<br>CACCACGGGACCCGACCTATCGCGCCCCGCACTTATTAGCGT |
| D'L1 | +29 | CGACTCCGCCCCCGCGAGTAGCGACGGCCGTGTGCC<br>GCTGAGGCGGGGGCGCTCATCGCTGCCGGCACACGG |
| D'P0 | -173 | GAGTCGTAAAGACCCAGTATTACGTGGTGCCC<br>CTCAGCATTTCTGGGTCATAATGCACCACGGG |
| GC | | GGCCGCATCGAACGCACACCCCCATCCGGTGGTCCGTGTGGAGGTC<br>CCGGCGTAGCTTGCGTGTGGGGGTAGGCCACCAGGCACACCTCCAG |

[a] The glycoprotein C (gC) sequence shown maps in the 5' transcribed non coding gene domain. The position of the α genes is shown in Fig.1. The locations of binding sites in gD and pBR322 (12); α0 and α4 (22,23,36); αTIF (40); gC (50) and $\gamma_2 42$ (55) and details of the procedures used in footprinting the α4 protein are in the references cited. Y: pyrimidine; R: purine; N: any nucleotide. D' refers to the $\gamma_2 42$ gene mapping in the DNA fragment BamHI D'' P and L refer to sequences from the promoter and 5' transcribed non coding sequences of this gene. The numbers refer to nucleotide sequence at the 5' end of the DNA fragment in reference to the transcription initiation site at +1.

### The Function of the α4 Protein in HSV Gene Regulation

The studies done to date indicate that α4 proteins regulate HSV gene expression both positively and negatively. The evidence for positive regulation is genetic and, to a more limited extent, biochemical (8,11,18,41, 43,51,52). Thus mutants with ts lesions in the α4 gene do not express β and γ genes at the non permissive temperatures (10,17,46,57). Cell lines expressing the α4 protein are capable of expressing β and γ genes introduced into these cells (1,2,42), and studies with an α4 gene with a ts lesion have shown that the expression of HSV-1 genes in these cells is dependent on the presence of functional α4 proteins (1,2). A slight in vitro enhancement of the transcription of the gD gene template upon the addition of partially purified α4 protein has also been reported (4,43).

Several lines of evidence have suggested that α4 also regulates genes negatively. Negative regulation of the α genes has been ascribed to the α4 proteins on the basis of genetic studies showing that ts mutants in the α4 gene shifted from permissive to non permissive temperature at a time after α4 protein synthesis had been turned off resume the synthesis of the protein (10,51). Consistent with this evidence, deletion analyses have suggested that the 3' binding site in the α4 gene may play a role in the autoregulation of the α4 gene in Vero cells (39). More recent studies have suggested that α4 protein may regulate negatively not only α genes (14,38, 39,42) but also γ genes expressed late in infection (1). The characteristics which determine the net effect of the α4 protein on the expression of a particular gene are not known, but most likely involve the binding site and its position relative to the binding sites of other transcriptional factors. Thus the binding of the α4 protein to the transcription initiation site (α4 gene) or adjacent to the CCAAT sequence (α0 gene) may affect either the direct binding of the host cell factors or their interactions with other elements of the transcriptional apparatus. The interaction of this protein with viral and host cell transcriptional factors is likely to be the major focus of future studies on the regulation of HSV gene transcription.

### CONCLUSIONS

The focus of this chapter has been on HSV-1 transacting factors that operate early in infection. Each of the trans-acting factors, αTIF and α4, requires for its function specific cis-acting sites in the viral DNA. It has been known for many years, however, that infection with HSV-1 can result in the induction of cellular genes (27,37) or of non HSV genes introduced into cells by transfection (16,45,54,56). In the case of the αTIF, sequences homologous to its cis-site have been found in a retrovirus long terminal repeat, in the SV40 72 bp repeat, and in the promoter regulatory domains of a number of inducible cellular genes (9,19,26). There is as yet less information on the inducibility of cellular genes by the α4 protein. Both the mechanism of induction and the range of genes inducible by these viral trans-acting factors remains to be determined. It should be noted however that HSV rapidly shuts off host gene expression by turning off the synthesis of host proteins (13). Since host shut off and expression of cellular genes or of genes resident in the cell are competing processes, and since HSV-1 ultimately destroys the cell in which it multiplies, the extent of expression of the induced host genes will probably be minimal and inconsequential. This may not be the case for cells abortively infected with HSV and in which the shut off of host gene expression may be transient. In such cells, the expression of the induced non HSV genes may be preeminent. This remains, however, to be tested.

## ACKNOWLEDGEMENTS

These study were aided by grants from the National Cancer Institute (CA08494 and CA19264) and the National Institute for Allergy and Infectious Diseases (AI124009), the United States Public Health Service, and from the American Cancer Society (MV-2W). T.M.K. (CA09241), J.L.C. McK. (CA09241), N.M. (AI07099) and D.S. (GM7281) were U.S. Public Health trainees during the conduct of these studies. P.M-N. was a Damon Runyon Foundation Fellow.

## REFERENCES

1. Arsenakis, M., Campadelli-Fiume, G., and Roizman, B. (1988): J. Virol. (in press).
2. Arsenakis, M., Hubenthal-Voss, J., Campadelli-Fiume, G., Pereira, L., and Roizman, B. (1986): J. Virol., 60: 674-682.
3. Batterson, W., and Roizman, B. (1983): J. Virol., 46: 371-377.
4. Beard, P., Faber, S., Wilcox, K.W., Pizer, L.I. (1986): Proc. Natl. Acad. Sci. USA, 83: 4016-4020.
5. Bzik, D.J., and Preston, C.M. (1986): Nucleic Acids Res., 14: 929-943.
6. Campbell, M.E.M., Palfreyman, J.W., and Preston, C.M. (1984): J. Mol. Biol., 180: 1-19.
7. Church, G.M., Ephrussi, A., Gilbert, W., and Tonegawa, S. (1985): Nature, 313: 798-801.

8. DeLuca, N.A., McCarthy, A.M., and Schaffer, P.A. (1985): J. Virol. 56: 558–570.

9. Dhar, R., McClements, W.L., Enquist, L.W., and Vande Woude, G.F. (1980): Proc. Natl. Acad. Sci. USA, 77: 3937–3941.

10. Dixon, R.A., and Schaffer, P.A. (1980): J. Virol., 36: 189–203.

11. Everett, R.D. (1984): EMBO J., 3: 3134–3141.

12. Faber, S.W., and Wilcox, K.W. (1986): Nucleic Acids Res., 14: 6067–6083.

13. Fenwick, M., Morse, L.S., and Roizman, B. (1979): J. Virol., 29: 825–827.

14. Gelman, I.H., and Silverstein, S. (1987): J. Virol., 61: 2286–2296.

15. Heine, J.W., Honess, R.W., Cassai, E., and Roizman, B. (1974): J. Virol., 14: 640–651.

16. Herz, C., and Roizman, B. (1983): Cell, 33: 145–151.

17. Honess, R.W., and Roizman, B, (1974): J. Virol., 14: 8–19.

18. Honess, R.W., and Roizman, B. (1975): Proc. Natl. Acad. Sci. USA, 72: 1276–1280.

19. Kristie, T.M., Batterson, W., Mackem, S., and Roizman, B. (1983): In: Enhancers and Eukaryotic Gene Expression, edited by Y. Gluzman, and T. Shenk, pp. 141–151.

20. Kristie, T.M., Michael, N., Spector, D., and Roizman, B. (1987): In; Mechanisms of Control of Gene Expression, UCLA Symposia on Molecular and Cellular Biology, edited by B., Cullen, L.P., Gage, M.A.Q., Siddiqui, A-M., Skalka, and H., Weissmann, Alan R. Liss Inc., New York.

21. Kristie, T.M., and Roizman, B. (1984): Proc. Natl. Acad. Sci. USA, 81: 4065–4069.

22. Kristie, T.M., and Roizman, B. (1986): Proc. Natl. Acad. Sci. USA, 83: 3218–3222.

23. Kristie, T.M., and Roizman, B. (1986): Proc. Natl. Acad. Sci. USA, 83: 4700–4704.

24. Kristie, T.M., and Roizman, B (1987): Proc. Natl. Acad. Sci. USA, 84: 71–75.

25. Kristie, T.M., and Roizman, B. (1988): J. Virol. (in press).

26. Laimins, L.A., Khoury, G., Gorman, C., Howard, B., and Gruss, P. (1982): Proc. Natl. Acad. Sci. USA, 79: 6453–6457.

27. LaThangue, N.B., Shriver, K., Dawson, C., and Chan, W.L. (1984): EMBO J., 3: 267–277.

28. Mackem, S., and Roizman, B. (1982): Proc. Natl. Acad. Sci. USA, 79: 4917–4921.

29. Mackem, S., and Roizman, B. (1982): J. Virol., 43: 1015–1023.

30. Mackem, S., and Roizman, B. (1982): J. Virol., 44: 939–949.

31. Mavromara-Nazos, P., Silver, S., Hubenthal-Voss, J., McKnight, J.L.C., and Roizman, B. (1986): Virology, 149: 152–164.
32. McGeoch, D.J., Dolan, A., Donald, S., and Brauer, D.H.K. (1986): Nucleic Acids Res., 14: 1727–1745.
33. McKnight, J.L.C., Kristie, T., Silver, S., Pellet, P.E., Mavromara-Nazos, P., Campadelli-Fiume, G., Arsenakis, M., and Roizman, B. (1986): In: Cancer Cells 4, Control of Gene Expression and Replication, edited by M., Botchan, T.,Grodzicker, and P., Sharp, pp. 163–173. Cold Spring Harbor Laboratories, Cold Spring Harbor, New York.
34. McKnight, J.L.C., Kristie, T.M., and Roizman, B. (1987): Proc. Natl. Acad. Sci. USA, (in press).
35. McKnight, J.L.C., Pellet, P.E., Jenkins, F.J. and Roizman, B. (1987): J. Virol., 61: 992–1001.
36. Muller, M.T. (1987): J. Virol., 61: 858–865.
37. Notarianni, E.L., and Preston, C.M. (1982): Virology, 123: 113–122.
38. O'Hare, P., and Hayward, G.S. (1985): J. Virol., 56: 723–733.
39. O'Hare, P., and Hayward, G.S. (1987): J. Virol., 61: 190–199.
40. Pellet, P.E., McKnight, J.L.C., Jenkins, F., and Roizman, B. (1985): Proc. Natl. Acad. Sci. USA, 82: 5870–5874.
41. Pereira, L., Wolff, M.H., Fenwick, M., and Roizman, B. (1977): Virology, 77: 733–749.
42. Persson, R.H., Bacchetti, S., and Smiley, J.R. (1985): J. Virol., 54: 414–421.
43. Pizer, L.I., Tedder, D.G., Betz, J.L., Wilcox, K.W., and Beard, P. (1986): J. Virol., 60: 950–959.
44. Post, L.E., Mackem, S., and Roizman, B. (1981): Cell, 24: 555–565.
45. Post, L.E., Norrild, B., Simpson, T., and Roizman, B. (1982): Mol. Cell. Biol., 2: 233–240.
46. Preston, C.M. (1979): J. Virol., 29: 275–284.
47. Preston, C.M., Cordingley, M.G., and Stow, N.D. (1984): J. Virol., 50: 708–716.
48. Preston, C.M., and Notarianni, E.L. (1983): Virology, 131: 492–501.
49. Pruijn, G.J.M., van Driel, W., and van der Vliet, P.C. (1986): Nature, 322: 656–659.
50. Roizman, B. (1979): Ann. Rev. Genet., 13: 25–57.
51. Roizman, B., and Batterson, W. (1985): In: Virology, edited by B., Fields, pp. 497–526. Raven Press, New York.
52. Sandri-Goldin, R.M., Goldin, A.L., Holland, L.E., Glorioso, J.C., and Levine, M. (1983): Mol. Cell. Biol., 3: 2028–2044.
53. Sen, R., and Baltimore, D. (1986): Cell, 46: 705–716.

54. Shih, M-F., Arsenakis, M., Tiollais, P., and Roizman B. (1984): Proc. Natl. Acad. Sci. USA, 81: 5867-5870.
55. Silver, S., and Roizman, B. (1985): Mol. Cell. Biol., 5: 518-528.
56. Smiley, J.R., Smibert, C., and Everett, R. (1987): J. Virol., 61: 2368-2377.
57. Watson, R.J., and Clements, J.P. (1980): Nature, 285: 329-330.
58. Wilcox, K.W., Kohn, A., Sklyanskaya, E., and Roizman, B. (1980): J. Virol., 33: 167-182.

# General and Molecular Biology of Papillomaviruses

P.M. Howley

*Laboratory of Tumor Virus Biology*
*National Cancer Institute, Bethesda, Maryland, USA*

The papillomaviruses are a group of small DNA viruses which induce squamous epithelial tumors (warts and papillomas). The first papillomavirus described was the cottontail rabbit papillomavirus. Subsequently, papillomaviruses have been isolated and characterized from other vertebrate species, including man. Standard virologic approaches to the study of these viruses have been limited, however, due to the lack of a tissue culture system for their in vitro propagation. This failure may, in part, be due to the fact that the productive functions of the papillomaviruses are expressed only in fully differentiated squamous epithelial cells. To date, tissue culture systems for keratinocytes have not permitted the full expression of the papillomavirus life cycle.

The papillomaviruses were originally grouped together with the polyomaviruses to form the family of viruses called the papovaviruses (36). The papillomaviruses, however, are larger than the polyomaviruses (55 nm compared with 40 nm) and contain larger genomes (8 kb pairs compared with 5 kb pairs). Members of the polyomavirus genus, such as SV40 and the murine polyomavirus, have been studied in great detail, largely due to the fact that they are easily propagated in the laboratory. Prior to the advent of recombinant DNA technology, studies with the papillomaviruses were limited due to the inability to propagate the virus in tissue culture. This technology, however, has permitted the molecular cloning of a number of papillomavirus genomes which provided sufficient quantities of viral DNA to begin a systematic study of the papillomaviruses and also provided a standardization of the viral genomic reagents.

## Squamous Epithelial Cell Tropism

The productive functions of the papillomaviruses, including vegetative viral DNA synthesis and the expression of late viral genes, occur only in the fully differentiated squamous epithelial cells of the wart. Vegetative viral DNA synthesis has been detected by in situ hybridization techniques only in the squamous epithelial cells of the stratum spinosum and of the granular layer of the epidermis, but not in the basal layer nor in the underlying dermal fibroblasts (22). Viral capsid protein production and virus assembly occur only in the super stratum spinosum and in the granular layer where epithelial cells are terminally differentiated. Investigators generally believe that the viral genome is present in the epithelial cells of the basal layer and it is generally thought that the expression of specific viral genes in the basal layer and in the lower layers of the epidermis is responsible for proliferation of the epithelial cells characteristic of a wart or a papilloma. As the cells of the epidermis migrate upward through the stratum spinosum into the granular layer, they undergo a program of differentiation. The control of papillomavirus late gene expression, therefore, appears tightly linked to the state of differentiation of the squamous epithelial cells. The molecular basis for this control is not yet known.

## Plurality of Human Viral "Genotypes"

There are no serologic reagents yet available to distinguish the various HPVs. Different HPV types are, therefore, distinguished on the basis of their DNA. An HPV type is considered a new type if it shares less than 50% DNA homology with each of the other HPV types defined. To date 46 different HPVs have been described (Table 1).

## GENOMIC ORGANIZATION

### Sequence Analysis

To date, 14 papillomavirus genomes have been completely or partially sequenced. These include the genomes of several animal papillomaviruses and the following HPV genomes: HPV-1, HPV-5, HPV-6, HPV-8, HPV-11, HPV-16, HPV-18, HPV-31, HPV-33 (3).

Papillomavirus genomes are double-stranded closed circular molecules containing approximately 8000 base pairs. All of open reading frames (ORFs) greater than approximately 400 bases in size are located on one strand. All of the detectable polyadenylated RNAs in transformed cells as well as in productively infected cells of those viruses which have been studied are transcribed from a single strand (12). In addition to the coding regions each viral genome contains transcription and replication control regions.

### TABLE 1. Human Papillomaviruses

| Virus Type | Clinical Association | Reference(s) |
|---|---|---|
| HPV-1 | Plantar warts | 13,17 |
| HPV-2 | Verruca vulgaris | 39 |
| HPV-3 | Flat warts | 41 |
| HPV-4 | Plantar warts | 16,21 |
| HPV-5 | Macular lesions in EV[a] | 38 |
| HPV-6 | Genital warts & laryngeal papillomas | 18 |
| HPV-7 | Common warts in meat handlers | 40,42 |
| HPV-8 | Macular lesions in EV | 38,46 |
| HPV-9 | Macular lesions in EV | 28 |
| HPV-10 | Flat warts | 29 |
| HPV-11 | Laryngeal papillomas & genital warts | 15 |
| HPV-12 | Macular lesions in EV | 29 |
| HPV-13 | Oral focal epithelial hyperplasia | 45 |
| HPV-14 | Macular lesions in EV | 59 |
| HPV-15 | Macular lesions in EV | 27 |
| HPV-16 | Cervical dysplasia, Bowenoid papulosis, and cervical carcinoma | 64 |
| HPV-17 | Macular lesions in EV | 27 |
| HPV-18 | Cervical dysplasia and carcinoma | 64 |
| HPV-19 | Macular lesions in EV | 14,27 |
| HPV-20 | Macular lesions in EV | 14,27 |
| HPV-21 | Macular lesions in EV | 27 |
| HPV-22 | Macular lesions in EV | 27 |
| HPV-23 | Macular lesions in EV | 27 |
| HPV-24 | Macular lesions in EV | 27 |
| HPV-25 | Macular lesions in EV | 14,41 |
| HPV-26 | Flat warts | 40,43 |
| HPV-27 | Verruca vulgaris | K. Zachov et al., unpubl. |
| HPV-28 | Flat warts | M. Favre et al., unpubl. |
| HPV-29 | Verruca vulgaris | M. Favre et al., unpubl. |
| HPV-30 | Genital warts and laryngeal carcinoma | 25 |
| HPV-31 | Cervical dysplasia | 31 |
| HPV-33 | Genital intraepithelial neoplasia and cervical carcinomas | 6 |

[a]) Epidermodysplasia verruciformis
Types 32 and 34-41 have also been described at meetings, but full descriptions have not appeared in press.

## Transforming Papillomaviruses

There is a subgroup of papillomaviruses whose members are capable of inducing fibroblastic tumors when inoculated into hamsters. This subgroup of viruses includes the bovine papillomaviruses types 1 and 2, the deer papillomavirus, the ovine papillomavirus, and the European elk papillomavirus. With the exception of the ovine papillomavirus, each of these viruses has been demonstrated to be capable of transforming susceptible rodent cells in culture. Transformation of susceptible rodent cells by these papillomaviruses has provided a biologic system for studying the latent, non-productive infection of cells by the papillomaviruses. The most extensively studied of the papillomaviruses is the bovine papillomavirus type 1 (BPV-1) which has served as the prototype papillomavirus for the study of the molecular biology and genetics of the group of viruses (24). BPV-1 is associated with cutaneous fibropapillomas in cattle and can induce fibroblastic tumors in a variety of foreign hosts, including horses, hamsters, and rabbits. In cell lines established from BPV-1 induced tumors, and in cell lines establisheed in vitro from transformation by either the virus or its cloned DNA, the BPV-1 genome is stably maintained as a multicopy nuclear plasmid (30).

## Genomic Organization of BPV-1

A linearized map of the genomic organization of BPV-1 is depicted in Fig. 1 (9). The major ORFs are shown by open boxes and are labeled with numbers and the letters E or L. The E ORFs are located within the 69% transforming segment of the BPV-1 genome or within the analogous regions of the other papillomavirus genomes (32). The L ORFs map within a region only transcribed for BPV-1 in the differentiated keratinocytes of a bovine fibropapilloma or within the analogous regions of the other papillomavirus genomes (12). The numbers at the 5' and 3' ends of the ORFs refer to the first nucleotide of the ORF and to the nucleotide preceding the stop codon, respectively. The positions of the first AUG codon are indicated by the dashed vertical line. Probable polyadenylation sites are indicated by triangles with the letter A (4).

## Papillomavirus Gene Functions

The known papillomavirus gene functions are listed below in Table 2. Most functions have been mapped in BPV-1 which has served as the prototype for the genetic analysis of the papillomaviruses.

FIG. 1.

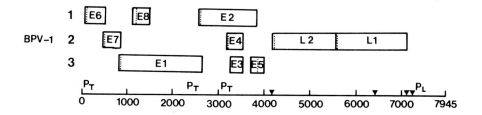

**TABLE 2.** Papillomavirus Gene Functions

| Open Reading Frames | Function(s) Assigned | Virus | Reference(s) |
|---|---|---|---|
| E1 (5′) | Modulator of DNA replication | BPV-1 | (35) |
| E1 (3′) | Replication | BPV-1 | (34,35,52) |
| E2 | Transregulation of transcription; probable indirect effects on replication and transformation | BPV-1 HPV-16 | (56,57) (47) |
| E3 | None yet assigned | -- | |
| E4 | Abundant cytoplasmatic protein in warts | HPV-1a | (11) |
| E5 | Transformation | BPV-1 | (10,19, 49,62) |
| E6 | Transformation, plasmid copy number control | BPV-1 | (7,54,61) |
| E7 | Plasmid copy number control | BPV-1 | (7,34) |
| E8 | None yet assigned | -- | |
| L1 | Major capsid protein | BPV-1 | (12,48) |
| L2 | Minor capsid protein | HPV-1a | (26) |

## Two Independent Transforming Genes (E5 and E6)

Several laboratories have identified different regions of the BPV-1 genome that influence viral transforming functions (10,19,52,54,61). There are two independent transforming genes in BPV-1 which correspond to the E5 and E6 ORFs, respectively. The proteins encoded by each of these genes have each been recently identified. The E5 protein consists of 44 amino acids, is strikingly hydrophobic, and is localized in the nuclear and cytoplasmic membranes (53); the E6 protein is cysteine rich and has been localized to the nucleus as well as to membrane fractions (2).

Transformation assays using NIH 3T3 cells have also recently been developed for the HPVs associated with human cervical carcinoma, i.e., HPV-16 (60,63). The genes responsible for this transformation are currently being mapped.

## TRANSCRIPTION

### The Promoters

BPV-1 transformed cells contain multiple viral RNA species which vary in size from approximately 1000 to approximately 4000 bases (20). Because of the low abundance of these transcripts, precise mapping of the viral RNAs was difficult using standard hybridization and nuclease digestion techniques. Two recent studies involving either the electron microscopic analysis of RNAs in transformed cells have revealed that multiple discrete species of viral RNAs are generated by differential splicing (58,61). All of the RNAs present in the transformed cells appear to be polyadenylated at the same site, base 4203 (see Fig. 1) (61). There are a minimum of five distinct promoters functional in transformed cells and a distinct promoter located in the viral control region which appears to function only in terminally differentiated cells as a late promoter (4). The location of known promoters are indicated in Fig. 2 by arrows and labeled $P_n$ where n is the nucleotide position of the major promoter active in the transformed cells. These promoters are also active in the fibromatous portion of a BPV-1 induced fibropapilloma in cattle (4). $P_L$ is the major promoter active in the fibropapilloma (4). LCR refers to the long control region of the viral genome containing transcription and replication control sequences (4).

### Transcriptional Enhancers

The bovine papillomavirus contains transcriptional regulatory sequences which act in cis to augment trans-

cription from heterologous promoter elements. One
transcriptional enhancer is located 3' to the polyadenylation site of the genes expressed in BPV–1 transformed cells between the bases 4390 and 4451 (33). This
element referred to as the "distal enhancer" is able to
substitute for the SV40 72 base pair repeat enhancer in
a sensitive assay for SV40 large T antigen expression
and can increase the efficiency of stable transformation of the herpes TK gene (8,33). Recent studies,
however, have shown that this is not a cis essential
element for BPV–1 DNA mediated transformation or for
stable extrachromosomal plasmid maintenance (23).

Transcriptional regulatory elements have also been
mapped to the 1.0 kb LCR of the BPV–1 genome using an
enhancer dependent expression vector for chloramphenicol acetyl transferase (57).

FIG. 2

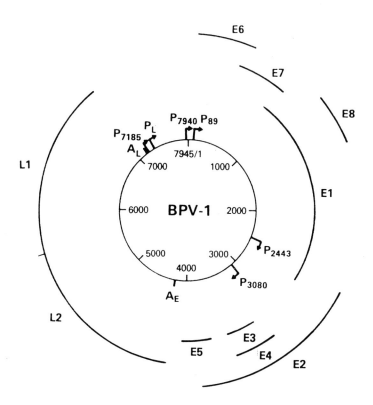

The LCR can act as an E2 conditional enhancer in that it functions to augment transcription in a position and orientation independent manner from a heterologous promoter but only in the presence of the viral E2 gene product (57). Genetic dissection of the LCR reveals two E2 responsive elements (E2REs), one mapping in the vicinity of P7185 and PL (Fig. 2) and the other just upstream of the promoters, P7940 and P89 (56). One characteristic of these elements is the presence of the sequence motif ACC(N)6GGT several times in each of the E2REs. Recent studies have revealed that the viral E2 protein has DNA binding characteristics and binds specifically to this motif (1,37). It is presumed that the binding of E2 to these motifs is involved in transcriptional transactivation (56).

### Transactivation by the Viral E2 Gene Product

The full E2 gene product is a specific DNA binding protein (1,37). It is a transcriptional transactivator which functions through two responsive elements (E2REs) located in the viral LCR (56). This was shown first for BPV-1 (57) and more recently for HPV-16 (47); E2 transactivation is likely a general characteristic of all papillomaviruses.

Genetic studies in the full genome background have implicated the E2 gene product as having a role in transformation and plasmid maintenance. BPV-1 mutants affected in the E2 ORF are dramatically decreased in their efficiencies of focus formation on mouse cells (10,19,28). Transformants selected by virtue of their morphologic transformed phenotype induced by these E2 mutants usually contain the viral DNA in an integrated state indicating a role for the E2 gene product in plasmid maintenance. It seems likely that the role of E2 in the viral functions of transformation and plasmid maintenance may be indirect, through the activation of the LCR enhancer element. The LCR enhancer element functions in the virus on the 5' promoters upstream from the cap site at base 89 (56). Activation of this element by the E2 gene product leads to the expression of the 5' ORFs including E6, E6/E7, and E1 which have been shown to have an effect on transformation and plasmid maintenance (see Table 2).

### PAPILLOMAVIRUSES AND CARCINOGENIC PROGRESSION

### Animal Models

The Shope papillomavirus induces benign cutaneous papillomas in rabbits which frequently progress to invasive squamous cell carcinomas. Such malignant progression is more frequent and more rapid in lesions painted with a cocarcinogen such as coaltar or methylcholanthrene (50,51). The role of cofactors in malignant progression of papillomavirus induced lesions is a general one and may be important in those cancers associated with papillomaviruses in humans.

## Human Ano-Genital Carcinomas

A subset of the human papillomaviruses has now been associated with ano-genital lesions (64). In general, HPV-6 and HPV-11 have been associated with benign lesions and with lesions which are less likely to progress to carcinoma. HPV types 16, 18, 31, and 33 are found in the invasive carcinomas, as well as dysplasias and in situ carcinomas which may progress to malignancy (64).

## Molecular Biology

In general, HPV-16 and HPV-18 DNAs are found as extra chromosomal molecules in benign lesions and integrated in malignant lesions. Integration generally occurs in a manner which disrupts the integrity of the E2 ORF of these viruses thus releasing the LCR promoters from the control imparted by the viral E2 gene product (5,47,55). Although integrated, the viral genomes are usually transcriptionally active; the E6 and E7 are the genes which are expressed (5,55). The predicted structural features of the HPV-16 and HPV-18 E6 gene products are similar to that of the BPV-1 E6 gene product which is a proven viral oncogene. It has been postulated that its unregulated expression in cervical carcinomas may play a role in carcinogenic progression.

## REFERENCES

1. Androphy, E., Lowy, D., and Schiller, J. (1987): Nature, 325: 70-73.
2. Androphy, E.J., Schiller, J.T., and Lowy, D.R. (1985): Science, 230: 442-445.
3. Baker, C.C. (1987): In: Genetic Maps, edited by S. O'Brien, Cold Spring Harbor, New York (in press).
4. Baker, C.C., and Howley, P.M. (1987): EMBO J. (in press).
5. Baker, C.C., Phelps, W.C., Lindgren, V., Braun, M.J., Gonda, M.A., and Howley, P.M. (1987): J. Virol., 61: 962-971.
6. Beaudenon, S., Kremsdorf, D., Croissant, O., Jablonska, S., Wain-Hobson, S., and Orth, G. (1986): Nature, 321: 246-249.
7. Berg, L.J., Singh, K., and Botchan, M. (1986): Mol. Cell. Biol., 6: 559-569.

8. Campo, M.S., Spandidos, D.A., Lang, J., and Wilkie, N.M. (1983): Nature, 303: 77-80.
9. Chen, E.Y., Howley, P.M., Levinson, A.D., and Seeburg, P.H. (1982): Nature, 299: 529-534.
10. DiMaio, D., Guralski, D., and Schiller, J.T. (1986): Proc. Natl. Acad. Sci. USA, 83: 1797-1801.
11. Doorbar, J., Campbell, D., Grand, R.J.A., and Gallimore, P.H. (1986): EMBO J., 5: 355-362.
12. Engel, L.W., Heilman, C.A., and Howley, P.M. (1983): J. Virol., 47: 516-528.
13. Favre, M., Orth, G., Croissant, O., and Yaniv, M. (1975): Proc. Natl. Acad. Sci. USA, 72: 4810-4814.
14. Gassenmaier, A., Lammel, M., and Pfister, H. (1984): J. Virol., 52: 1019-1023.
15. Gissmann, L., Diehl, V., Schultz-Coulon, H., and zur Hausen, H. (1982): J. Virol., 44: 393-400.
16. Gissmann, L., Pfister, H., and zur Hausen, H. (1977): Virology, 7: 569-580.
17. Gissmann, L., and zur Hausen, H. (1976): Proc. Natl. Acad. Sci. USA, 73: 1310-1313.
18. Gissmann, L., and zur Hausen, H. (1980): J. Cancer, 25: 605-609.
19. Groff, D.E., and Lancaster, W.D. (1986): Virology, 150: 221-230.
20. Heilman, C.A., Engel, L., Lowy, D.R., and Howley. P.M. (1982): Virology, 119: 22-34.
21. Heilman, C.A., Law, M.F., Israel, M.A., and Howley, P.M. (1980): J. Virol., 35: 395-407.
22. Howley, P.M. (1982): Am. J. Pathol., 113: 414-421.
23. Howley, P.M., Schenborn, E.T., Lund, E., Byrne, J.C., and Dahlberg, J.E. (1985): Mol. Cell. Biol., 5: 3310-3315.
24. Howley, P.M., and Schlegel, R. (1987): In: Papova-viridae. 2. The Papillomaviruses, edited by N.P. Salzman and P.M. Howley, pp. 141-163, Plenum Press, New York.
25. Kahn, T., Schwarz, E., and zur Hausen, H. (1987): Int. J. Cancer (in press).
26. Komly, C.A., Breitburd, F., Croissant, O., and Streeck, R.E. (1986): J. Virol., 60: 813-816.
27. Kremsdorf, D., Favre, M., Jablonska, S., Obalek, S., Rueda, L.A., Lutzner, M., Blanchet-Bardon, D., van Voorst Vader, P.C., and Orth, G. (1984): J. Virol., 52: 1013-1018.
28. Kremsdorf, D., Jablonska, S., Favre, M., and Orth, G. (1982): J. Virol., 43: 436-447.
29. Kremsdorf, D., Jablonska, S., Favre, M., and Orth, G. (1982): J. Virol., 48: 340-351.
30. Law, M.F., Lowy, D.R., Dvoretzky, I., and Howley, P.M. (1981): Proc. Natl. Acad. Sci. USA, 78: 2727-2731.

31. Lorincz, A.T., Lancaster, W.D., and Tample, G.F. (1986): J. Virol., 58: 225-229.
32. Lowy, D.R., Dvoretzky, I., Shober, R., Law, M.F., Engel, L., and Howley, P.M. (1980): Nature, 287: 72-74.
33. Lusky, M., Berg, L., Weiher, H., and Botchan, M. (1983): Mol. Cell. Biol., 3: 1108-1122.
34. Lusky, M., and Botchan, M.R. (1985): J. Virol., 53: 955-965.
35. Lusky, M., and Botchan, M.R. (1986): J. Virol., 60: 729-742.
36. Melnick, J.L. (1962): Science, 135: 1128-1130.
37. Moskaluk, C., and Bastia, D. (1987): Proc. Natl. Acad. Sci. USA, 84: 1215-1218.
38. Orth, G., Favre, M., Breitburd, F., Croissant, O., Jablonska, S., Obalek, S., Jarzabek-Chorzelska, M., and Rzesa, G. (1980): Cold Spring Harbor Conference on Cell Proliferation, 7: 259-282.
39. Orth, G., Favre, M., and Croissant, O. (1977): J. Virol., 24: 108-120.
40. Orth, G., Jablonska, S., Favre, M., Croissant, O., Jarzabek-Chorzelska, M., and Jibard, N. (1981): J. Invest. Dermatol., 76: 97-102.
41. Orth, G., Jablonska, S., Favre, M., Croissant, O., Jarzabek-Chorzelska, M., and Rzesa, G. (1978): Proc. Natl. Acad. Sci. USA, 75: 1537-1541.
42. Ostrow, R.S., Kryzyek, R., Pass, F., and Faras, A.J. (1981): Virology, 108: 21-27.
43. Ostrow, R.S., Zachov, K.R., Thompson, O., and Faras, A.J. (1984): J. Invest. Dermatol., 82: 362-366.
44. Petterson, U., Ahola, H., Stenlund, A., and Moreno-Lopez, J. (1987): In: Papovaviridae. 2. The Papillomaviruses, edited by N.P. Salzman, and P.M. Howley, pp. 67-107, Plenum Press, New York.
45. Pfister, H., Hettich, I., Runne, U., Gissmann, L., and Chilf, G.N. (1983): J. Virol., 47: 363-366.
46. Pfister, H., Nurnberger, F., Gissmann, L., and zur Hausen, H. (1981): Int. J. Cancer, 27: 645-650.
47. Phelps, W.C., and Howley, P.M. (1987): J. Virol (in press).
48. Pilacinski, W.P., Glassman, D.L., Krzyzek, R.A., Sadowski, P.L., and Robbins, A.K. (1984): Biotechnology, 1: 356-360.
49. Rabson, M.S., Yee, C., Yang, Y.C., and Howley, P.M. (1986): J. Virol., 60: 626-634.
50. Rous, P., and Beard, J.W. (1935): J. Exp. Med., 62: 523-548.
51. Rous, P., and Kidd, J.G. (1936): Science, 83: 468-469.
52. Sarver, N., Rabson, M.S., Yang, Y.C., Byrne, J.C., and Howley, P.M. (1984): J. Virol., 52: 377-388.
53. Schlegel, R., Wade-Glass, M., Rabson, M.S., and

Yang, Y.C. (1986): Science, 233: 464–466.

54. Schiller, J.T., Vass, W.C., and Lowy, D.R. (1984): Proc. Natl. Acad. Sci. USA, 81: 7880–7884.

55. Schwarz, E., Freese, U.K., Gissmann, L., Mayer, W., Roggenbuck, B., Stremlau, A., and zur Hausen, H. (1985): Nature, 314: 111–114.

56. Spalholz, B.A., Lambert, P.F., Yee, C.L., and Howley, P.M. (1987): J. Virol. (in press).

57. Spalholz, B.A., Yang, Y.-C., and Howley, P.M. (1985): Cell, 42: 183–191.

58. Stenlund, A., Zabielski, J., Ahola, H., Moreno-Lopez, J., and Pettersson, U. (1985): J. Mol. Biol., 182: 541–554.

59. Tsumori, T., Yutsudo, M., Nakano, Y., Tanigaki, T., Kitamura, H., and Hakura, A. (1983): J. Gen. Virol., 64: 967–969.

60. Tsunokawa, Y., Takebe, N., Kasamatsu, T., Terada, M., and Sugimura, T. (1986): Proc. Natl. Acad. Sci. USA, 83: 2200–2203.

61. Yang, Y.C., Okayama, H., and Howley, P.M. (1985a): Proc. Natl. Acad. Sci. USA, 82: 1030–1034.

62. Yang, Y.C., Spalholz, B.A., Rabson, M.S., and Howley, P.M. (1985b): Nature, 318: 575–577.

63. Yasumoto, S., Burkhardt, A.L., Doniger, J., and DiPaolo, J.A. (1986): J. Virol., 57: 572–577.

64. zur Hausen, H., and Schneider, A. (1987): In: Papovaviridae. 2. The Papillomaviruses, edited by N.P. Salzman, and P.M. Howley, pp. 245–259, Plenum Press, New York.

# Structural, Antigenic and Molecular Analysis of Bovine and Human Papillomaviruses

G. Della Torre, R. Donghi, M. Muttini,
P.O. De Campos Lima, M.A. Pierotti and G. Della Porta

*Division of Experimental Oncology A,*
*Istituto Nazionale Tumori*
*Milan, Italy*

Epidemiological studies indicate that an infectious agent with a long latency is involved in the etiology of human cervical carcinomas (11). The human papillomaviruses (HPVs) appear to be convincing candidates for such a role. As for other virological diseases, a serological assay could provide an effective way to type an HPV infection in individual patients. This approach is hampered by the lack of a cell culture system capable to propagate the virus and to produce sufficient amounts of viral antigens of the multiple types of HPV (18). However, a group-specific antigen common to most HPVs infecting various species has been demonstrated (12). Antisera from patients and from immunized animals recognize this antigen displayed also by a PV from a different species (1,12), indicating a close relationship among various PVs due to the existence of well conserved sequences in viral genomes (10). To date, the group-specific antigen more easily available to test humoral antibody response to HPV and to assess a serological association of HPV with genital lesions derives from bovine papilloma virus (BPV) (1).

More recently, the availability of molecular probes relative to the different HPVs has permitted a more direct approach based on the detection and the characterization of HPV DNA sequences. Molecular analysis has revealed that this group of viruses is remarkably heterogeneous and that only certain HPV types are consistently associated with specific benign or malignant genital lesions (9). Although functional studies on the role of the viral DNA in malignant progression are at an early stage, the characterization of specific HPV DNAs in genital lesions has already revealed features of considerable diagnostic and research value.

Here, we present and discuss the characterization of

BPV proteins used in a serological assay to detect specific anti-HPV antibodies in patients sera. Preliminary results of a molecular analysis of the DNA from benign and malignant genital lesions using HPVs molecular probes are also reported.

### Serological Analysis of Patients with Benign and Malignant Genital Lesions and Characterization of the Target BPV Proteins

Sera from 74 women with lesions of the uterine cervix and vulva (43 condylomata, 11 intraepithelial neoplasias and 20 invasive carcinomas) and from 12 healthy controls were examined by direct or indirect radioimmunological assay (RIA) for IgG antibodies to the group-specific antigen of BPV. As already reported by others (1,13), virions were isolated from a pool of bovine fibropapillomas, purified by a single CsCl gradient centrifugation and used, as target, after treatment with detergent to disclose the group-specific antigen masked inside the virion. The positive control was a rabbit antiserum against disrupted BPV virions with normal rabbit serum as a negative control. The specificity of the assay was ascertained also by testing the immune serum against whole virions not displaying group-specific antigens.

In a direct RIA, all patients and control sera showed low levels of specific antibodies and the mean value of their binding indexes at 1:100 dilution was 8.2, 7, 7.5 and 7.8 for condyloma, intraepithelial neoplasia and carcinoma patients and healthy women, respectively. In an indirect RIA, all patients and control sera were able to inhibit the binding of a specific immune serum and their mean percentage of inhibition was 19.7%, 22.6%, 17% and 18.8% for condyloma, intraepithelial neoplasia and carcinoma patients and healthy individuals, respectively. Therefore, no significant differences were found in the frequency or level of antibodies between each of the 3 groups of patients and the group of normal controls. These results are in contrast with the serological findings of Baird (1), but agree with those obtained by Di Luca et al. (5), and seem to exclude a serological correlation between HPV and genital lesions at least for the humoral response against the group-specific antigen. A possible explanation could be the weak immunogenicity of the group-specific antigen in natural conditions and/or the topological localization of the virus in the outer portion of the mucosal epithelium, where it is sequestered from the immune system. To establish wether a viral component was recognized by antibodies in sera of patients, three of the RIA-positive sera were analyzed by Western blotting technique. The protein patterns obtained suggest that the sera recognized the viral protein of 55 KD corresponding to the main capsid component, but also nonviral proteins contaminating the viral preparation (data not shown). Since keratinocytes are the source of the BPV virions used as target antigen, a rabbit anti-keratin serum was initially tested by RIA on isolated BPV virions to verify the purity of the viral preparation. As shown in Figure 1, the reactivity of the anti-keratin serum was high and comparable to the reactivity of a rabbit anti-BPV serum.

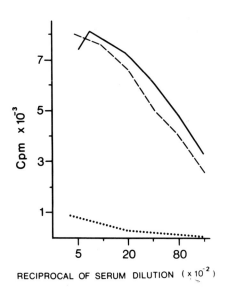

**FIG. 1.** Binding activity of a rabbit anti-BPV serum (———), a rabbit anti-keratin serum (----) and a normal rabbit serum (....) on dissociated BPV particles revealed by goat anti-rabbit $^{125}$I labelled immunoglobulins.

This result could be explained by the presence of free keratins in the viral preparation or by cross-reactions between viral proteins and keratins. To investigate this issue, we further purified the BPV virions and analyzed their ability to react with anti-keratin monoclonal antibodies.

The viral preparation was iodinated and gel filtered under nondissociating conditions on a Sephadex G-150 column to obtain in the void volume the recovery of intact virions and to separate free proteins, both of viral and tissue origin. The iodinated polypeptides contained in the void volume fractions were reacted with the specific immune serum or with the anti-keratin serum, and the immunoprecipitates were analyzed by SDS-PAGE under reducing conditions. A complete identity between the polypeptides identified by the anti-BPV and the anti-keratin antibodies was observed (data not shown), thus supporting the concept of a cross-reactivity between BPV antigens and keratin. Table 1 summarizes the results obtained by reacting BPV proteins with several mouse monoclonal antibodies to intermediate filament proteins: anti-keratin antibodies with different tissue and keratin specificities, anti-desmin (DES) and anti-vimentin (VIM) antibodies and an antibody recognizing an antigenic determinant common to all classes of the intermediate filaments (PAN). RIA was used to evaluate the amount of the antibody bound to dissociated virions, the Western blotting technique to visualize antigenic proteins among the electrophoretically separated and denatured viral proteins, and the radioimmuno-precipitation (RIP) to analyze the protein composition of intact virions after their immunological recognition.

**TABLE 1.** Reactivity of BPV Proteins with Mouse Monoclonal Antibodies to Intermediate Filament Proteins

| | Antibody | RIA (°) | Western blotting | RIP (*) |
|---|---|---|---|---|
| A N T I — K E R A T I N | E-12 | ++ | 55KD | + |
| | KL-1 | +++ | 55KD | + |
| | AE1-AE3 | + | 55KD | + |
| | H-11 | + | − | + |
| | 10-11 | + | − | + |
| | CK-2 | − | − | − |
| | CAM 5-2 | − | − | − |
| | VIM | ++ | − | + |
| | DES | − | − | + |
| | PAN | ++ | − | + |

(°): + = Binding index at serum dilution of 1:250 was 5-15; ++ = 15-25; +++ = 25-35.

(*): + = 76, 57 and 28 KD proteins identified in the autoradiograms.

We observed that almost all the antibodies tested were able to bind virions in RIA and RIP, whereas some of them recognize the main capsid 55KD protein, as revealed by Western blotting technique. The absence of reactivity of unrelated mouse monoclonal antibodies proved the specificity of the immunological reactions. Fig. 2 exemplifies the patterns of reactivity typically obtained with the three different techniques with anticytokeratin antibodies.

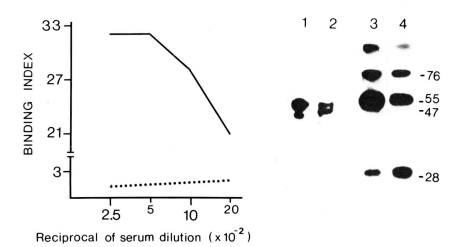

**FIG. 2.** Analysis of the reactivity of the mouse anti-keratin monoclonal antibody KL-I on BPV by different techniques. Left side: binding indexes of KL-I increasing dilutions with dissociated BPV particles (———) or bovine serum albumin (......) measured by goat anti-mouse $^{125}$I labelled immunoglobulins. Right side: Western blotting of SDS-PAGE of BPV proteins. KL-1 monoclonal antibody (lane 1) and rabbit anti-BPV serum (lane 2) were developed by the relative anti-immunoglobulins. SDS-PAGE of purified $^{125}$I labelled BPV particles immunoprecipitated with KL-1 monoclonal antibody (lane 3 ) or rabbit anti-BPV serum (lane 4).

It is interesting to note that the same viral polypeptides were recognized, both in Western blotting technique and in RIP, by the rabbit anti-BPV serum and the anticytokeratin monoclonal antibodies. Although the possibility of a cross-reaction between the 55 KD viral protein and keratins requires further verification, it is tempting to speculate that their immunological relatedness may be related to the peculiarity of papillomaviruses to replicate only in terminally differentiated keratinocytes.

## Molecular Heterogeneity of HPV Sequences in Benign and Malignant Genital Lesions

A molecular analysis to identify HPV DNA sequences directly in neoplastic as well as in precancerous lesions appears particularly suitable to explore the role of HPVs in tumor development. In fact, it has been reported that the risk of genital neoplasia is associated with HPV-16 or HPV-18 types infection (2,4,7). Their DNA can be found also in a certain proportion of condylomata and intraepithelial neoplasias of lower grades, which usually harbor DNA of other HPV types (HPV-6 or HPV-11), suggesting that the biological evolution of benign or premalignant lesions may depend on the HPV type (3). The physical state of HPV-16 or HPV-18 DNA appears to vary with the degree of malignancy (2,8,17), and structurally modified genomes of these types can be detected in carcinomas (2,15). These findings, together with the demonstration of expressed HPV-16 or HPV-18 genomes in cell lines established from carcinomas (2,16,19), would imply an involvement of virally encoded or regulated molecules in neoplastic onset and/or progression.

We studied the molecular complexity of HPV in pathological specimens using HPV-16 sequences as probe.

A first level of complexity is represented by the physical form of HPV-16 DNA, which can be detected as free nuclear episomes or as integrated sequences in the host chromosomes. DNA obtained from a flat cervical condyloma, digested with Bam HI and hybridized with HPV-16 probe, as shown in lane 3 of Fig. 3, appeared as a single band of 7.9 Kb comigrating with the native linearized HPV-16 DNA (lane 5), which strongly suggests that the HPV exists in this premalignant lesion as free viral genomes.

Conversely, as shown in lane 4 of the same figure, the DNA from a cervical carcinoma generated a hybridization smearing over a substantial region of the gel, thus indicating the integration of viral genomes. The large band of 7.9 kb can be interpreted as episomal HPV DNA, as integrated tandem repeats or as both. The analysis of undigested viral DNA confirmed the presence of free episomes in the carcinoma DNA (lane 2) comigrating with the band of the nicked circular HPV 16 DNA of the flat condyloma (FII in lane 1). To determine whether HPV oligomeric episomes were also present in the carcinoma DNA, the latter was digested with Hind III (a noncutting enzyme for HPV-16) and subjected to a two-dimensional gel electrophoresis that permits the separation of integrated from free viral sequences. In Fig. 4 the viral sequences appear resolved as a continuous trail of cellular DNA, representing the integrated forms, and as discrete spots of free oligomers of variable size.

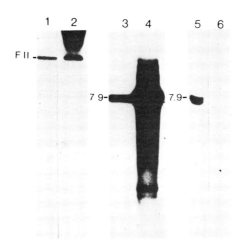

**FIG. 3.** Southern blot hybridization of HPV-16 probe on un-digested or Bam HI digested DNA from a flat condyloma (lanes 1, 3) and an invasive cervical carcinoma (lanes 2, 4). FII marks the nicked circular HPV-16 DNA present in the undigested DNA of condyloma or carcinoma. HPV-16 DNA (lane 5) and HeLa cell DNA (lane 6) cleaved with Bam HI were applied as controls.

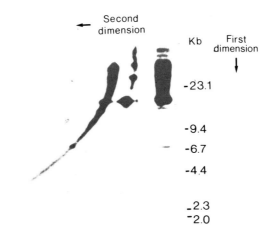

**FIG. 4.** Analysis of the physical state of HPV-16 DNA in a cervical carcinoma DNA. The tumor DNA (the same as in Fig. 3) was digested with Hind III and then separated by two-dimensional gel electrophoresis. The first dimension was run in 0.4% agarose (right side) and the second one in 1% agarose (left side); blotted DNA was hybridized with HPV-16 probe. The position of molecular weight markers (λ DNA Hind III fragments) are indicated.

To summarize, the analysis of the physical form of HPV-16 indicated that the virus was present only as free episomal DNA in the flat condyloma, whereas in the examined carcinoma it existed as free oligomeric episomes as well as DNA integrated in the host cells genoma, most likely with a prevalence of tandem repeats.

The next examples deal with another level of the molecular complexity found in HPV DNA from malignant genital lesions. Basically, two patterns of viral DNA can be distinguished with bands of a molecular weight higher or lower than the 7.9 kb HPV-16 linear form, respectively. Fig. 5 shows the patterns of the viral sequences from an anal PV-associated intraepithelial neoplasia (lane 2) and from an invasive cervical carcinoma (lanes 3 and 4) after digestion of the samples with the linearizing enzyme Bam HI. They represent examples of rearranged viral genomes with a larger size than that of the prototype HPV-16, which are most likely due to duplication of some viral regions. The pattern observed with the anal tumor DNA without digestion (lane 1) is consistent with viral genomes present as oligomers, whereas in the cervical carcinoma the virus seems to exist also in an integrated form, as can be deduced from the smearing observed in lane 3 after a longer exposure of the autoradiogram.

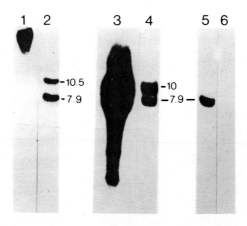

**FIG. 5.** Southern blot hybridization of HPV-16 probe on undigested (lane 1) and Bam HI digested (lane 2) DNA from an anal PV-associated intraepithelial neoplasia and on Bam HI digested DNA from an invasive vulvar carcinoma (lanes 3 and 4 after high and low exposure, respectively). Bam HI digested HPV-16 (lane 5) and HeLa cells DNA (lane 6) were applied as controls.

Another type of HPV-16 rearrangement can result from deletion of viral sequences, as reported in the examples of Fig. 6. The DNAs from two PV-associated VIN III were examined after digestion with Bam HI. The first sample in lane 1 yielded two bands of 6.4 and 3.4 kb, respectively, consistent with the virus being present as episomal DNA. The second VIN III case was resolved at low exposure in a single band of 7.1 kb (lane 3), which indicates a deletion of about 800 bp from the viral genome. Also in this case a higher exposure revealed that part of the virus was probably integrated in the genomic DNA (lane 2).

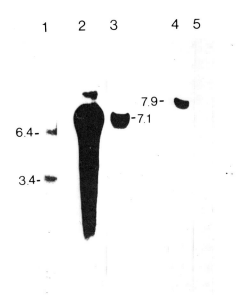

**FIG. 6.** Southern blot hybridization of HPV-16 probe on Bam HI digested DNA from PV-associated VIN III of two different patients (lane 1; lanes 2 and 3 after high and low exposure, respectively). Bam HI digested HPV-16 (lane 4) and HeLa cells DNA (lane 5) were applied as controls.

Finally, the potential correlation between the molecular complexity of HPV sequences and the nature of different genital lesions is indicated from the results reported in Fig. 7. The hybridization patterns of HPV 16 were examined in the DNA from three different lesions that coexisted in the same patient: a condyloma (lane 1), a VIN III (lane 2) and an early vulvar carcinoma (lane 3). After digestion with Bam HI, all the samples showed a band of 7.9 kb similar to that of the HPV-16 prototype. However, an anomalous band of 2.8 kb was additionally detected in the condyloma, it changed its size in the VIN III (2.6 kb), and apparently disappeared in the vulvar cancer. In parallel, also the physical form of the virus was changed, passing from pure free episomes in the benign lesion to a pattern compatible with an integration in the VIN III and the carcinoma.

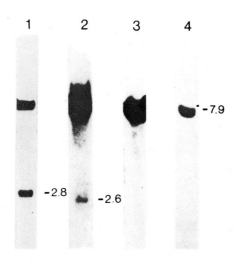

**FIG. 7.** Southern blot hybridization of HPV–16 probe on DNA from three different areas of a PV–associated early vulvar carcinoma (multicentric) (lane 1: condyloma; lane 2: VIN III; lane 3: carcinoma). Bam HI digested HPV–16 DNA (lane 4) was applied as a control.

This example demonstrates the general finding that HPV–16 is found almost exclusively as free episomes in condylomata and, at least partially, is integrated in carcinomas. Thus, the transition of the viral physical form from the episomal to an integrational state appears to be correlated with the progression from a benign to a malignant form of genital lesions. In addition, different distinct rearrangements of HPV–16 sequences can be detected in synchronous histologically different genital lesions.

A detailed analysis of the mechanisms leading to the reported molecular complexity of the HPV genome in tumor DNA should be carried out to explore possible interactions of viral sequences with cellular genes (oncogenes) following chromosomal integration (6,14) and to reveal whether the rearrangement of the viral sequence is due to duplication or deletion of specific and consistent viral genes. These approaches will eventually provide an understanding of the pathogenetic role of HPV in genital lesions.

## ACKNOWLEDGEMENTS

We thank our colleagues G. Pasquini, G. Raineri and M. Azzini for the excellent technical, secretarial and photographic assistance.

## REFERENCES

1. Baird, P.J. (1983): Lancet, ii: 17–18.
2. Boshart, M., Gissmann, L., Ikenberg,H., Kleinheinz, A., Scheurlen, W., and zur Hausen, H. (1984): EMBO J., 3: 1151–1157.
3. Brescia, R.J., Jenson, A.B., Lancaster, W.D., and Kurman, R.J. (1986): Human Pathol., 17: 552–559.
4. Crum, C.P., Ikenberg, H., Richart, R.M., and Gissmann, L. (1984): N. Engl. J. Med., 310: 880–883.
5. Di Luca, D., Rotola, A., Pilotti, S., Monini, P., Caselli, E., Rilke, F., and Cassai, E. (1987): Int. J. Cancer, 40: 763–769.
6. Durst, M., Croce, C.M., Gissmann, L., Schwarz, E., and Huebner, K. (1987): Proc. Natl. Acad. Sci. USA, 84: 1070–1074.
7. Durst, M., Gissmann, L., Ikenberg, H., and zur Hausen, H. (1983): Proc. Natl. Acad. Sci. USA, 80: 3812–3915.
8. Durst, M., Kleinheinz, A., Hotz, M., and Gissmann, L. (1985): J. Gen. Virol., 66: 1515–1522.
9. Gissmann, L. (1984): Cancer Surv., 3: 161–181.
10. Heilman, C.A., Law, M.-F., Israel, M.A., and Howley, P.M. (1980): J. Virol., 36: 395–407.
11. Howley, P.M. (1987): In: Important Advances in Oncology 1987, edited by V.T. Jr. DeVita, S. Hellman, and S.A. Rosenberg, pp. 55–73. J.B. Lippincot Co., Philadelphia.
12. Jenson, A.B., Rosenthal, J.D., Olson, C., Pass, F., Lancaster, W.D., and Shah, K. (1980): J. Natl. Cancer Inst., 64: 495–500.
13. Lancaster, W.D., Olson, C., and Meinke, W. (1976): J. Virol., 17: 824–831.
14. Popescu, N.C., DiPaolo, J.A., and Amsbaugh, S.C. (1987): Cytogenet. Cell Genet., 44: 58–62.
15. Scheurlen, W., Stremlau, A., Gissmann, L., Hohn, D., Zenner, H.-P., and zur Hausen, H. (1986): Int. J. Cancer, 38: 671–676.
16. Schneider-Gadicke, A., and Schwarz, E. (1986): EMBO J., 5: 2285–2292.
17. Scholl, S.M., Kingsley Pillers, E.M., Robinson, R.E., and Farrel, P.J. (1985): Int. J. Cancer, 35: 215–218.

18. Taichman, L.B., Breitburd, F., Croissant, O., and Orth, G. (1984): J. Invest. Dermatol., 83: 2s-6s.
19. Yee, C., Krishnan-Hewlett, I., Baker, C.C., Schlegel, R., and Howley, P.M. (1985): Am. J. Pathol., 119: 361-366.

# Implication of Papillomaviruses in Non-Genital Tumours

E-M. de Villiers

*Deutsches Krebsforschungszentrum*
*Heidelberg, F.R.G.*

Human papilloma viruses are generally divided into two groups – those that cause disease of the mucosa and those that afflict epidermal tissue. Of the latter group, some viruses are closely associated with distinct clinical disease, e.g. HPV 2 with verrucae vulgares, HPV 3 with verrucae planae and the so called epidermodysplasia verruciformis group of viruses (HPV 5, 8, 9, 12, 14, 15, 17, 19 – 25, 36) (10). Although most of the viruses belonging to this group can be found in benign lesions, lesions containing HPV 5 or 8 show a remarkable tendency to progress to malignant tumours especially at sites of solar exposure. The same applies to HPV 14, 17 and 20, but to date reported to occur at a lower frequency (9,11). Belonging to the group of human papilloma viruses which normally afflict the mucosal tissue are HPV 6, 11, 13, 16, 18, 31, 32, 33, 35, 39, and 42 (3,7,9,12). Of these, the molecular biological and epidemiological role of HPV 6, 11, 16, and 18 in genital lesions have been extensively studied (12). HPV 6 and 11 are associated with benign genital proliferations and HPV 16 and 18 with premalignant and malignant genital lesions.

In this series we report on the prevalence of these 4 virustypes (or of closely related subtypes) in a series of lesions originating from the skin, head and neck area (cutaneous and mucosal), as well as the respiratory and digestive tracts.

The methods we used, were as follows:

1. Total cellular DNA was radioactively labelled using $^{32}$P-TTP and hybridized under stringent conditions (Tm -20°C) to DNAs of various human papillomaviruses (5).
2. $^{32}$P-HPV-DNA was hybridized under stringent conditions (Tm -20°C) to cellular DNA digested with a specific restriction enzyme.

3. $^{32}$P-HPV-18-DNA was hybridized under relaxed conditions (Tm -30°C) to cellular DNA digested with either Bam HI or Eco RI restriction enzymes.

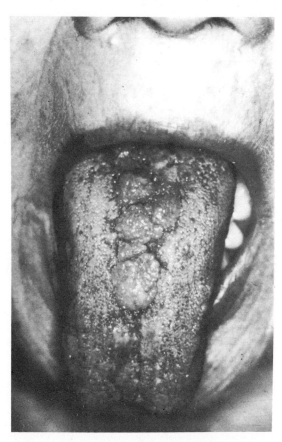

**FIG. 1.** A tongue papilloma (WV-4276) harbouring HPV 11 DNA (photo kindly provided by Dr. Neumann, University of Munster).

All biopsies were, in the first instance, screened using the first method mentioned. Most of the positive results were confirmed by applying method 2 using a restriction enzyme which would yield a typical digestion pattern of the HPV in question. Biopsies with negative results after the first test, were all screened under relaxed conditions with HPV 18, a positive result indicating the presence of papillomavirus-related sequences. To minimize non-specific cross-hybridization with cellular sequences, the clone of HPV 18 without the control region of the genome (1,1 kb Bam HI fragment) was used in this test.

Table 1 summarizes the biopsies tested.

**TABLE 1**

| Sites of Biopsies | Benign | Malignant |
|---|---|---|
| Head and Neck | 206 | 253 |
| Skin | 295 | 65 |
| Digestive Tract | 19 | 99 |
| Lung | 0 | 45 |
| Total | 520 | 462 |

## HEAD AND NECK TUMOURS

Papillomavirus sequences could be detected in rough-ly 50% of papillomatous proliferations in the mouth. Of these, 18% contained HPV 6 or HPV 11 sequences. An example of a tongue papilloma harbouring HPV 11 can be seen in Fig. 1.

Fig. 2 shows the patterns of HPV 11 DNA after Pst I and Hinc II restriction enzyme digestion, isolated from a nasal papilloma.

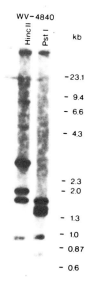

**FIG. 2.** HPV 11 DNA in the DNA from a nasal papilloma (Pst I and Hinc II digestion).

Of all laryngeal papillomas tested, 75% harboured either HPV 6 or HPV 11 DNA. HPV 18 DNA was found in a histologically identified fibrolipoma of the parotis. HPV 18-related sequences were identified in a persisting,highly proliferative inverted papilloma of the upper jaw, in another tongue papilloma and two oral papillomatous proliferations. A squamous epithelial carcinoma of the supraglottis contained HPV 18-related sequences.

An interesting case was a papillomatous tumour on the face of a patient which contained HPV 11-related sequences. Histologically it contained numerous atypical cells, but it was not possible to give a definite classification.

Looking at papillomatous lesions of the mouth and laryngeal papillomas, we find a very high percentage (up to 75%) containing HPV DNA sequences, the majority being either HPV 6 or HPV 11. However, examining about 120 other benign tumours in the head and neck region, we find only the single case mentioned to contain papilloma virus sequences. In the malignant tumours of this region HPV DNA could be demonstrated in only 3.5% of biopsies tested. This does not correlate at all with other reports (1,4,8), although the methods applied here could be regarded as more sensitive than in situ hybridization or antigenic staining of histological sections.

### TUMOURS OF THE DIGESTIVE TRACT

Nineteen benign lesions and 99 malignant tumours were tested. The benign lesions mostly included intestinal polyps, although six oesophageal papillomas were tested as well. The majority of malignant tumours were stomach, colon and rectal carcinomas.

HPV 18-related sequences could be detected in one oesophageal papilloma, 2 of 46 oesophageal carcinomas, 2 of 18 stomach carcinomas, one of 20 colon carcinomas and one of 10 rectal carcinomas. The HPV-related sequences from one stomach carcinoma and the oesophageal papilloma were cloned and on analysis found to consist of a fragment with a size of 1,3 kb which could be allocated to the transforming (E6-E7) region of the HPV 18 genome.

### SKIN TUMOURS

As we mentioned at the beginning, this study only reports on the presence of HPV 6, 11, 16, and 18 (or 18-related sequences) in the tumours tested. Although no tumours of cutaneous origin (except the papillomatous lesion of the face mentioned earlier) contained HPV 6 or 11 sequences, a few tumours were shown to contain either HPV 16 or HPV 18-related sequences. HPV 16 DNA was found in a biopsy of an epidermal naevus on the foot (Fig. 3) and in a squamous cell carcinoma in a patient with arsenic keratoses. HPV 18-related sequences were identified in seborrhoic warts and 2 cases of psoriasis.

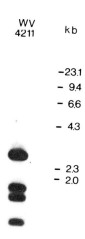

WV
4211   kb

−23.1
− 9.4
− 6.6

− 4.3

− 2.3
− 2.0

**FIG. 3.** HPV 16 DNA (typical Pst I digestion pattern) in the cellular DNA from an epidermal naevus.

Although some of the viruses of the cutaneous group have been found to be present in tumours of mucosal origin, e.g. HPV 2 in a tongue carcinoma (6); HPV 3-related and HPV 5-related sequences in condylomata acuminata, as well as HPV-2 and HPV-5 related sequences in Bowen's disease (4, unpublished results); HPV 1, 2, and 10 have been reported in single case of condylomata acuminata (10); HPV 7 DNA have been found in several cases of oral papillomatous in immunosuppressed patients (unpublished results), viruses known to cause mucosal lesions have not been reported to cause skin proliferations.

## WHAT ARE THE IMPLICATIONS
## OF THESE FINDINGS DESCRIBED ABOVE?

A large number of a very wide variety of histological types of benign and malignant lesions have been screened for the presence of DNA sequences of papillomaviruses normally associated with genital tumours. The presence of HPV 6, 11, 16 and 18 in tumours of the head and neck region as well as the digestive tract could well be expected, as most tissues are mucosal, and, considering certain human habits, the spreading of these viruses into or via the oral cavity is feasible. Regarding the causal factors in the etiology of tumour development (with the exception of oral papillomatosis and laryngeal papillomas), the role of these viruses found here remains, at present, unclear. This applies to results concerning the skin tumours as well. We do, however, not exclude the possibility that other, as yet unknown papillomaviruses could be the causal agents of the as yet negative proliferative lesions.

## REFERENCES

1. Abramson, A.L., Brandsma, J., Steinberg, B., and Winkler, B. (1985): Arch, Otolaryngol., 111: 709–715.
2. Adler-Storthz, K., Newland, J.R., Tessin, B.A., Yeudall, W.A., and Shillitoe, E.J. (1986): J. Oral Pathol., 15: 230–233.
3. Beaudenon, S., Praetorius, F., Kremsdorf, D., Lutzner, M., Worsaae, N., Pehau-Arnaudet, G., and Orth, G. (1987): J. Invest. Dermatol. (in press).
4. Brandsma, J.L., Steinberg, B.M., Abramson, A.B., and Winkler, B. (1986): Cancer Res., 6: 2185–2188.
5. de Villiers, E-M., Schneider, A., Gross, G., and zur Hausen, H. (1986): Med. Microbiol. Immunol., 17: 281–286.
6. de Villiers, E-M., Weidauer, H., Otto, H., and zur Hausen, H. (1985): Int. J. Cancer, 36: 575–578.
7. Lorincz, A.T., Lancaster, W.D., and Tample, G.F. (1986): J. Virol., 58: 225–229.
8. Milde, K., and Loening, T. (1986): J. Oral. Pathol., 15: 292–296.
9. Orth, G.: Personal communication.
10. Pfister, H. (1986): Zbl. Haut, 152: 193–202.
11. Yutsudo, M., Shimakage, T., and Hakura, A. (1985): Virology, 144: 295–298.
12. zur Hausen, H., and Schneider, A.: In: The Papillomaviruses, edited by P.M. Howley, and N.P. Salzman (in press).

# Laryngeal Papillomatosis

## A. Bomholt

*ENT Department, Roskilde Hospital, Roskilde, Denmark*

The first account of laryngeal papillomas has been attributed to Marcellus Donalus, who in the 17th century reported on "warts in the throat" (21). More than 200 years later, McKenzie (16) distinguished this condition from other laryngeal tumours and used the term papilloma. Although papilloma of the larynx is probably the most commonly used term, synonyms such as multiple laryngeal papillomatosis, recurrent respiratory papillomatosis, squamous papillomas of the larynx, juvenile and adult laryngeal papillomatosis and upper airway papillomatosis are common in the literature. The suffix-tosis indicated that more than one papillomatous lesion is present.

### ETIOLOGY

Ever since the experiments reported by Ullman in 1923 (20), laryngeal papillomas have been believed to have a viral etiology. Using a filtrable agent, Ullman was apparently able to transplant growth of papilloma to both skin and mucous membranes. The papilloma virus etiology (HPV-6, HPV-11) seems now to have been conclusively substantiated by hybridization technique (17).

The mode of transmission has not yet been definitively established. In cases of juvenile onset papillomas, intrapartum infection during fetal passage through an infected birth canal is a possibility that has been supported by the demonstration of a relationship between condylomas and laryngeal papillomas (18). However, the incidence of condylomas is probably increasing, at least in our area, whereas the incidence of juvenile laryngeal papillomatosis appears to be unchanged. Another point to be considered is that cases of siblings with laryngeal papillomas have never been reported.

The mode of transmission is unknown also in cases of

adult onset papillomas. The predominance of affected males has been explained by Strong et al. (19) to be derived from oral contact with infected genitalia. If this hypothesis was correct, there would be an accumulation of laryngeal papillomas among people living in close contact with infected subjects, which does not appear to be the case.

In 1983, Batsakis et al. (2) claimed that activation of a persistent viral infection coupled to an unknown promotor is the etiological basis for laryngeal papillomas. The observation that juvenile onset papillomatosis may recur after a quiescent period of several years following puberty supports this hypothesis (5). Although the "promotor" has never been defined, the following observations indicate that it might be part of the hormonal system: absence of papillomas during pregnancy, male predominance, and the fact that onset of papillomas just before or during puberty is rare (5,6). Also, the hormonal sensitivity of the larynx should not be disregarded.

## JUVENILE ONSET – ADULT ONSET

Laryngeal papillomatosis is often divided into a juvenile and an adult type according to onset before or after puberty. It is, however, a question whether such a division should be maintained. It is generally accepted that histological similarity, if not identity, exists among papillomas occurring in childhood and those with adult onset (1), and ultrastructural observations support this view (13). The incidence and sex ratio have been demonstrated to be identical for both types of papillomas (5,6) (see later) and they both have the same papilloma virus etiology (17). In children the disease occasionally takes a more serious course, which might indicate two different entities. However, the different luminal conditions of the juvenile and adult larynges should be taken into consideration and the seemingly different biological behaviour of papillomas in children and in adults should be regarded in the light of differences in immunocompetence and hormonal status. Some studies have reported similarities and no principal differences in clinical behaviour among adult patients with juvenile and adult onset (6,9). All these observations speak in favour of the hypothesis that laryngeal papillomas with juvenile and adult onset are one and the same disease.

## PATHOLOGY OF PAPILLOMAS

The lesions are most frequently encountered on the true vocal cords, the anterior commissure and the false vocal cords, but spread of lesions to the epiglottis is not uncommon. More rarely, the lesions extend to the supra and/or subglottic spaces.

The papillomas vary in colour from light pink to red and appears as glistening, elevated, mulberry-like nodular masses. The size ranges from small nodules to the bulk of a cherry.

The fact that papillomas occur either as solitary lesions or as multiple lesions makes some investigators consider them as separate entities. However, progression from a state of solitary lesion to a state of multiple lesions (papillomatosis) and vice-versa is not infrequently observed (6). As long as no distinctly different etiology has been demonstrated, solitary and multiple lesions must be regarded as one condition with varying clinical behaviour.

Microscopically, the papilloma is composed of a thickened squamous epithelium covering a stromal core. The thickening of the epithelium is primarily caused by an increased number of cells belonging to the spinous cell layer. The basal cells are bordered by a distinct basement membrane. Varying degrees of atypia may be found, especially in adults, and mitosis may be present.

The stromal core is composed of a vascular connective tissue with multiple extensions towards the surface. A mild inflammatory infiltration is often observed.

## DIAGNOSIS AND TREATMENT

Because of the characteristic laryngeal appearance, a tentative diagnosis is usually easy to establish in younger individuals by indirect laryngoscopy. In older patients it is more obvious to fear a malignant condition. However, a definite diagnosis can be established by histological examination of tumour tissue.

The principal treatment of laryngeal papillomas is still surgery, either microsurgical removal or evaporization by means of carbondioxide laser technique. The latter is claimed by some to be superior to the former. It is evident that the laser technique offers certain advantages, but a curative effect or even a positive effect on the recurrence pattern has as yet not been demonstrated (6).

The main purposes of surgery are to confirm the diagnosis, to maintain free airways and voice and to control or even cure the disease. The latter continues to be elusive, and Clark's statement in 1980 that papillomas will not respond to treatment until their period of active growth has passed, might be valid even today (15).

Several topical and systemic medications have been proposed. These include: steroid hormons, antibiotics

(aureomycin), antimetabolites (5-fluorouracil), bleomycin, idoxuridine, podophyllum, various types of
vaccine and, recently, interferon. Most of these agents
have been abandoned. The only successful adjuvant
therapy, based on clinical (4,11,12,15), histological
(8), and ultra-structural studies (7), appears to be
interferon.

## SYMPTOMS

The most common symptom in laryngeal papillomas is
hoarseness, affecting almost all patients. In infants,
aphonia and even inspiratory stridor may occasionally
be observed. Acute airway obstruction requiring emer-
gency tracheostomy is rare in the developed countries.

## CLINICAL COURSE

It seems to be a general impression that laryngeal
papillomatosis, especially in cases with juvenile
onset, is a severe disease, which has a relentless
propensity to recur, lacks behavioural predictability,
and is difficult to control (10,11,15,19).

This serious impression may arise from the fact that
most major studies reported over the last 30 years deal
with selected series and therefore reflect the usual
practice at the large well-reputed institutions rather
than the natural history of laryngeal papillomatosis.

In epidemiological studies from the Copenhagen
region (1,744,000 inhabitants), comprising all patients
treated for laryngeal papillomas from 1980 through
1983, the general impression was that laryngeal papillomatosis has a good prognosis and low morbidity (5,6).

For the group with juvenile onset (23 patients), it
could be concluded that the condition in most cases
will subside before puberty. Eleven children, either
younger that 15 years of age or disease-free before
puberty, underwent, on an average, 4 direct laryngoscopies (range 1-21 years); the median duration of
disease was 2 years (range 1-10 years). In five cases,
the disease persisted into adult age. The study showed
that regression before puberty did not ensure complete
recovery. Seven of the adult patients with juvenile
onset experienced relapse from 6 to 22 years after
puberty (median 21 years) (5).

In the group with adult onset (74 patients), the
median duration of disease was 2 years (range 1-32
years) and the median number of direct laryngoscopies
was 6 (range 1-32) (6).

The risk of malignant degeneration without prior
irradiation to the neck is a subject of discussion (1).
In some large series, malignant degeneration was noted
in adult patients up to several years after onset

(3,10). A recent epidemiological study showed an incidence of benign papillomas versus malignant degeneration of laryngeal papillomas of 10:1 (6).

Malignant degeneration of juvenile onset papillomas has also been reported after prior irradiation to the neck. Consequently, irradiation therapy was abandoned several years ago. A few cases of malignant degeneration of long-standing diffuse papillomatous growth involving the bronchi have been reported without prior irradiation (5).

## INCIDENCE

Since McKenzie (16) over 100 years ago reported laryngeal papillomas to be the most common benign tumour of the larynx, this statement has been repeated in several studies. Reliable data on the incidence, however, have not been reported until recently. The reason seems to be that the major studies have dealt with selected series of patients often collected over a period of 15-30 years. Bjork and Weber (3) concluded from their study that laryngeal papillomas show male predominance and that there is an equal distribution among children and adults.

In the epidemiological studies from the Copenhagen region, the male/female ratio was almost 3:1 and an incidence of 0.7/100,000 was found (5,6). The incidence of juvenile onset laryngeal papillomas was 0.7/100,000 in the at risk population aged 0-14 years. A similar incidence was found for adult onset laryngeal papillomas in the at risk population over 15 years of age.

The prevalence, as expressed by the number of patients undergoing direct laryngoscopy from 1980 through 1983, was 2.6/100,000. As opposed to other studies, our data indicated that adult onset laryngeal papillomas constitute a more serious diagnostic and therapeutic problem than do juvenile onset laryngeal papillomas. Whether or not a real change in disease behaviour has taken place could not be substantiated. In some studies, however, a change in incidence during the study period has been attributed to extrinsic factors (3,14). Variations in incidence from country to country cannot be excluded, and the introduction of microsurgery in the 1960s may have had an impact on the clinical course.

## CONCLUSION

Laryngeal papilloma of the larynx is a benign epithelial neoplasm, which has been conclusively demonstrated to have a viral etiology. Available data indicate that laryngeal papillomas with juvenile and adult onset are the same disease and that solitary and multiple papillomas cannot be considered different entities. On the whole, laryngeal papillomatosis seems to have a good prognosis. Only in a few cases the disease may take a more serious course. In adult patients, malignant degeneration constitutes a risk, emphasizing the importance of repeating direct and indirect laryngoscopy.

## REFERENCES

1. Batsakis, J.G., editor (1979): Tumors of the Head and Neck, 2nd ed., Williams and Wilkins Co., Baltimore.
2. Batsakis, J.G., Reymon, A.K., and Rice, D.M. (1983): Head Neck Surg., 5: 332-344.
3. Bjorg, H., and Weber, C. (1957): Acta Otolaryngol., 46: 499-516.
4. Bomholt, A. (1983): Arch. Otolaryngol., 109: 550-552.
5. Bomholt, A. (1987): Submitted to Acta Otolaryngol.
6. Bomholt, A. (1987): Submitted to Acta Otolaryngol.
7. Bomholt, A., and Horn, T. (1985): Acta Otolaryngol., 100: 304-308.
8. Bomholt, A., Ostergaard, B., and Horn, T. (1986): Acta Otolaryngol., 102: 131-135.
9. Capper, J.W.R., Bailey. C.M., and Michaels, L. (1983): Clin. Otolaryngol., 8: 109-119.
10. Dedo, H.H., and Jackler, R.K. (1982): Ann. Otol. Rhinol. Laryngol., 91: 425-430.
11. Goepfert, H., Guttermann, J.U., Dichtel, W.J., Sessions, R.B., Cangir, A., and Sulek, M. (1982): Ann. Otol. Rhinol. Laryngol., 91: 431-436.
12. Haglund, S., Lundquist, P.G., Cantell, K., and Strander, H. (1981): Acta Otolaryngol., 107: 327-332.
13. Horn, T., and Bomholt, A. (1985): Acta Otolaryngol., 99: 649-654.
14. Klos, J. (1979): Ann. Otol. Rhinol. Laryngol., 79: 1132-1138.
15. McCabe, B.F., and Clark, K.F. (1983): Ann. Otol. Rhinol. Laryngol., 92: 2-7.
16. McKenzie, M. (1871): Lindsay and Blakiston, Philadelphia.
17. Mounts, P., Shah, K.V., and Kashima, H. (1982): Proc. Natl. Acad. Sci. USA, 79: 5425-5429.
18. Quick, C.A., Kryzek, R.A., Watts, S.L., and Faras, A.J. (1980): Ann. Otol. Rhinol. Laryngol., 89: 467-471.
19. Strong, M.S., Vaughn, C.W., Healy, G.B., Cooperband, S.R., and Clement, M.A.C.P. (1976): Ann. Otol. Rhinol. Laryngol., 85: 508-516.
20. Ullman, E.V. (1923): Acta Otolaryngol., 5: 317-338.
21. Webb, W.W. (1956): Laryngoscope, 6: 871-918.

# Sexually Transmitted Diseases: An Overview of Clinical Manifestations and Long Term Sequelae of Herpesvirus and Human Papillomavirus Infections

C.A. Benson[1] and G.D. Wilbanks[2]

[1]Section of Infectious Disease, Department of Medicine;
[2]Department of Obstetrics and Gynecology
Rush Medical College
Rush Presbyterian St. Luke's Medical Center
Chicago, Illinois, USA

Sexually transmitted diseases affect more than 10 million persons per year in the United States. Data from the World Health Organization suggest that a proportional number of patients are affected in other western countries. Those most commonly at risk fall within the 15 to 29 year age group. Complications resulting from sexually transmitted diseases may interfere with the reproductive capacity of infected individuals, and may result in excess morbidity or mortality of offspring or of patients later in adult life.

There are more than 30 different organisms that produce sexually transmitted diseases (Table 1). The most common etiologic agents reported in the United States are Neisseria gonorrhoeae, Chlamydia trachomatis, and Herpes simplex virus (HSV). Syphilis, genital condylomata, chancroid, and lymphogranuloma venereum remain prominent sexually transmitted diseases worldwide. The clinical syndromes most often caused by sexually transmitted pathogens include vulvovaginitis, mucopurulent cervicitis, urethritis, genital ulcers or condylomata, proctitis, and pelvic inflammatory disease. While many sexually transmitted pathogens cause well recognized syndromes localized to the genital region, the importance of extragenital manifestations of disease cannot be overemphasized. Recent international experience with infection due to human immunodeficiency virus (HIV) and hepatitis B virus underscores the importance of the ability of sexually transmitted organisms to cause devastating systemic disease. The primary focus of this symposium is the role of

Herpesviruses and human papillomavirus (HPV), common sexually transmitted pathogens, in carcinogenesis of the human genital tract. The scope of this discussion will be limited to the clinical manifestations and sequelae of disease due to these organisms.

**TABLE 1.** Etiologic Agents of Sexually Transmitted Diseases

BACTERIA:

Neisseria gonorrhoeae
Neisseria meningitidis
Hemophilus ducreyii
Calymmatobacterium granulomatis
Gardnerella vaginalis
Mobiluncus curtisii
Mobiluncus mulieris
Shigella species
Salmonella species
Campylobacter species
Group B streptococci
Listeria monocytogenes
Bacteroides spp.
Anaerobic Gram positive cocci

CHLAMIDIA/MYCOPLASMA:

Chlamydia trachomatis
(includes LGV strains
L1-L3)

Mycoplasma hominis
Mycoplasma genitalium
Ureaplasma urealyticum


SPIROCHETES:

Treponema pallidum

VIRUSES:

Herpes simplex type 1
Herpes simplex type 2
Cytomegalovirus
Eptein-Barr virus
Human papillomavirus
Pox virus
Hepatitis A
Hepatitis B
Non-A Non-B hepatitis virus
Human immunodeficiency virus

FUNGI:

Candida species

ECTOPARASITES:

Phthirus pubis
Sarcoptes scabei

ENDOPARASITES:

Entamoeba histolytica
Giardia lamblia
Cryptosporidium species
Isospora belli
Trichomonas vaginalis

While the exact incidence of genital infection due to HSV is unknown, recent data suggest that it is clearly increasing. Since 1975, the reported incidence of genital HSV infection increased by 12% in the United

Kingdom (4, 15). There are an estimated 250,000 to 600,000 new cases in the United States per year (7,57). Adler-Storthz et al., report a 50% increase in the incidence of HSV type 2 infection during their four year study period (2). Supplanting syphilis, HSV infection is now the most common cause of genital ulcers in patients seen in sexually transmitted disease clinics in developed countries (57).

Approximately 70% of genital HSV infections are caused by HSV type 2, the remainder by HSV type 1 (16,17,57). The reverse is true of oral-labial HSV infection. While infection with these two virus types may be clinically indistinguishable, they do demonstrate distinct epidemiologic and physicochemical differences. Transmission of the virus occurs through contact of virus-containing secretions with skin or mucosal surfaces. Infectivity is high with up to 80% of patients developing infection after a single contact (44,57). Both horizontal and vertical transmission have been documented during asymptomatic viral shedding, which occurs in up to five percent of infected individuals (27,51). Approximately 50% of all genital HSV infections are asymptomatic (51,57).

Primary disease in a previously uninfected individual is characterized by an incubation period averaging four to seven days (mean 5.8, range one to 45 days) (16,17). Prodromal symptoms of malaise, fever and headache are followed by the development of exquisitely painful clusters of vesiculopustular lesions on an erythematous base, usually localized to the vulva, vagina or perineum in women and to the penis in men. The lesions rapidly enlarge, coalesce and ulcerate, creating shallow-based ulcers. Herpetic cervicitis may be the sole manifestation of initial infection in women and HSV can be isolated from the cervix in 65% to 88% of women during first episodes of infection (16,17). Crusting of external lesions and healing of all lesions generally occurs over a 14 to 21 day period although healing may be prolonged in some (16,17). Symptomatic primary infection may be accompanied by pharyngitis, aseptic meningitis or sacral radiculomyelitis with sacral plexus autonomic dysfunction causing urinary retention, constipation or impotence (16). Symptomatic first episodes of genital HSV infection in patients who have had prior HSV-1 oral-labial infections or previous asymptomatic genital infections are less often associated with systemic symptoms, are less severe, and heal more quickly than those in patients who have never had prior HSV infection (17,49).

In addition to prolonged painful primary episodes, both HSV-1 and HSV-2 produce latent infection with a propensity to recur. Genital HSV-2 infection is more likely to reactivate and recurs more frequently than does genital HSV-1 infection (49). Prospective studies report 55% of patients with HSV-1 and 80% with HSV-2 genital infections will have recurrent episodes within the first 12 months following primary infection (17). While recurrences do not follow a uniform pattern with regard to frequency, the median number of yearly clinical episodes is five to eight (16,17). Recurrent episodes are usually characterized by milder symptoms of shorter duration (mean 9.3 to 10.6 days) with lesions confined to approximately one tenth the area of involvement present with primary infection (16). Asymptomatic viral shedding is detectable in from 0.25 to 8% of infected patients (16). The duration is usually short (mean 3.2 days) and viral titers are low.

The diagnosis of genital HSV infection is often a clinical one, although supportive laboratory studies are available. The most reliable and sensitive diagnostic test for HSV infection is virus culture. Cultures are most likely to yield virus when obtained from lesions in the early vesiculopustular stage (15,16). Eighty to 95% of cultures obtained from such lesions will be positive; the yield is diminished to less than 20% once lesions ulcerate and crust (15-17). Cytologic smears from clinical specimens may demonstrate multinucleated giant cells. Immunocytochemical techniques, such as immunofluorescent staining of lesion scrapings with monoclonal antibodies, decrease the time to confirm the diagnosis, however, the sensitivity of these techniques ranges from 70 to 80% when compared with virus culture and more extensive experience is needed before they can become diagnostic standards (15,25,57). Serologic techniques are generally of little diagnostic utility. Seroconversion or a four-fold rise in antibody titer to HSV-1 or HSV-2 can be expected only during a true primary HSV infection (16,17).

Of more importance perhaps than the often extreme discomfort and inconvenience of primary and recurrent genital episodes are the potential complications and long term impact of genital infection due to HSV. Extragenital manifestations of disease occur in up to 28% of patients with primary genital herpes infection (16). These include neck stiffness, headache, aseptic meningitis, transverse myelitis, cutaneous dissemination, and direct extension of disease causing endometritis, pelvic inflammatory disease, pelvic cellulitis or suppurative lymphadenitis (16). Disseminated neonatal HSV infection, although rare, may result from congenital transmission, or more commonly, when infants are delivered through an infected birth canal. Transmission has been reported during primary and recurrent maternal genital infection and during asymptomatic cervical shedding of virus (54).

Another perhaps less well-recognized long term

complication of genital HSV infection is the possible oncogenic transformation of infected tissue by this virus. A seroepidemiologic relationship has been suggested between genital HSV infection and cervical carcinoma in women (1,6,14). A high percentage of patients with invasive cervical carcinoma have antibody to HSV-2 in contrast to a lower percentage of control patients (1,6,14). Aurelian et al. have demonstrated antibody to ICP10/Ag-4, an HSV-2 induced protein, in 49.6% of women with cervical intraepithelial neoplasia (CIN), 63% of women with cervical carcinoma in situ (CIS), 72.7% of women with invasive cervical carcinoma, and in only 11.7% of normal controls (5). In a prospective study of 209 women, loss of antibody was demonstrated after successful surgical removal of tumor and antibody reappeared with tumor recurrence (5).

Further in vivo and in vitro studies have demonstrated the oncogenic potential of HSV-2. Chen et al. showed that cervical carcinoma could be induced in 50% of mice after repeated intravaginal inoculation with inactivated HSV-2 and could be prevented by administration of a glycoprotein subunit vaccine (12). On a more basic level, the BglII N DNA fragment of HSV-2 has been shown to malignantly transform cells in vitro (60). This fragment encodes for a 38-kd protein which has been seroepidemiologically associated with cervical carcinoma (60). The 38-kd protein is thought to play a role in the transformation process, however, it has not been consistently identified in malignantly transformed cells (60).

Studies utilizing immunocytochemical and DNA hybridization techniques have demonstrated HSV-2 antigen and DNA in tumor tissue from women with cervical carcinoma. Eglin et al. demonstrated RNA complementary to HSV-2 DNA in 65% of biopsies from patients with CIN and in none of internally paired benign epithelial biopsies (22). Prakash et al. demonstrated HSV-2 DNA in 15% of biopsied invasive cervical neoplasms and in only 7% of benign cervical lesions (48). Park et al. showed HSV-2 DNA in one of eight cervical carcinoma biopsy specimens (47). While these data are not overwhelmingly convincing, they do suggest that HSV may act as a cofactor, initiator or potentiator in the development of cervical carcinoma.

Lastly, the economic and social impact of HSV genital infections is significant. For example, of the estimated 0.5 million cases per year of genital HSV infection in the United States, two to five percent require hospitalization for an associated complication. This fraction may be higher in underdeveloped countries where access to medical care is limited. Congenital and neonatal disease is associated with an unacceptably high morbidity and mortality and the risk of neonatal transmission obviates the need for ceasarian section delivery. Further, it is difficult to assess the impact that fear of transmission or acquisition of infection has had or will have on future relationships of infected individuals.

Of the remaining Herpesviruses, both cytomegalovirus (CMV) and Epstein-Barr virus (EBV) can be sexually transmitted, although this is not their principle mode of transmission. Neither of these agents produce localized genital syndromes, however, they can be excreted for prolonged periods in saliva and genital secretions, providing routes of viral transmission through intimate contact (3,43). Most healthy individuals infected with these viruses are asymptomatic. Of the 20% who develop symptomatic disease, mononucleosis is the most common clinical manifestation (3,31,43). Symptoms and signs include fever, fatigue, myalgias, pharyngitis, lymphadenopathy, splenomegaly, atypical lymphocytosis, hepatic dysfunction, and occasionally skin rash, pneumonitis, myopericarditis, or neurologic dysfunction (3,31,43). Splenomegaly and exudative pharyngitis are more common during EBV induced mononucleosis in contrast to CMV associated disease. While fever, fatigue and viral shedding may be prolonged, most individuals recover without sequelae over a three to six week period (3,31,43). The diagnosis can be made, in patients with a clinically compatible illness, by culture and/or specific serology.

As with HSV, both CMV and EBV are capable of maintaining latent infection and producing reactivation disease. The clinical importance of primary or reactivation infection with CMV in the normal host is confined to pregnancy. Primary infection during pregnancy is transmitted to up to 50% of fetuses and clinically apparent CMV disease is present in 10% of infected newborns (26,56). Additionally, sensorineural deafness and intellectual and behavioral disorders have been noted in 10% of offspring with subclinical neonatal infection (29). The risk of congenital transmission is reduced during reactivation disease due to partial protection imparted by passive transfer of maternal antibody. The clinical importance of primary or reactivation infection with EBV in the normal host lies in the ability of this virus to immortalize and transform lymphocytes, processes thought to play a role in the pathogenesis of nasopharyngeal carcinoma, Burkitt's lymphoma, and other lymphoproliferative disorders (43). In the immunocompromised host, severe multisystem disease and aggressive lymphoproliferative disease may result from either primary or reactivation infection with CMV and EBV, respectively. Lastly, the roles of these viruses in human genital malignancies are not as well recognized as those of HSV and HPV and will be reviewed in another portion of this volume.

HPV is a non-enveloped DNA virus of the Papovavirus family. Several types of this virus produce genital warts, a sexually transmitted disease with a rising worldwide incidence. As it is not a reportable disease in the United States, its incidence and prevalence are difficult to ascertain. In a study from Rochester, Minnesota, the number of cases diagnosed increased each year from 1950 to 1975 (13). The highest annual incidence of 106.5 cases per 100,000 population was reported from 1975 through 1978 (13). British investigators have noted an increase in men from 39.8 to 66.9 cases and in women from 20.3 to 34.6 cases per 100,000 population between 1971 and 1978, making HPV infection the fourth most common sexually transmitted disease in the United Kingdom (4). Patients between ages 15 and 29 who have had multiple sexual partners appear to be at highest risk (11). The infectivity rate of the virus is approximately 65% following an incubation period ranging from three weeks to eight months, with a mean of three months after contact with an infected partner (46).

HPV infects squamous epithelial cells of mucosal and cutaneous surfaces. Productive infection is manifested histopathologically by an increase in the stratum spinosum (acanthosis), degenerative cytoplasmic vacuolization (koilocytosis), nuclear alteration and pyknosis, and production of excess keratin, resulting in the clinical appearance of genital warts (28,30). Flat condylomata of the cervix, vaginal wall, or within the urethra, often visible only with a colposcope, have a thickened white epithelium with finger-like projections, each of which contains a dilated capillary loop (41). These lesions also histologically demonstrate the characteristic pattern of acanthosis, koilocytosis and dyskeratosis (41).

Genital warts usually first appear at the site of inoculation, which includes the frenum, coronal sulcus and inner prepuce of the penis in men and the posterior introitus and adjacent labia in women (46,53). They may be visible on or within the urethra, vagina, anus, adjacent perineum, or cervix in from six to 20% of patients (46,53). Of particular diagnostic import, flat condylomata may be visible only with the aid of the colposcope (41,42). Bladder condylomata have been described but are uncommon. Anal condylomata are common in homosexual men (46,53). Other than occasional irritative or obstructive symptoms engendered by the location of the lesions, most patients are asymptomatic.

The diagnosis of genital condylomata is dependent on the characteristic appearance of the lesions. When uncertainty is fostered by the presence of atypical lesions or flat condylomata associated with cervical dysplasia, histologic examination of sampled tissue will show acanthosis, koilocytosis, pyknosis, and hyperkeratinization. The association of flat condylomata with cervical intraepithelial neoplasia (CIN) is substantial, as further discussion will emphasize, and the two lesions may be histologically difficult to differentiate from one another. Papanicolaou (PAP) smear may show koilocytes suggestive of condylomata or dysplasia in the absence of visible lesions. In such situations, colposcopic examination to localize lesions is necessary. Men with meatal or distal intraurethral warts may require cystourethroscopy to exclude proximal intraurethral or bladder lesions, which may serve as reservoirs for repeated transmission of virus. External lesions should be treated prior to internal examination to prevent spread of virus to intraurethral or bladder structures. Serologic studies are not routinely available and the virus cannot be propagated in vitro.

The natural history and clinical course of HPV infection has received considerable attention. An illustrative study by De Brux et al., analyzing 764 cervical HPV lesions, reported that 26.8% of lesions regressed, 52.9% persisted and 20.3% progressed to more extensive involvement or dysplasia over an 18 month period (19,58). It is this natural history, demonstrating the proclivity of HPV, like other DNA viruses, to establish latent, persistent, or recurrent infection, that has engendered concern over the possible correlation between cervical, vulvar or penile HPV infection and malignant transformation of genital condylomata.

The concept of cervical carcinoma, and possibly vulvar and penile carcinoma, as sexually transmitted diseases, is a relatively recent one. An epidemiologic association has been noted between sexual activity and the occurrence of cervical carcinoma. Early studies reported a near non-existent incidence of cervical carcinoma in celibate women compared with sexually active women (55). The risk of cervical carcinoma appears to increase with an increase in the number of sexual partners reported by affected women (55). This association led investigators to begin their search for a sexually transmitted etiology by focusing on the role of the male partner. Certain "male factors" have been implicated in the pathogenesis of cervical carcinoma. "High risk" male partners may be those who have had multiple sexual partners, those with penile condylomata or penile carcinoma, those who have semen levels high in arginine-rich basic protein and those who have been previously married to or sexually involved with women who had cervical carcinoma (8,10,32,39,50,55). Women sexually active with such "high risk" male partners may have a significantly higher risk of subsequently developing cervical carcinoma (55).

With the advent of immunocytochemical and molecular virologic techniques, HPV has emerged from these earlier studies as another likely contender in the search for an oncogenic sexually transmitted pathogen. Kurman et al., studied 322 cases of cervical dysplasia and carcinoma in situ (CIS) using immunoperoxidase staining for HPV structural proteins (33). They found HPV structural proteins in 43% of mildly dysplastic (CIN I) lesions, 15% of moderate dysplastic (CIN II) lesions, 17% of severely dysplastic (CIN III) lesions, and 10% of lesions with CIS (33). In five of the 12 high grade lesions (CIN III/CIS) studied, areas of moderate dysplasia containing HPV structural proteins were found merging into areas of high grade dysplasia. This suggested a clear morphologic transition possibly induced by HPV.

In-situ hybridization studies have further demonstrated HPV DNA within both dysplastic and frankly malignant cervical lesions. Durst et al., using a HPV-16 DNA probe, identified HPV-16 DNA in from 34.8 to 61.6% of cervical cancer biopsy specimens obtained from patients living in different geographic locales (21). They also demonstrated HPV-16 DNA sequences in biopsy samples taken from vulvar and penile carcinomas (21). Only two of 33 benign condylomata adjacent to dysplastic lesions were positive for HPV-16 DNA sequences while most were positive for HPV-6 and HPV-11 sequences. The investigators concluded that the predominance of HPV-16 in malignant tumors made contamination from benign condylomata containing HPV-6 and 11 unlikely. Of 111 dysplastic or malignant cervical lesions studied by Lorincz et al., 101 (90.9%) had one or more HPV DNA sequences identified within biopsy samples (36). Sixty four of the 67 lesions recorded as cervical cancers contained HPV DNA sequences (36). Of the HPV DNA sequences identified within these lesions, 53.4% were HPV-16 or HPV-18; the remainder were recorded as HPV-6 or as yet uncharacterized sequences. Of note, 10 specimens were obtained from women with lymph node metastases and three of these 10 specimens had identical HPV sequences identified in both the primary and metastatic lesions (36). In a study by Syrjanen et al., of 343 women with HPV associated cervical condylomata and CIN, followed with serial PAP smears and punch biopsies, 25.1% of lesions regressed, 60.9 % persisted and 14% progressed over a mean period of 18 $\pm$ 15 months (58). Of the total number of lesions reported, 4.1% progressed to CIS. The lesions that progressed during follow-up were those containing HPV-16 or 18 DNA sequences. Of note, these investigators found HPV DNA sequences in 63.6% of punch biopsy specimens taken from histologically normal tissue adjacent to areas of HPV associated CIN. This finding was confirmed by MacNab et

al., who found HPV-16 DNA sequences in eight of 11
(73%) samples of normal tissue taken from within two to
five centimeters of genital cancers (38). Both studies
concluded that HPV associated lesions are capable of
malignant transformation and progression. Table 2
summarizes data from additional recent studies demonstrating HPV DNA sequences in biopsies of CIN and in
situ or invasive genital malignancies.

**TABLE 2.** Studies Utilizing DNA Hybridization Techniques
to Identify Human Papillomavirus Sequences in
Dysplastic or Neoplastic Genital Tissue

| AUTHOR | HPV DNA SEQUENCES | |
|---|---|---|
| | CIN | CIS/INVASIVE CA |
| Durst et al. (21) | | 11/18 |
| | | 8/23 |
| | | 2/7  (vulvar) |
| | | 1/4  (penile) |
| Crum et al. (18) | 7/10 | |
| Wagner et al. (63) | 4/13 | |
| | 15/22 | |
| Syrjanen et al. (58) | 29/49 | |
| Fukushima et al. (23) | 15/18 | 3/17 |
| Lehn (35) | | 4/6 |
| Lorincz et al. (36) | 37/44 | 64/67 |
| Prakash et al. (48) | 6/12 | 13/20 |
| Scholl et al. (52) | 3/4 | 5/11 |
| Wagner et al. (62) | | 68/101 |
| Burk et al. (9) | 5/11 | 16/17 |
| de Villiers et al. (20) | | 18/45 |
| Lancaster et al. (34) | | 13/13 (primary) |
| | | 3/13 (metastases) |
| Lorincz et al. (37) | 12/13 | |
| MacNab et al. (38) | | 21/25 |
| Tomita et al. (59) | | 17/30 |
| Tsunokawa et al. (61) | | 5/9 |
| McCance et al. (40) | | 27/53 (penile) |
| Gal et al. (24) | | 5/8  (anal) |

The data here reviewed support the concept that HPV
associated cervical dysplasias may consist of a diverse
group of lesions induced by a number of HPV types of
varying oncogenic propensity. A subset of HPV types,
specifically HPV-16 and HPV-18, may act alone or in
conjunction with other factors such as HSV infection,
to induce malignant transformation. Our current inabi-

lity to rapidly identify the HPV type involved and the uncertainty as to whether other types of HPV can induce neoplastic transformation as well, dictates that treatment of genital condylomata include a search for and treatment of other dysplastic lesions.

In conclusion, as this brief discussion of Herpesvirus and Human Papillomavirus infection illustrates, the scope of sexually transmitted infection transcends the morbidity associated with local genital disease and extends to extragenital and long term consequences. The diagnosis of well recognized syndromes associated with sexually transmitted pathogens remains challenging. Recognition, treatment, and prevention of their sequelae are of paramount importance, as the remainder of this volume will emphasize.

## REFERENCES

1. Adam, E., Kaufman, R.H., Adler-Storthz, K., Melnick, J.L., and Dreesman, G.R. (1985): Int. J. Cancer, 35: 19-26.
2. Adler-Storthz, K., Dreesman, G.R., Kaufman, R.H., Melnick, J.L., and Adam, E. (1985): Am. J. Obstet. Gynecol., 151: 582-586.
3. Alford, C.A., and Britt, W.J. (1985): In: Virology, edited by B.N. Fields, D.M. Knipe, R.M., Chanock, J.L. Melnick, B. Roizman, and R.E. Shope, pp. 629-660. Raven Press, New York.
4. Annual Report of the Chief Medical Officer of the Department of Health and Social Security, 1979 (1981): Br. J. Vener. Dis., 57: 402-405.
5. Aurelian, L., Kessler, I.I., Rosenshein, N.B., and Barbour, G. (1981): Cancer, 48 (2 Suppl.): 455-471.
6. Aurelian, L., Schumann, B., Marcus, R.L., and Davis, H.J. (1973): Science, 181: 161-164.
7. Becker, T.M., Blount, J.H., and Guinan, M.E. (1986): JAMA, 253: 1601-1603.
8. Buckly, J.D., Harris, R.W., and Doll, R. (1981): Lancet, ii: 1010-1014.
9. Burk, R.D., Kadish, A.S., Calderin, S., and Romney, S.L. (1986): Am. J. Obstet. Gynecol., 154: 982-989.
10. Campion, M.J., Singer, A., Clarkson, P.K., and McCance, D.J. (1985): Lancet, i: 943-946.
11. Centers for Disease Control (1983): Morb. Mort. Week. Rep., 32: 306-308.
12. Chen, M.H., Dong, C.Y., Liu, Z.H., Skinner, G.R., and Hartley, C.E. (1983): Vaccine, 1: 13-16.
13. Chuang, T-Y., Perry, H.O., Kurland, L.T., and Ilstrup, D.M. (1984): Arch. Dermatol., 120: 469-475.
14. Coleman, D.V., Morse, A.R., Beckwith, P., Anderson,

M.C., Gardner, S.D., Knowles, W.A., and Skinner
G.R. (1983): Br. J. Obstet. Gynaecol., 90: 421–
427.

15. Corey, L. (1986): Diagn. Microbiol. Infect. Dis., 4
(3 Suppl.): 111S–119S.

16. Corey, L., Adams, H.G., Brown, Z.A., and Holmes,
K.K. (1983): Ann. Intern. Med., 98: 958–972.

17. Corey, L., and Spear, P.G. (1986): N. Engl. J.
Med., 314: 686–691, 749–757.

18. Crum, C.P., Ikenberg, H., Richart, R.M., and
Gissmann, L. (1984): N. Engl. J. Med., 310:
880–883.

19. De Brux, J., Orth, G., Croissant, O., Cochard, B.,
and Ionesco, M. (1983): Bull. Cancer, 70: 410–
422.

20. de Villiers, E.M., Schneider, A., Gross, G., and
zur Hausen, H. (1986): Med. Microbiol. Immunol.,
174: 281–286.

21. Durst, M., Gissmann, L., Ikenberg, H., and zur
Hausen, H. (1983): Proc. Natl. Acad. Sci. USA,
80: 3812–3815.

22. Eglin, R.P., Kitchener, H.C., MacLean, A.B.,
Denholm, R.B., Cordiner, J.W., and Sharp, F.
(1984): Br. J. Obstet. Gynaecol., 91: 265–269.

23. Fukushima, M., Okagaki, T., Twiggs, L.B., Clark,
B.A., Zachow, K.R., Ostrow, R.S., and Faras, A.J.
(1985): Cancer Res., 45: 3252–3255.

24. Gal, A.A., Meyer, P.R., and Taylor, C.R. (1987):
JAMA, 257: 337–340.

25. Goldstein, L.C., Corey, L., McDougall, J.K.,
Tolentino, E., and Nowinski, R.C. (1983): J.
Infect. Dis., 147: 829–837.

26. Grant, S., Edmond, E., Syme, J. (1981): J. Infect.
Dis., 143: 24–31.

27. Growdon, W.A., Apodaca, L., Cragun, J., Peterson,
E.M., and de la Maza, L.M. (1987): JAMA, 257:
508–511.

28. Grussendorf, E.I., and zur Hausen, H. (1979): Arch.
Dermatol. Res., 264: 55–63.

29. Hanshaw, J.B., Scheiner, A.P., Moxley, A.W., Gaev,
L., Abel, V., and Scheiner, B. (1976): N. Engl.
J. Med., 295: 468–470.

30. Howley, P.M. (1982): Arch. Pathol. Lab. Med., 106:
429–432.

31. Klemola, E., von Essen, R., Henle, G., and Henle,
W. (1970): J. Infect. Dis., 121: 608–614.

32. Klemola, E., von Essen, R., and Wagner, O. (1969):
Ann. Intern. Med., 71: 11–19.

33. Kurman, R., Jenson, A., and Lancaster, W. (1983):
Am. J. Surg. Pathol., 7: 39–52.

34. Lancaster, W.D., Castellano, C., Santos, C.,
Delgado, G., Kurman, R.J., and Jenson, A.B.
(1986): Am. J. Obstet. Gynecol., 154: 115–119.

35. Lehn, H., Krieg, P., and Sauer, G. (1985): Proc. Natl. Acad. Sci. USA, 82: 5540–5544.
36. Lorincz, A., Temple, G., Santos, C., Castellano, C., Lemos, L., Delgado, G., Petrilli, E., Hummel, S., Kurman, R., Jenson, A.B., and Lancaster, W.D. (1985): Gynecol. Oncol., 20: 252.
37. Lorincz, A.T., Temple, G.F., Patterson, J.A., Jenson, A.B., Kurman, R.J., and Lancaster, W.D. (1986): Obstet. Gynecol., 68: 508–512.
38. MacNab, J.C.M., Walkinshaw, S.A., Cordiner, J.W., and Clements, J.B. (1986): N. Engl. J. Med., 315: 1052–1058.
39. Martinez, I. (1969): Cancer, 24: 777–780.
40. McCance, D.J., Kalache, A., Ashdown, K., Andrade, L., Menezes, F., Smith, P., and Doll, R. (1986): Int. J. Cancer, 37: 55–59.
41. Meisels, A., Fortin, R., and Roy, M. (1977): Acta Cytol., 21: 379–390.
42. Meisels, A., Morin, C., and Casas-Cordero, M. (1982): Int. J. Gynecol. Pathol., 1: 75–94.
43. Miller, G. (1985): In: Virology, edited by B.N. Fields, D.M. Knipe, R.M. Chanock, J.L. Melnick, B. Roizman, and R.E. Shope. pp. 563–589. Raven Press, New York.
44. Nahmias, A.J., Dowdle, W.R., Naib, Z.M., Josey, W.E., McClone, D., and Domescik, G. (1969): Br. J. Vener. Dis., 45: 294–298.
45. Ng, A.B., Reagan, J.W., and Yen, S.S. (1970): Obstet. Gynecol., 36: 645–651.
46. Oriel, J.D. (1971): Br. J. Vener. Dis., 46: 37–42.
47. Park, M., Kitchener, H.C., and MacNab, J.C. (1983): EMBO J., 2: 1029–1034.
48. Prakash, S.S., Reeves, W.C., Sisson, G.R., Brenes, M., Godoy, J., Bacchetti, S., de Britton, R.C., and Rawls, W.E. (1985): Int. J. Cancer, 35: 51–57.
49. Reeves, W.C., Corey, L., Adams, H.G., Vontver, L.A., and Holmes, K.K. (1981): N. Engl. J. Med., 305: 315–319.
50. Reid, B.L., French, P.W., Singer, A., Hagan, B.E., and Coppleson, M. (1978): Lancet, ii: 60–64.
51. Rooney, J.F., Felser, J.M., Ostrove, J.M., and Straus, S.E. (1986): N. Engl. J. Med., 314: 1561–1564.
52. Scholl, S.M., Pillers, E.M., Robinson, R.E., and Farrel, P.J. (1985): Int. J. Cancer, 35: 215–218.
53. Shah, K.V. (1985): In: Virology, edited by B.N. Fields, D.M. Kripe, R.M. Chanock, J.L. Melnick, B. Roizman, and R.E. Shope. pp. 371–392. Raven Press, New York.
54. Sher, J., Bottom, E., Desmond, E., and Simons, W. (1982): Am. J. Obstet. Gynecol., 144: 906–909.
55. Singer, A., and French, P. (1984): In: Cancer of

the Uterine Cervix. Biochemical and Clinical Aspects, edited by D.C.H. McBrien, and T.F. Slater, pp. 5–20. Harcourt Brace Jovanovich, New York.

56. Stagno, S., Pass, R.F., Dworsky, M.E., Henderson, R.E., Moore, E.G., Walton, P.D., and Alford, C.A. (1982): N. Engl. J. Med., 306: 945–949.

57. Straus, S.E., Rooney, J.F., Sever, J.L., Seidlin, M., Nusimoff-Lehrman, S., and Cremer, K. (1985): Ann. Intern. Med., 103: 404–419.

58. Syrjanen, K., Vayrynen, M., Mantyjarvi, R., Parkkinen, S., Saarikoski, S., Syrjanen, S., and Castren, O. (1985): In: Papillomaviruses: Molecular and Clinical Aspects, edited by P.M. Howley, and T.R. Broker, pp. 31–45. Alan R. Liss, Inc., New York.

59. Tomita, Y., Kubota, K., Kasai, T., Sekiya, S., Takamizawa, H., and Simizu, B. (1986): Intervirology, 25: 151–157.

60. Trimble, J.J., Gay, H., and Docherty, J.J. (1986): J. Reprod. Med., 31(5 Suppl.): 399–409.

61. Tsunokawa, Y., Takebe, N., Nozawa, S., Kasamatzu, T., Gissmann, L., zur Hausen, H., Terada, M., and Sugimura, T. (1986): Int. J. Cancer, 37: 499–503.

62. Wagner, D., de Villiers, E.M., and Gissmann, L. (1985): Geburts. Frauenh., 45: 226–231.

63. Wagner, D., Ikenberg, H., Boehm, N., and Gissmann, L. (1984): Obstet. Gynecol., 64: 767–772.

# Is There Today an Epidemic Outbreak of Cancer of the Uterine Cervix?

## M. Hakama[1] and K. Louhivuori[2]

*[1]Department of Public Health,*
*University of Tampere, Tampere, Finland*
*[2]Finland and Finnish Cancer Registry, Helsinki, Finland*

The question in the title implies that there should be an increase in the overall incidence of and mortality from cervical cancer. The background for such a trend could be general changes in sexual mores allowing a higher prevalence of sexually transmitted infections. Therefore the purpose of this paper is to assess at the population level the credibility of the hypothesis of sexually transmitted viruses being causes of cervical cancer. Such an assessment would be very indirect independently whether the answer to the question in the little will be positive or negative.

The link between viral infections and cervical cancer on population level could be made more specific. First, there should have occurred a recent change in the incidence trend and the trends should not simply follow a long term pattern. Second, one might expect the changes in the trends appearing first and be more substantial at young ages.

There is no good overall data worldwide on the mortality and morbidity of cervical cancer. Especially the long term trends are not well known. The five Nordic countries, Denmark, Finland, Iceland, Norway and Sweden have a rather uniform cancer registration system with long background (9). The registration started in Denmark in 1940's and in the other Nordic countries in the 1950's. Also the death statistics have long tradition. Therefore the Nordic Countries represent an area with long enough trends for the risk of cervical cancer known with reasonable degree of validity.

## EFFECT OF SCREENING ON THE TRENDS

The trends for invasive cervical cancer are affected also by the extent of the screening practised in the

population and not only by the changes in the etiological exposures. The detailed data on the intensity and
coverage of mass screenings for cervical cancer are not
available in general. Again, in the Nordic countries
the extent of the cytological screening programmes is
well known (5).

The screening programmes in the Nordic countries are
specificly organized to consist several essential
elements: An organized programme (7) defines the target
population, the individuals to be screened, as well as
the ages and frequencies of screening. Such a programme
utilized personal invitations with given times and
places for screening and the programme gives personal
information for the results of screening even when the
smear is negative. Furthermore, an organized programme
has a considerable extent of quality control in taking
of the smears, making of the diagnosis and evaluating
the effects of the programme.

In three of the Nordic countries, Finland (5),
Iceland (10) and Sweden (19), there is a nationwide
organized screening programme whereas in Denmark (11)
only half and in Norway (18) only a small proportion of
the population is covered by an organized programme.
Cytological smears are, however, frequently taken also
outside the organized system by private gynaecologists
and elsewhere. These spontaneous smears are more frequent than the organized smears in all the Nordic
countries except in Iceland.

There are different cervical screening policies in
the Nordic countries within the organized programmes.
In Finland, Iceland and Sweden a nationwide population
based organized programme has been in operation at
least since early 1970's. The recommended age groups to
be covered are 30 to 55 years in Finland, 25 to 69
years in Iceland and 30 to 49 years in Sweden. The
screening intervals recommended are 5 years in Finland,
2 to 3 years in Iceland and 4 years in Sweden. In
Denmark the recommendations vary by county and in
Norway only 5 per cent of the population was covered by
an organized programme.

There was a strong correlation between the extent of
the organized screening programme and changes in the
risk of cervical cancer (5). The incidence rates show a
substantial downward trend. In Finland about 400 cases
of cervical cancer were diagnosed annually before the
establishing of the screening programme (6). In early
1980's the annual number has been less than 200 (3,4).
Also the changes in the incidence of invasive cervical
cancer by age correlated with the intensity of the
screening programme (6). Up to the age of 50 years the
reduction in the age-specific incidence was 70 per cent
or more from 1950's to 1970's. Most substantial reduction in the incidence occurred between 1967 and 1974.

Outside that period the changes were smaller and less regular. There was practically no change in the incidence of cervical cancer at age 60 and over.

The time trends for the incidence of cervical cancer correlated with the organized screening programmes also in the other Nordic countries (5). The reduction in the risk was steepest in Iceland, Finland and Sweden, intermediate in Denmark. In Norway the incidence rates for cervical cancer increased up to late 1970's.

In some countries, e.g. in England and in the U.S.A., there was a decreasing trend in the mortality from uterine cancer already before introducing of the mass screenings for cervical cancer (13). Such trends may be indicating decrease in the risk of the disease, improvement of results of treatment or changes in diagnostic criteria. Whatever were the causes for the observed decreasing trends, similar changes were not observed for the time trends for incidence of cervical cancer in the Nordic countries. In fact, there was an increase in the risk of invasive cervical cancer before the introducing of the screening programmes (5). The increase was most substantial in Iceland, it was seen for Norway until late 1970's and it could be demonstrated also for Denmark, Finland and Sweden by an analysis based on birth cohorts.

## EVIDENCE OF OUTBREAK DUE TO CHANGES IN ETIOLOGY

The proposed recent outbreak of invasive cervical cancer is difficult to evaluate because of the confounding effects of cytological screening. In Finland as well as in the other Nordic countries there has been a rapidly decreasing trend in the incidence of cervical cancer which has slowed down during the recent years. The stabilization of the decreasing trend may indicate either a recent outbreak of cervical cancer or it may indicate obtaining of the ultimate expected risk of disease due to the screening programme.

No screening programme will eradicate the invasive disease. Because the programme is gradually introduced then the effect will also appear gradually, i.e. there is a decreasing trend in incidence. The incidence rates should ultimately stabilize to the level of the expected residual risk in the population. The determinants of this residual risk are: 1) the risk between two screening for those with a negative smear at first screening, 2) the risk among those not attending the programme, and 3) the proportion of the nonattenders in the population. The Finnish organized mass screening system provided estimation of those parameters and they were estimated in early 1970's on basis of first 70,000 women attending the programme twice (8). The predicted ultimate reduction in the risk of invasive disease with full maturation of the programme was about 60 per cent. The observed incidence rate in early 1980's is 65 per cent less than the rates before the screening programme (3,4). Because of the similarity of the predicted and observed reduction in risk it is likely that the stabilization of the rates simply indicates that the ultimate effect of the screening programme was obtained. Therefore the change in the trends do not imply that there were an outbreak of invasive cervical cancer. Even a slight increase in the incidence may indicate a continuation of a long term trend and not necessarily a recent outbreak of the disease.

The other prerequisity for an outbreak was an increase in the risk to appear first and to be more substantial at young ages. The risk of cervical cancer is small at ages less than 30. The incidence rates at age 20-29 years have been relatively stable and none of the Nordic countries showed a substantial increase in the rates around 1980 (2-4,14-16,21-24). Therefore there is neither a strong indication of an outbreak of cervical cancer at young ages.

Most of the evidence on an outbreak of cervical cancer comes from the observations on an increase in the preinvasive cervical lesions at young ages. First, the numbers of preinvasive lesions depend both on the risk and on the extent of screening. Some of the increase is due to more frequent screening. Second, the diagnosis of dysplasia is an evidence for both the proposed cause, the exposure, the viral infection and the proposed effect, the outcome, the malignancy. Therefore it is not self evident that the numbers of virus induced dysplasias will result in invasive cervical cancer. Third, even if there is a true increase of dysplasias at young ages which will transform invasive cervical cancer, it will not follow that women at those young ages should be screened. Screening is aimed at prevention of invasive disease and it is sufficient to screen at ages shortly before the preinvasive lesion will surface invasive cancer. The low risk of cervical cancer at ages under 25 or even under 30 indicate that screening under those ages will result in few prevented cancers only. Given the risk in Finland, even an increase in the risk by factor two would result in less than 100 annual cases of invasive cervical cancer for the total Italian female population aged 25-29. Therefore the cost-effectiveness is very low as compared to screening of women over 30.

There are alarming observations on the outbreak of preinvasive cervical lesions especially at young ages and even indications of increase of invasive disease (1,12,17). However, some of the observations may be biassed and due to more frequent screening and changes in the diagnostic accuracy (20). Even if true, the implications of such an increase should be carefully assessed. The significance of the increased risk is not in the present numbers, but they may indicate an increased risk of cervical cancer carried by the present young cohorts to ages with substantially higher risk and consequently more frequent cases of cervical cancer. In several countries cervical cancer is one of the commonest female cancers and the risk of invasive disease should be carefully monitored. If the population based figures, i.e. the incidence and mortality rates, show an increasing trend at ages with high risk resulting in a substantial number of new cases of cervical cancer, the health policy should obviously be changed accordingly.

## CONCLUSION

In summary, one of the best information sources for the long term risks of invasive cervical cancer is provided by the Nordic Cancer Registries. If there were an epidemic outbreak of cancer of the uterine cervix due to sexually transmitted viral infections the trends of incidence of invasive cervical cancer should fulfil two criteria. First, there should be a change in the long term trend in the incidence of invasive disease even after adjusting for the confounding effects of the large scale mass screenings. Second, such changes should first appear and should be more substantial at young ages. Neither of these prerequisities seems to be evidently true in the Nordic countries. Therefore the Nordic trends do not give much credibility for an hypothesis of an epidemic outbreak of cervical cancer.

## REFERENCES

1. Armstrong, B., and Holman, D. (1981): Med. J. Aust., 1: 460-462.
2. Danish Cancer Registry - Institute of Cancer Epidemiology (1985): Cancer Incidence in Denmark 1981 and 1982. Danish Cancer Society, Kobenhavn.
3. Finnish Cancer Registry - The Institute for Statistical and Epidemiological Cancer Research (1985): Cancer Incidence in Finland 1981. Cancer Society of Finland publication No. 33, Helsinki.
4. Finnish Cancer Registry - The Institute for Statistical and Epidemiological Cancer Research (1986): Cancer Incidence in Finland 1982. Cancer Society of Finland publication No. 34, Helsinki.
5. Hakama, M. (1982): In; Trends in Cancer Incidence: Causes and Practical Implications, edited by K. Magnus, pp. 279-292. Hemisphere Publishing Corporation, New York.
6. Hakama, M. (1985): Maturitas, 7: 3-10.

7. Hakama, M., Chamberlain, J., Day, N.E., Miller, A.B., and Prorok, P.C. (1985): Br. J. Cancer, 52: 669–673.

8. Hakama, M., and Rasanen-Virtanen, U. (1976): Am. J. Epidemiol., 103: 512–517.

9. Hakulinen, T., Andersen, A., Malker, B., Pukkala, E., Schou, G., and Tulinius, H. (1986): Acta Pathol. Microbiol. Immunol. Scand. 94A (suppl. 288).

10. Johannesson, G.E., Geirsson, G., Day, N., and Tulinius, H. (1982): Acta Obstet. Gynecol. Scand. (Suppl.), 61: 199–203.

11. Lynge, E. (1983): Int. J. Epidemiol., 12: 405–413.

12. MacGregor, J.E., and Teper, S. (1978): Lancet, ii: 774–776.

13. Miller, A.B. (1986): In: Screening for Cancer of the Uterine Cervix, edited by M. Hakama, A.B. Miller, and N.E. Day, pp. 149–160, IARC Scientific Publications No. 76, Lyon.

14. National Board of Health and Welfare. Cancer Registry (1984): Cancer Incidence in Sweden 1981. Schmidts Boktryckeri AB, Helsingborg.

15. National Board of Health and Welfare. Cancer Registry (1984): Cancer Incidence in Sweden 1982. Schmidts Boktryckeri AB, Helsingborg.

16. National Board of Health and Welfare. Cancer Registry (1986): Cancer Incidence in Sweden 1983. Schmidts Boktryckeri AB, Helsingborg.

17. Parkin, D.M., Nguyen-Dinh, X., and Day, N.E. (1985): Br. J. Obstet. Gynaecol., 92: 150–157.

18. Pedersen, E., Hoeg, K., and Kolstad, P. (1971): Acta Obstet. Gynecol. Scand. (Suppl.), 11.

19. Petterson, F., Bjorkholm, E., and Naslund, I. (1985): Int. J. Epidemiol., 14: 521–527.

20. Saxen, E.A. (1982): In: Trends in Cancer Incidence: Causes and Practical Implications, edited by K. Magnus, pp. 5–16. Hemisphere Publishing Corporation, New York.

21. The Cancer Registry of Norway (1983): Incidence of Cancer in Norway 1981. Oslo.

22. The Cancer Registry of Norway (1984): Incidence of Cancer in Norway 1982. Oslo.

23. The Cancer Registry of Norway (1985): Incidence of Cancer in Norway 1983. Oslo.

24. The Cancer Registry of Norway (1985): Incidence of Cancer in Norway 1984. Oslo.

# Epidemiological Studies Implicating Human Papillomavirus in the Causation of Carcinoma of the Lower Genital Tract

## N. Munoz and F.X. Bosch

*Unit of Field and Intervention Studies*
*International Agency for Research on Cancer*
*Lyon, France*

There is strong epidemiological evidence suggesting that a sexually transmitted infectious agent is involved in the causation of cervical cancer; however, conclusive evidence implicating any one type of agent is still lacking. An association with herpes simplex type 2 (HSV-2) was originally proposed about 20 years ago, but, despite the fact that past exposure to the virus can be measured serologically, no relationship has been definitively established. In a recent prospective study, in which adjustment for other risk factors for cervical cancer was made, no relationship between HSV-2 infection and subsequent cervical cancer was found, but the number of cases identified during the study period was still too small to allow any definitive conclusions to be drawn (61). A later study has suggested an association between HSV-2 infection and the recently observed increase in cervical intraepithelial neoplasia (CIN) among young women in Australia (1).

During the last decade, attention has been focused on the possible role of human papilloma viruses (HPV). In the late 1970s, it was recognized that morphological features previously interpreted on smears and biopsies as dysplasia were in fact manifestations of an HPV infection of the cervix (33). The subsequent cloning of HPV genomes in bacteria permitted the assessment of exposure to specific types of HPV. To date, close to 50 different types of HPV have been described, and at least 12 of them have been associated with lesions of the genital tract (20). Several methods have been used to assess exposure to HPV. They are, in ascending order of sensitivity and specificity: colposcopy, cytology and histology, electron microscopy, immunoperoxidase staining of HPV capsid antigen, and HPV-DNA typing.

Serological tests are not yet available (18). The best
assessment of HPV exposure and the most precise diagnosis of the associated lesion should be obtained by
combining colposcopy, cyto-histology and DNA typing.

Although there is some epidemiological evidence
suggesting an association between HPV and genital
cancer, to date, no convincing epidemiological study
has been reported in which the relationship to HPV has
been assessed in conjunction with recognized risk
factors for genital cancer. Some studies of this type
are, however, under way, and these are described below.
In the first part of this report, the available evidence suggesting an association between HPV and genital
cancer is reviewed and discussed.

## HPV AND CERVICAL NEOPLASIA

The available epidemiological evidence linking HPV
to cervical neoplasia can be summarized as follows:
1. prevalence surveys of HPV in various population
   groups (with cervical cancer, with preneoplastic
   lesions and with normal cervix);
2. longitudinal studies of women with HPV infections;
3. other studies: laboratory studies and studies on
   sexual transmission of HPV;
4. on-going epidemiological studies on HPV and cervical
   cancer.

### Prevalence Surveys of HPV

Only studies in which exposure to HPV was assessed
by DNA-DNA hybridization tests, the most sensitive and
specific method, and in which the histologic type was
specified are considered below.

**Invasive squamous and adenosquamous cell carcinoma.**
Table 1 summarizes most of the studies reported to
date in which Southern blot hybridization was used
(except in one of the studies from FRG in which reverse
blot was used (11)) to identify the HPV-DNA types in
the tissue specimens.

In all these studies HPV-16 has been the type most
commonly detected; its prevalence ranges from 15.4% in
the USA (14) to 92.0% in the UK (29). Large variations
within a given country are also observed. However, the
number of cases in each series is rather small.

In one of these studies (28), HPV-16 was found not
only in 84% of 25 genital tumoral tissues but also in
72% of clinically and histologically normal tissues
within 2-5 cm of the tumours. In the study from Japan
(66), an analysis of HPV type by age suggested that the
prevalence of HPV-16 was higher in women with cervical
cancer (all cell types) under 60 (44%) than in women

over 60 years of age (18%). However, results from a more recent study from the UK (31) suggest that HPV-16 positivity increases with age not only among women with invasive cervical cancer, but also among control women. Moreover, after adjusting for age, the presence of HPV-16 DNA was not a discriminant factor between cases and controls.

**TABLE 1.** Prevalence of Type-Specific HPV-DNA in Invasive Squamous Cell and Adenosquamous Carcinoma of the Cervix

| Country | Ref. | No. of Cases | HPV-DNA Type Identified (%) | | | | | |
|---|---|---|---|---|---|---|---|---|
| | | | 16 | 18 | 16/18 | 31 | 6/11 | Total |
| FRG | (12) | 18 | 61.1 | | | | | 72.2* |
| FRG | (3) | 13 | | 15.4 | | | | |
| FRG | (11) | 17 | 47.1 | 6.0 | | | 6.0 | 52.9** |
| UK | (52) | 11 | 45.5 | | | | | |
| UK | (29) | 13 | 92.0 | | | | 0.0 | |
| UK | (28) | 8 | 87.5 | 12.5 | | | | |
| UK | (31) | 44 | 66.0 | | | | | |
| USA | (14) | 13 | 15.4 | | | | | 15.4*** |
| USA | (27) | 39 | | | 56.0 | 5.0 | 0.0 | 82.0**** |
| USA (sq) | (54) | 19 | 68.4 | 0.0 | | | | |
| USA (adsq) | (54) | 11 | 27.3 | 54.5 | | | | |
| Japan | (66) | 53 | 36.0 | 3.8 | | | | |
| Panama | (44) | 20 | 60.0 | | | | | |
| Brazil | (30) | 19 | 42.0 | 0.0 | | | 0.0 | |

sq = squamous carcinomas; adsq = adenosquamous carcinomas
* positive to any of HPV 6,8,9,10,11 or 16.
** positive to any of HPV 6,11,16,18
*** positive to any of HPV 1,2,3,4,5,6 or 16.
**** positive to any of HPV 6,11,16,18,31 or other unknown types.
Note: Two reports (3,12) do not specify the histology of the cases; (31) includes two cases of adenosquamous carcinomas; (14) includes one case of adenosquamous carcinoma and three undifferentiated carcinomas; (66) includes three adenosquamous carcinomas, and in (44) the clinical stage of the cases is given ranging from I to IV.

HPV-18 is the second most common HPV type in all series, except in a group of 11 adenosquamous carcinomas in which it was the most common type (54). HPV-31 was reported in 5% of 39 carcinomas from the USA (27) and HPV-6/11 in 6% of 17 carcinomas from the FRG (11). The prevalence of all HPV types ranges from 15.4% (14) to 82.0% in the USA (27).

The wide ranges in the prevalence of HPV-16, HPV-18 and total HPV are disturbing. Although in all these studies the most sensitive and specific test was used to determine the presence of HPV-DNA (Southern and reverse blot), it is not possible to determine whether the differences in prevalence of the various HPV types are real or not. The large variations in the prevalence of HPV-16 and HPV-18 might be partially explained by chance variation inherent in the small numbers of cases examined in the different studies and by the very selective character of the case series. However, the direction of the selection bias of the cases cannot be assessed from the published reports, as basic information such as age, socio-economic class and source of the patients and clinical stage of the tumours is not given in any of the studies.

The presence of HPV-DNA in apparently normal tissue surrounding the tumour adds to the difficulty of establishing a linkage between specific histological lesions and HPV types, particularly if DNA extraction techniques are used. The use of in-situ hybridization techniques might be of help in locating viral DNA in a sample that includes normal cells, HPV-infected cells and neoplastic cells. Furthermore, the biological meaning of the presence of HPV-DNA in normal tissue and the factors that relate to tumoral progression are still unknown.

**Adenocarcinoma.**
Table 2 summarizes all case series so far reported.

**TABLE 2.** Prevalence of Type-Specific HPV-DNA in Adenocarcinoma of the Cervix

| Country | Ref. | No.of Cases | HPV-DNA Type Identified (%) | | | |
|---------|------|-------------|------|------|-------|------|
|         |      |             | 16 | 18 | 16/18 | 6/11 |
| FRG   | (11) | 6  | 33.3 | 0.0  |      | 0.0 |
| USA   | (14) | 4  | 25.0 |      |      | 0.0 |
| USA   | (27) | 6  |      |      | 66.6 | 0.0 |
| USA   | (54) | 12 | 8.3  | 33.3 |      |     |
| Japan | (66) | 3  | 0.0  | 33.3 |      |     |

Although the numbers involved in these studies are very small, the relatively high proportion of adenocarcinomas positive for HPV-16 and-18 is puzzling if we consider that adenocarcinomas appear to have different epidemiological characteristics from squamous-cell carcinomas. The association with sexual factors seen for squamous-cell carcinomas appears to be less important for adenocarcinoma, since women with adenocarcinoma are more likely to be single, less likely to have been separated or divorced and have had fewer pregnancies than women with squamous-cell carcinomas (22,35,36).

## Precancerous lesions.

The prevalence of different HPV types in all degrees of CIN are given in Table 3.

**TABLE** 3. Prevalence of Type Specific HPV-DNA in CIN Lesions of the Cervix

| Country | Ref. | No.of Cases | HPV-DNA Type Identified (%) | | | | | | Hybrid. Test |
|---------|------|-------------|------|------|-------|-----|------|--------|------|
| | | | 16 | 18 | 16/18 | 31 | 6/11 | Total* | |
| FRG | (12) | 29 (T) | 13.8 | 0.0 | | | | 44.8 | S. Blot |
| FRG | (11) | 80 (T) | 30.0 | 2.5 | | | 15.0 | 48.8 | S. Blot |
| FRG | (62) | 35 (S) | | | 54.3 | | 22.9 | 82.9 | FISH |
| FRG | (50) | 67 (S) | | | 46.0 | | 28.0 | | FISH |
| UK | (29) | 78 (T) | 62.0 | | | | 28.0 | | S. Blot |
| UK | (63) | 17 (S) | | | | | 12.0 | | Dot |
| UK | (52) | 7 (T) | 42.9 | | | | | | S. Blot |
| UK | (56) | 27 (S) | 29.6 | 0.0 | | | 7.4 | 44.4 | S. Blot |
| USA | (27) | 26 (T) | | | | 34.6 | 19.2 | 3.8 | 84.6 | S. Blot |
| USA | (8) | 18 (T) | 83.3 | | | | 0.0 | | S. Blot |
| USA | (14) | **12 (T) | 50.0 | | | | 38.9 | 66.6 | S. Blot |
| Panama | (44) | 12 (T) | 25.0 | | | | | | S. Blot |

T = Tissue; S = Scrapes
FISH = filter in situ hybridization; S. Blot = Southern blot
* Total includes positives to HPV-DNA 6,11,16,18 and other unidentified types.
**total number of samples analyzed varies for each column.

HPV-16 was the predominant type in all the populations, ranging from 13.8% in FRG (12) to 83.3% in one of the USA series (8). HPV-6 and -11 were the second most common types in the FRG and in the UK (11,29,50, 62) and in one study from the USA (14). Note that four different hybridization tests for HPV-DNA were used in these studies. Interpretation of the observed differences in the prevalence of the different HPV types in CIN lesions is more difficult than for cancerous lesions because:

- All degrees of CIN lesion were included in most of these studies and it is possible that a considerable proportion of CIN lesions, especially of CIN I and CIN II, are in fact HPV infections. Therefore, the exposure of interest (in this case to HPV) may have been misclassified as the disease under study (in this case CIN lesions).

- Two different types of specimen were used in the studies summarized in Table 3: tissue samples and cervical scrapes. It has been suggested that cervical scrapes provide more representative samples than

biopsies, since cells from the entire cervical surface are so obtained, while in biopsies only a very
small tissue fragment is examined (27,62). A third
sampling technique was used in another study, in
which cells were obtained by cervico-vaginal lavage
and analysed using the Southern blot hybridization
technique for HPV-6, -11, -16 and -18. The results
were compared with standard Papanicolaou smears.
HPV-DNA was identified in 75% of women with dysplastic or carcinoma in-situ lesions and in 29% of women
with a normal Pap. If used alone, this technique
clearly precludes any interpretation about the site
of origin of the HPV identified (4).

Finally, the sensitivity and specificity of the different hybridization techniques (available and under
development) used in the studies reported are likely
to be different; moreover, these differences might be
related to the status of the virus or the viral DNA
in the specimen (16). In a small validation study,
results using the Southern blot technique were compared with those obtained with the in-situ hybridization method. Twenty samples were analysed by both
techniques; three positive results were detected by
Southern blot that were not detected using the in-
situ method, and in one case the opposite occurred.
The Kappa value for concordance of the two tests was
0.53. The interpretation of the authors was that the
two techniques might complement each other. The estimated limit of detection for HPV-DNA using the in-
situ hybridization technique was around 5 viral
genome copies per cell; that for the Southern blot
technique was as low as one viral genome copy in 20
cells (40). In another small study, Souther blot
hybridization was compared to the in-situ technique
in tissue sections in 18 samples of histologically
proven CIN lesions. In 6 cases, the Southern Blot was
positive and the in-situ was negative, and on only
one occasion was the reverse true. The kappa value
for concordance was 0.16 (8).

**Normal uterine cervix.**
Studies of various groups of women without cervical
neoplasia (or presumed not to have it) are listed in
Table 4.
Some of these groups consist of women attending
family planning clinics, venereal disease clinics or
gynaecological departments, others constitute special
groups, such as prostitutes; however, in the vast majority of cases, details were not given concerning their
source. In only one of these studies, was information
on the age of the patients given (31). Three types of
DNA hybridization tests were used. The prevalence of

HPV-16 ranges from 0 to 38.5% in small studies in the UK (7, 52). In the UK, women with smears showing non specific inflammatory changes had a higher prevalence of HPV-16 (15.3%) than women with normal smears (8.7%) (56). In Panama, no positive result for HPV-16 was found among 17 tissue samples from normal cervix (44); but, in an ongoing case-control study, 45% of the controls were positive for HPV-16 or -18 (47), while, in a separate study, 23% of 120 prostitutes were positive for HPV-16 or -18 (46).

**TABLE 4.** Prevalence of Type Specific HPV-DNA in Normal Cervix

| Country | Ref. | No.of Cases | HPV-DNA Type Identified (%) | | | | Hybrid. Test |
|---------|------|-------------|------|-------|------|-------|--------------|
| | | | 16 | 16/18 | 6/11 | Other | |
| FRG | (3) | 15 | | 0.0 | | | S. blot |
| FRG | (62) | 36 | | 0.0 | 11.0 | | FISH |
| FRG | (50) | 229 | | 2.0 | 0.4 | | FISH |
| UK | (29) | 17 | 18.0 | | 0.0 | | S. blot |
| UK | (52) | 12 | 0.0 | | | | S. blot |
| UK | (7) | 13 | 38.5 | | | | S. blot |
| UK | (63) | 19 (VD) | | | 10.5 | | Dot |
| UK | (63) | 18 (FP) | | | 0.0 | | Dot |
| UK | (56) | 98 (I) | 15.3 | | 2.0 | 7.0 | S. blot |
| UK | (56) | 104 (N) | 8.7 | | 0.0 | 2.9 | S. blot |
| UK | (31) | 26 (T) | 34.6 | | | | S. blot |
| USA | (27) | 9 (B) | 0.0 | | | | S. blot |
| USA | (27) | 191 (S) | | 0.0 | 0.5 | 10.5 | S. blot |
| Panama | (44) | 17 | 0.0 | | | | S. blot |
| Panama | (47) | 51 | | | 45.0 | | Dot |
| Panama | (46) | 120 (P) | | | 23.0 | | Dot |

VD = women from venereal disease clinic; FP = women from family planning clinic; I = women withinflammation in smears but normal at biopsy; N = women with normal smears; T = women under treatment for benign gynaecological disorders; B = women normal at biopsy; S = women from a screening clinic; P = prostitutes.

FISH = filter in-situ hybridization; S. blot = Southern blot.

The results of these studies should be interpreted in the light of the following considerations:

- The small number of subjects studied.

- The very selective nature of the groups studied. Most of the studies include women with normal cytology as controls, and therefore women with signs of HPV infection are likely to be excluded, resulting in an underestimation of the prevalence of HPV in these reference groups. In addition, the study subjects

were selected from several sources, and available
results indicate that the prevalence of HPV type
varies with the source. For example, in one of the UK
studies, women with normal cytology recruited from a
family planning clinic had a prevalence of 0 for
HPV-6 and -11, while women with normal cytology
recruited from a sexually transmitted disease clinic
had a prevalence of 10.5% (63).

- Information on the age of the patients was given in
  only one of these studies, which suggests that the
  positivity for HPV-16 increases with age (31). Should
  this finding be confirmed in larger studies of different populations, failure to adjust for age might
  explain some of the observed differences in prevalence rates among the populations studied and between
  women with abnormal and normal cervices.

- As discussed in section 3, the various hybridization
  tests used for assessing type specific exposure to
  HPV differ in sensitivity and specificity. It is thus
  necessary to conduct validation studies in which
  samples from normal subjects, HPV infected subjects
  and patients with cancer are analysed under experimental conditions using the various techniques
  available.

### Longitudinal Studies on HPV and Cervical Cancer

Longitudinal studies on women with HPV infection
have the advantage over cross-sectional surveys of
providing information on the presence of the putative
risk factor (HPV markers) before the occurrence of the
disease (CIN or invasive cancer) and of providing
direct estimates of the magnitude of the risk associated with exposure to HPV types.

In this section, we briefly review three follow-up
studies that have defined HPV exposure on the basis of
non-type-specific cytological signs of HPV infection,
and two studies in which DNA hybridization techniques
were used for HPV typing.

**Longitudinal studies in which HPV exposure was
determined cytologically.**

In one of the earliest studies, 2,466 women in
France with condylomatous lesions of the cervix were
followed up for an average period of 42 months by
cytology and/or biopsy. The presence of HPV was confirmed in a small sub-sample (57 cases) by the immunoperoxidase test. The progression rate, related to the
degree of nuclear atypia, was 10% for CIN I lesions and
17% for CIN II lesions (10). However, the endpoint and
time of progression were not specified.

In a larger retrospective cohort study in Canada, 5,416 women with ordinary, mostly flat condylomas but without signs of dysplasia or carcinoma in-situ, were followed up for a minimum of 1.5 years and a maximum of 8.5 years. The progression rate to dysplasia or neoplasia was 6.2%. The average time interval was related to the severity of the lesion: 2.75 years for progression to dysplasia and six years for progression to invasive cancer. The progression rate in another group of 453 women with atypical condyloma was 13% within 1.7 – 2.2 years (34).

In the third study, a cohort of 846 women in Australia with cytological evidence of HPV infection without dysplasia in smears taken during 1979 were followed by cytology for six years with an average of three smears per woman. Thirty women developed histologically verified carcinoma in-situ over the six-year period. The observed figure of 30 was compared with an expected number of 1.9, which was estimated on the basis of published incidence data for carcinoma in-situ in a state adjacent to the one from which the cohort was derived, which is clearly underestimated and inadequate (37).

In these three studies, the assessment of exposure to the putative risk factor (HPV types) was not specific with regard to HPV type, and in at least a fraction of the cases the exposure might have been confused with the endpoint (especially in the first study (10)).

**Follow-up studies in which HPV exposure was determined by DNA hybridization.**

In a small study in the UK, 100 women under 30 years of age with CIN I diagnosed in three consecutive smears within of a 16-week period and colposcopic examination were followed every four months for 19 to 30 months by colposcopy and cytology. Two months after recruitment, cervical scrapes were tested for HPV-6 and HPV-16 by filter DNA-DNA hybridization. On entry, 46 women were HPV-6 positive and 39 HPV-16 positive. In 26 women, the lesions progressed to histologically confirmed CIN III; 22 of these (85%) had positive results for HPV-16, while only one was positive only to HPV-6 (5).

Although the strict criteria for inclusion for a woman in this study prevent generalization of the results, this might be considered the most suggestive evidence available for a greater potential for progression of HPV-16-related cervical lesions than of HPV-6 related lesions.

In an ongoing study in Finland, 418 women have been enrolled in whom cytological changes consistent with HPV infections had been found in routine cervical Papanicolaou smears. On entry to the study, a diagnosis is established by colposcopy and biopsy, and each woman is followed up every six months by colposcopy and either cytology or biopsy. HPV in the biopsy material is being typed by in-situ DNA hybridization. In a preliminary analysis of 56 women for whom results of HPV-DNA typing were given, four had HPV-6, 30 HPV-11, 11 HPV-16 and 11 HPV-18. The progression rates to more advanced CIN lesions were 0 for HPV-6, 13.3% for HPV-11, 45.5% for HPV-16 and 27.3% for HPV-18. The preliminary results of this study, although suggesting a greater potential for progression of cervical lesions in the presence of HPV-16 and HPV-18, are difficult to interpret because cervical biopsies taken on entry and during the follow-up might have altered the natural history of the disease, and because a proper statistical analysis taking into account relevant variables such as lenght of follow-up for each woman, has not yet been performed (55).

## Other Studies

### HPV-DNA in cell lines from cervical cancer.
Cell lines derived from squamous-cell carcinomas and adenocarcinomas of the cervix have been shown to contain HPV-16 and -18 (3,53,58,65) and to be similar with regard to the integration and transcription of HPV-DNA (51).

### Transforming activity of HPV.
Two reports have documented the transforming activity of HPV-16 in vitro. In one, HPV-16 DNA obtained from a cervical adenocarcinoma induced malignant transformation of NIH 3T3 cells (57). In the second, NIH 3T3 cells were transfected with molecularly cloned HPV-16 DNA originally isolated from cervical carcinoma cells (64). In both cases, the transformed cells were highly tumorigenic to nude mice.
Cytological changes identical to those observed in condylomas associated with HPV-6 and HPV-11 were induced in a model in vivo, in which fragments of normal cervical tissue and of foreskins were grafted beneath the renal capsules of athymic mice after previous incubation with extracts of condyloma acuminata containing HPV-6 and -11 (24,25).

### Studies on sexual transmission of HPV infection.
The mode of transmission of the HPV types associated with genital cancers is not fully understood. Since most genital lesions contain very little infectious virus, repeated sexual contact is probably required. Transmission might also occur in utero or at birth. The importance of sexual transmission is illustrated by various studies of sexual partners. In one, 76% of the female sexual partners of 25 men with penile condylo

mata acuminata developed similar lesions of the genital tract, and there was good concurrence between the HPV-DNA types detected in each pair of sexual partners (6). In another study, the sexual partners of 21 male patients with Bowenoid papulosis and of 29 females with CIN lesions were investigated; HPV-16 was identified in both partners in 24% of the 50 couples. Since the male partners exhibited Bowenoid papulosis, these lesions might be one of the reservoirs for HPV-16 (17). In two studies of male partners of women with genital condylomata, 50-69% have been reported to have similar lesions in the penis (26,48).

HPV-5 or HPV-2 DNA has been found in the semen of three patients, two of whom had severe chronic wart disease (41).

## Ongoing Epidemiological Studies on HPV and Cervical Cancer

The available evidence linking HPV to cervical cancer is suggestive but by no means conclusive. Although the experimental data strongly suggested a role of certain HPV types in cervical neoplasia, the available epidemiological data are limited and difficult to interpret. There is, therefore, a great need for well-designed epidemiological studies in which epidemiologists work in close collaboration with laboratory scientists (virologists and molecular biologists). In such studies, special attention should be paid to the validity of the techniques used for assessing both HPV exposure and disease status. Hybridization tests for the identification of various types of HPV-DNA are at present the most reliable method of assessing HPV type-specific exposure; however, although several hybridization tests are available, very few validation studies of these tests have been reported. Finally, such epidemiological studies should investigate exposure to other known or suspected risk factors for cervical cancer and their possible interaction with HPV infection. Two studies that are under way are mentioned below.

In 1985, we initiated population-based case-control studies in nine provinces of Spain,* a country with very low incidence rates for cervical cancer, and in the city of Cali, Colombia, which has one of the highest incidence rates for this tumour. The study was designed to determine:
- how much of the ten-fold differential in risk between these two countries is due to female behaviour;

* Alava, Gerona, Guipouzcoa, Murcia, Navarra, Salamanca, Sevilla, Vizcaya and Zaragoza

– how much is due to male sexual behaviour;
– the role of specific types of HPV in the development of this tumour in the two populations.

For each country, the study will include 300 cases of cervical cancer (150 in-situ and 150 invasive cancers) and their respective male partners, and 300 controls and their respective male partners. All study subjects will be interviewed over a period of 18–24 months. The questionnaire elicits information on sexual behaviour, use of contraceptives, smoking habits, genital hygiene, screening history and previous history of gynaecological conditions. Exfoliated cells are being obtained from the uterine cervix of female cases and controls and from the urethra and external genitalia of their sexual partners. A standard cytological smear and a blood sample is also obtained. HPV-DNA markers will be sought in the cervical and urethral exfoliated cells and in fresh tissue samples from biopsies and surgical specimens collected from untreated cases. It is hoped that serological tests for HPV which are currently being developed will make possible the detection of past or present HPV infection in the women and in their male sexual partners. Antibodies to HSV-2, cytomegalovirus and human immunodeficiency virus and serum levels of beta-carotene, vitamin A and folic acid will also be measured.

The pilot phase of this study has demonstrated that cases can be found immediately after diagnosis and before treatment and that the expected number of incidence cases are being identified in each of the study centres. It also showed that the requirements of the protocol are acceptable to most of the study subjects and that the biological specimens collected are adequate for HPV typing.

A similar case-control study is being conducted in Panama, Costa Rica, Mexico and Bogota, Colombia (47). These studies should provide valuable information on the role of HPV in cervical cancer as well as on possible interactions between HPV and other recognized risk factors, such as smoking, use of oral contraceptives and other viral infections.

## HPV AND OTHER ANOGENITAL TUMOURS

### Cancer of the Penis

Table 5 summarizes the available information on the prevalence of HPV types in the penis in several population groups. In the only study on an asymptomatic population of blood donors in the FRG, a prevalence of 5.8% was reported for HPV 6/11, 16 and 18. Fifty-eight per cent of the 31 positive samples were positive to the four HPV types (19). In the same country, HPV-16 was found in 77% of biopsies from Bowenoid papulosis lesions (21) and in one of four carcinomas of the penis (12). Two studies from Brazil, a country with relatively high incidence rates of cancer of the penis, have been reported. In one, half of 53 cases were found to contain HPV-16 and 10% HPV-18 by Southern blod hybridization (30), while in the other study, 39% of 18 cases were shown to have HPV 18 and no case was found to contain HPV-16 (59).

**TABLE** 5. Prevalence of HPV-DNA in the Penis

| Country | Ref. | Study Population | No.of Cases | HPV-DNA Type Identified % | | | | Hybrid. Test |
|---------|------|------------------|-------------|------|------|------|-------|------|
| | | | | 16 | 18 | 6/11 | Total | |
| FRG | (19) | Blood donors | 530 | | | | 5.8 | FISH |
| FRG | (21) | Bowenoid pap. | 13 | 77.0 | | | | S. Blot |
| FRG | (12) | Squam. ca. | 4 | 25.0 | | | | S. Blot |
| Brazil | (30) | Squam. ca. | 53 | 49.0 | 9.4 | | | S. Blot |
| Brazil | (59) | Squam. ca. | 18 | 0.0 | 38.9 | 5.5 | | S. Blot |

FISH = filter in-situ hybridization; S. Blot = Southern blot

Studies on the prevalence of HPV in male genitalia are rendered particularly difficult because of the small number of cells recovered from the glands, the penile shaft or from the urethra (19).

Since the same HPV types are found in samples from penile and cervical cancers (a tumour five to 25 times more frequent than penile cancer), other sexually related factors (endogenous or exogenous) are clearly capable of modulating the process from HPV infection to neoplastic lesion. At the international level, a weak correlation exists between the age-adjusted incidence rates of the two tumours (60).

### Cancer of the Vulva and of the Vagina

An association between HPV and cancer of the vulva has long been suspected from case reports of giant condylomas progressing to carcinomas (23). A recent epidemiological study has shown that out of 362 women with squamous carcinomas of the vulva. 16.6% had coexisting condylomata, while no such lesion was reported in any of the 49 control women with non–squamous malignant tumours of the vulva (9). A few specimens from vulvar carcinomas have been analysed for HPV–DNA (Table 6): HPV–16 was the type most commonly found; HPV–18 and HPV–6 have also been detected in a few tumours (11). In one case of rapidly progressing verrucous carcinoma, HPV–6b was found repeatedly (45). In two specimens of carcinoma of the vagina analysed for HPV–DNA, HPV–6 was identified (39).

**TABLE 6.** Prevalence of HPV–DNA in Cancer of the Vulva and Vagina

| Country | Ref. | Diagnosis | No.of Cases | HPV–DNA Type Identified (%) | | |
|---------|------|-----------|-------------|------|------|------|
| | | | | 16 | 18 | 6 |
| FRG | (3) | Vulva ca. | 7 | 28.6 | 0.0 | |
| FRG | (11) | Vulva ca. | 7 | 57.0 | 33.3 | 33.3 |
| USA | (67) | Vulva ca. | 9 | | | 22.0 |
| USA | (45) | Vulva ca. | 1 | | | 100.0 |
| USA | (39) | Vagina ca. | 2 | | | 100.0 |

## Cancer of the Anus

Squamous carcinoma of the anus and of the rectum is a rare condition; however, relatively high rates have been reported especially among single men in San Francisco, where about a quarter of the adult population is believed to be homosexual (2). In Los Angeles, it was also found that the incidence of anal carcinoma appears to be increasing among single males (42,43). Dysplastic lesions with concurrent cytological signs of HPV infection have been found in the anorectal mucosa of 35–44% of homosexual men tested (13,32,38).

Squamous proliferative lesions of the anus in eight homosexual males were studied using immunohistochemical staining for HPV antigen: five cases were positive (three invasive verrucous carcinoma, one squamous carcinoma and one in–situ carcinoma) (15). HPV–16 has recently been reported in one of two anal carcinomas (49).

Although the evidence is scanty, there are some indications that squamous cancers of the anal canal might be related to sexual behaviour, that male homosexuals are at high risk, that dysplastic lesions of the anorectal junction are identifiable and might represent early stages of the neoplastic process, and that, in a large proportion of cases, these dysplastic lesions show concurrent signs of HPV infection.

## CONCLUSION

There is experimental evidence and some epidemiological data to suggest an association between HPV and cancers of the anogenital tract in both males and females. However, to date, no well designed epidemiological work has been reported in which the relationship between HPV and genital cancer has been assessed in conjunction with known or suspected risk factors for the cancer. Close collaboration between epidemiologists and laboratory scientists is needed to implement adequate studies.

## REFERENCES

1. Armstrong, B.K., Allen, O.V., Brennan, B.A., Fruzynski, I.A., de Klerk, N.H., Waters, E.D., Machin, J., and Gollow, M.M. (1986): Br. J. Cancer, 54: 669-675.
2. Austin, D.F. (1982): Natl. Cancer Inst. Monogr., 62: 89-90.
3. Boshart, M., Gissmann, L., Ikenberg, H., Kleinheinz, A., Scheurlen, W., and zur Hausen, H. (1984): EMBO J., 3: 1151-1157.
4. Burk, R.D., Kadish, A.S., Calderin, S., and Romney, S.L. (1986): Am. J. Obstet. Gynecol., 154: 982-989.
5. Campion, M.J., McCance, D.J., Cuzick, J., and Singer, A. (1986): Lancet, ii: 237-240.
6. Campion, M.J., Singer, A., Clarkson, P.K., and McCance, D.J. (1985): Lancet, i: 943-946.
7. Cox, M.F., Meanwell, C.A., Maitland, N.J., Blackledge, G., Scully, C., and Jordan, J.A. (1986): Lancet, ii: 157-158.
8. Crum, C.P., Nagai, N., Levine, R., and Silverstein, S. (1986): Am. J. Pathol., 123: 174-182.
9. Daling, J.R., Chu, J., Weiss, N.S., Emel, L., and Tamini, H.K. (1984): Br. J. Cancer, 50: 533-535.
10. De Brux, J., Orth, G., Croissant, O., Cochard, B., and Ionesco, M. (1983): Bull. Cancer, 70: 410-422.
11. De Villiers, E.M., Schneider, A., Gross, G., and zur Hausen, H. (1986): Med. Microbiol. Immunol., 174: 281-286.
12. Durst, M., Gissmann, L., Ikenberg, H., and zur Hausen, H. (1983): Proc. Natl. Acad. Sci. USA, 80: 3812-3815.
13. Frazer, I.H., Medley, G., Crapper, R.M., Brown, T.C., and Mackay, I.R. (1986): Lancet, ii: 657-660.
14. Fukushima, M., Okagaki, T., Twiggs, L.B., Clark, B.A., Zachow, K.R., Ostrow, R.S., and Faras, A.J. (1985): Cancer Res., 45: 3253-3255.

15. Gal, A.A., Meyer, P.R., and Taylor, C.R. (1987): J. Am. Med. Ass., 257: 337-340.
16. Gissmann, L.: Personal communication.
17. Gross, G., Ikenberg, H., de Villiers, E.M., Schneider, A., Wagner, D., and Gissmann, L. (1986): In: Viral Etiology of Cervical Cancer, 21 Banbury Report, edited by R. Peto, and H. zur Hausen, pp. 149-165, Cold Spring Harbor Laboratory, New York.
18. Grubb, G.S. (1986): Int. J. Epidemiol., 15: 1-7.
19. Grussendorf-Conen, E.I., de Villiers, E.M., and Gissmann, L. (1986): Lancet, ii: 1092.
20. Howley, P. (1986): N. Engl. J. Med., 315: 1089-1090.
21. Ikenberg, H., Gissmann, L., Gross, G., Grussendorf-Conen, E.I., and zur Hausen, H. (1983): Int. J. Cancer, 32: 563-565.
22. Korhonen, M.O. (1980): Gynecol. Oncol., 10: 312-317.
23. Kovi, J., Tillman, R.L., and Lee, S.M. (1974): Am. J. Clin. Pathol., 61: 702-710.
24. Kreider, J.W., Howett, M.K., Lill, N.L., Bartlett, G.L., Zaino, R.J., Sedlacek, T.V., and Mortel, R. (1986): J. Virol., 59: 369-376.
25. Kreider, J.W., Howett, M.K., Wolfe, S.A., Bartlett, G.L., Zaino, R.J., Sedlacek, T.V., and Mortel, R. (1985): Nature, 317: 639-641.
26. Levine, R.U., Crum, C.P., Herman, E., Silvers, D., Ferenczy, A., and Richart, R.M. (1984): Obstet. Gynecol., 64: 16-20.
27. Lorincz, A.T., Lancaster, W.D., Kurman, R.J., Bennett Jenson, A., and Temple, G.F. (1986): In: Viral Etiology of Cervical Cancer, 21 Banbury Report, edited by R. Peto, and H. zur Hausen, pp. 225-237, Cold Spring Harbor Laboratory, New York.
28. MacNab, J.C.M., Walkinshaw, S.A., Cordiner, J.W., and Clements, J.B. (1986): N. Engl. J. Med., 315: 1052-1058.
29. McCance, D.J., Campion, M.J., Clarkson, P.K., Chesters, P.M., Jenkins, D., and Singer, A. (1985): Br. J. Obstet. Gynecol., 92: 101-105.
30. McCance, D.J., Kalache, A., Ashdown, K., Andrade, L., Menezes, F., Smith, P., and Doll, R. (1986): Int. J. Cancer, 37: 55-59.
31. Meanwell, C.A., Cox, M.F., Blackledge, G., and Maitland, N.J. (1987): Lancet, i: 703-707.
32. Medley, G. (1984): Br. J. Vener. Dis., 60: 205.
33. Meisels, A., and Fortin, R. (1976): Acta Cytol., 20: 505-509.
34. Meisels, A., and Morin, C. (1986): In: Viral Etiology of Cervical Cancer, 21 Banbury Report, edited by R. Peto, and H. zur Hausen, pp. 115-119, Cold Spring Harbor Laboratory, New York.

35. Menczer, J., Modan, B., Oelsner, G., Sharon, Z., Steinitz, R., and Sampson, S. (1978): Cancer, 41: 2464-2467.
36. Milson, I., and Friberg, L.G. (1983): Cancer, 52: 942-947.
37. Mitchell, H., Drake, M., and Medley, G. (1986): Lancet, i: 573-575.
38. Nash, G., Allen, W., and Nash, S. (1986): J. Am. Med. Ass., 256: 873-876.
39. Okagaki, T., Clark, B.A., Zachow, K.R., Twiggs, L.B., Ostrow, R.S., Pass, F., and Faras, A.J. (1984): Arch. Pathol. Lab. Med., 108: 567-570.
40. Ostrow, R.S., Manias, D.A., Clark, B.A., Okagaki, T., Twiggs, L.B., and Faras, A.J. (1987): Cancer Res., 47: 649-653.
41. Ostrow, R.S., Zachow, K.R., Niimura, M., Okagaki, T., Muller, S., Bender, M., and Faras, A.J. (1986): Science, 231: 731-733.
42. Peters, R.K., and Mack, T.M. (1983): Br. J. Cancer, 48: 629-636.
43. Peters, R.K., Mack, T.M., and Bernstein, L. (1984): JNCI, 72: 609-615.
44. Prakash, S.S., Reeves, W.C., Sisson, G.R., Brenes, M., Godoy, J., Bacchetti, S., de Britton, R.C., and Rawls, W.E. (1985): Int. J. Cancer, 35: 51-57.
45. Rando, R.F., Sedlacek, T.V., Hunt, J., Bennet Jenson, A., Kurman, R.J., and Lancaster, W.D. (1986): Obstet. Gynecol., 67: 70S-75S.
46. Reeves, W.C.: Personal communication.
47. Reeves, W.C., and Brinton, L.: Personal communication.
48. Sand, P.K., Bowen, L.W., Blischke, S.O., and Ostergard, D.R. (1986): Obstet. Gynecol., 68: 679-681.
49. Scheurlen, W., Stremlau, A., Gissmann, L., Hohn, D., Zenner, H.P., and zur Hausen, H. (1986): Int. J. Cancer, 38: 671-676.
50. Schneider, A., Kraus, H., Schuhmann, R., and Gissmann, L. (1985): Int. J. Cancer, 35: 443-448.
51. Schneider-Gadicke, A., and Schwarz, E. (1986): EMBO J., 5: 2285-2292.
52. Scholl, S.M., Kingsley Pillers, E.M., Robinson, R.E., and Farrel, P.J. (1985): Int. J. Cancer, 35: 215-218.
53. Schwarz, E., Freese, U.K., Gissmann, L., Mayer, W., Roggenbuck, B., Stremlau, A., and zur Hausen, H. (1985): Nature, 314: 111-114.
54. Smotkin, D.: Personal communication.
55. Syrjanen, K., Mantyjarvi, R., Parkkinen, S., Vayrynen, M., Saarikoski, S., Syrjanen, S., and Castren, O. (1986): In; Viral Etiology of Cervical Cancer, 21 Banbury Report, edited by R.

Peto, and H. zur Hausen, pp. 167–177, Cold Spring Harbor Laboratory, New York.

56. Toon, P.G., Arrand, J.R., Wilson, L.P., and Sharp, D.S. (1986): Br. Med. J., 293: 1261–1264.
57. Tsunokawa, Y., Takebe, N., Kasamatsu, T., Terada, M., and Sugimura, T. (1986): Proc. Natl. Acad. Sci. USA, 83: 2200–2203.
58. Tsunokawa, Y., Takebe, N., Nozawa, S., Kasamatsu, T., Gissmann, L., zur Hausen, H., Terada, M., and Sugimura, T. (1986): Int. J. Cancer, 37: 499–503.
59. Villa, L.L., and Lopes, A. (1986): Int. J. Cancer, 37: 853–855.
60. Vines, J.J., and Ascunce, N. (1986): Oncologia, 9: 324–333.
61. Vonka, V., Kanka, J., Hirsch, I., Zavadova, H., Kromar, M., Suchankova, A., Rezacova, D., Broucek, J, Press, M., Domorazkova, E., Svoboda, B., Havrankova, A., and Jelinek, J. (1984): Int. J. Cancer, 33: 61–66.
62. Wagner, D., Ikenberg, H., Boehm, N., and Gissmann, L. (1984): Obstet. Gynecol., 64: 767–772.
63. Wickenden, C., Steele, A., Malcolm, A.D.B., and Coleman, D.V., (1985): Lancet, i: 65–67.
64. Yasumoto, S., Burkhardt, A.L., Doniger, J., and DiPaolo, J.A. (1986): J. Virol., 57: 572–577.
65. Yee, C., Krishnan-Hewlett, I., Baker, C.C., Schlegel, R., and Howley, P.M. (1985): Am. J. Pathol., 119: 361–366.
66. Yoshikawa, H., Matsukura, T., Yamamoto, E., Kawana, T., Mizuno, M., and Yoshike, K. (1985): Jpn. J. Cancer Res., 76: 667–671.
67. Zachow, K.R., Ostrow, R.S., Bender, M., Watts, S., Okagaki, T., Pass, F., and Faras, A.J. (1982): Nature, 300: 771–773.

# Xenografts of Human Tissues as a Model System for the Study of Co-Factors in Uterine Cervical Carcinogenesis

## J.W. Kreider and M.K. Howett

*Departments of Pathology and Microbiology, College of Medicine,*
*The Milton S. Hershey Medical Center,*
*The Pennsylvania State University,*
*Hershey, Pennsylvania, USA*

The molecular basis of uterine cervical carcinogenesis is poorly understood, but epidemiological studies have demonstrated that a number of factors contribute to increased risk for initiation and promotion. Some of these factors may include human papillomavirus and herpesvirus (15) infection, cigarette smoking (13,14) and hormonal stimulation (1). Because ethical considerations curtail many interventional studies in humans, it may never be possible to directly demonstrate the extent to which individual putative co-factors contribute to cervical carcinogenesis. Some aspects of this multifactorial complex may be evaluated in experimental animals, e.g. hydrocarbon carcinogenesis of murine cervix (4), but for some factors, e.g. human papillomaviruses, there are no satisfactory animal surrogates. The study of human papillomaviruses (HPVs) in the pathogenesis of human disease is confronted with a number of practical obstacles. With few exceptions, the HPVs replicate poorly in naturally-occurring lesions and cannot be produced in cell cultures or in other species. Further, there has not yet been developed a satisfactory system for HPV transformation of human cells in culture.

We recently described studies in which the spectrum of diseases induced by HPV-11 in human patients was reproduced in xenografts of human tissues which were grafted beneath the renal capsule of athymic mice. The lesions which resulted were histologically and biologically identical to those present in patients. Typical condylomata were induced in uterine cervix (8), foreskin, vulva, leg skin (5,6), and urethra and vocal cord (7).

We now describe preliminary studies on the development of a model system to test the potential contribution of a number of co-factors in cervical carcinogenesis. We evaluated the effects of joint infection of human cervix and skin xenografts with HPV-11 and HSV-2. Both of these viruses are common genital tract infections of man and zur Hausen (15) has suggested that they may act synergistically to produce malignant transformation of human cervix. As an ancillary project, we studied the effect of infection with HSV-2 on malignant transformation of Shope rabbit papilloma. We also developed methods for contact treatment of human skin grafts with benzo[a]pyrene and for determining whether resulting tumors were of human origin.

## JOINT INFECTION OF PAPILLOMAVIRUS LESIONS OF RABBIT AND MAN WITH HSV-2

### Shope Papillomavirus-Induced Papillomas and Carcinomas

Shope rabbit papillomas, after two years of growth, spontaneously convert to malignant, epidermoid carcinomas in more than one half of the animals (10). Factors responsible for the malignant change are unknown. We tested the hypothesis the HSV-2 infection of papillomas would increase the frequency of malignant change when compared to PBS-treated, contralateral controls on the same rabbits. Two independent experiments were performed. In the first, eleven female New Zealand White domestic rabbits were shaved on the dorsum and 2x2 cm sites on each flank were scarified and inoculated with 0.1 ml of a 10% (w/v) extract of cottontail rabbit papillomas. Papillomas appeared at these sites within 3 weeks. Between days 40-45, the left sided papillomas were injected with 0.1 ml of live HSV-2 (strain 333) containing $6x10^7$ pfu/ml. The right-sided papillomas were injected with PBS. Within 2-3 days, the HSV-2 injected papillomas became intensely inflammed, indurated, and sometimes scabby. The PBS-treated papillomas never developed inflammation. A few HSV-2 treated papillomas were biopsied at this point, but herpesvirus inclusions were rarely demonstrated. Some of the injected papillomas temporarily slowed growth rates, and one completely regressed. Most papillomas eventually formed cutaneous horns 4-5 cm long and 1-2 cm in diameter at the base. The rabbits were observed for a maximum of 2 years, or until the presentation of a malignancy. Carcinomas were first grossly recognizable as shallow ulcers with rolled margins at the periphery of the base of the papillomas. Animals with persistent ulcers were killed and an autopsy conducted. Overall survival, therefore, was determined by the time to appearance of malignancy. This period ranged from 287 to 503 days. At autopsy, multiple sections were obtained from the base of all papillomata, concentrating on the ulcerated foci when present. Tissue from one of the PBS-treated papillomas was lost due to accident and could not be evaluated. The results (Table 1) indicated that the frequency of carcinomatous change was not different between the PBS and the HSV-2 treated papillomas.

**TABLE 1.** Superinfection of Shope Rabbit Papilloma with HSV-2 and the Subsequent Development of Carcinomas

| Experiment | Treatment Groups | |
| --- | --- | --- |
| | PBS | HSV-2 |
| I | 6/10 | 4/11 |
| II | 3/7 | 2/7 |
| Totals | 9/17 | 6/18 |

The second experiment was initiated after completion of the first. Ten female rabbits were employed in a protocol which was identical to the original experiment. The results of this experiment were similar to the first except that 3 rabbits died of unrelated, spontaneous diseases at less than 170 days and were therefore not at risk for malignancy so they were excluded from the study. The incidence of malignant change in surviving uninjected and HSV-2 injected contralateral papillomas is presented in Table 1. The incidence of malignancies in the HSV-2 treated papillomas was not different from the incidence in the PBS-injected tumors. Even when the data from both experiments was pooled, there were still no significant differences. We examined HSV-2 injected papillomas for persistent herpes DNA. DNA was extracted from PBS and HSV-2 treated papillomas and examined by "dot blot" methods for the presence of Shope papillomavirus DNA and HSV-2 whole virus DNA and for Bg1 II N subfragment. Shope DNA was found in all 23 papillomas tested. We could not detect HSV-2 information in any of the tumors when whole virion was used as a probe, however when a DNA subfragment Bg1 II N was utilized, 2 tumors out of 10 that had received HSV-2 injections demonstrated persistence of HSV-2 information in the tumor. This is attributable to the greater sensitivity of the smaller probe. We concluded that superinfection of Shope rabbit papillomas with HSV-2 did not increase the frequency of malignant change and that some portions of the HSV-2 genome did persist in the papillomas.

### HSV-2 Superinfection of Experimentally-Induced Condylomata of Human Cervix and Foreskin

We have demonstrated that HSV-2 infection of human skin grafts on athymic mice produced cytopathic effects consisting of vesicle formation, syncitial cells, and numerous intranuclear inclusions which contained HSV capsid antigen, demonstrated with the immunoperoxidase technique. These observations demonstrated that human skin xenografts were fully susceptible to live HSV-2. Unfortunately, athymic mice were all killed by the live HSV, so in the current experiments, the virus was irradiated with ultraviolet light to destroy viral cytopathic effects without impairing cell transforming activity (2). Fragments of human cervix or human foreskin were infected with HPV-11 alone or in combination with UV-irradiated HSV-2 ($1\times10^7$ pfu/ml, irradiated with 46 erg/mm$^2$/s). Infected and control grafts were transplanted beneath the renal capsule of athymic mice. Cervical tissues were examined after 2-3 months (8) and foreskin after 3-4 months (6). We have used foreskin in lieu of uterine cervix in many experiments since it often is in better condition than cervix and has an especially robust response to HPV-11 infection. The results of our experiments (Table 2) demonstrated that HPV-11 morphologically transformed both cervix and foreskin. Superinfection with UV-irradiated HSV-2 did not improve the frequency of condylomatous transformation nor did it alter the morphology of the transformed tissues.

**TABLE 2.** Joint Infection of Human Tissues with HPV-11 and HSV-2

| Tissue Type | Treatment Groups | | | |
|---|---|---|---|---|
| | PBS | HPV-11 | HSV-2 | HPV-11+HSV-2 |
| Uterine cervix | 0/13 | 7/22 | 0/9 | 8/14 |
| Foreskin | 0/2 | 3/5 | 0/5 | 5/9 |

Treatment with nitrosomethylurea can facilitate biochemical transformation with HSV-2 (3). Since we found that treatment with HSV-2 alone or in combination with HPV-11 did not transform human skin or cervix beyond that which could be attributed to HPV-11, we used nitrosomethylurea in an attempt to potentiate morpho-

logical transformation. Chips of human cervix were
exposed to 0.04 mM nitrosomethylurea for one hour, and
then they were washed and treated with UV-irradiated
HSV-2 as previously described. They were then grafted
beneath the renal capsule. After 3 months, the animals
were killed and the grafts examined microscopically.
Only one tumor was found, and that was a lymphosarcoma,
presumably of spontaneous, murine origin. Therefore,
prior treatment with nitrosomethylurea did not improve
the negative results of HSV-2 treatment (Table 3).

**TABLE 3.** Failure of Nitrosomethylurea and UV-HSV-2
to Induce Tumors in Human Cervical Grafts Transplanted
beneath the Renal Capsule of Athymic Mice

| Treatments | No. Tumors/Total Grafts |
| --- | --- |
| None | 0/37 |
| NMU | 0/32 |
| UV-HSV-2 | 1/42 |
| UV-HSV-2 + NMU | 0/42 |

## ATTEMPTS TO TRANSFORM HUMAN SKIN XENOGRAFTS
## WITH BENZO[a]PYRENE

Prior to an assessment of the interaction of HPV and
co-factors in carcinogenesis, it was essential to
establish a reliable system for routine morphologic
alteration of human skin with a co-factor, e.g. a
chemical carcinogen. We now describe 2 experiments
which are preliminary attempts to establish such a
system. Human skin was obtained from a bank of cada-
veric tissues which were preserved in 10% glycerol and
stored in liquid nitrogen. These tissues were part of
the supply used at this institution for the treatment
of burned patients. The skin was from a single donor,
and was taken from various sites, especially trunk and
limbs. The tissues were rapidly thawed and grafted to
orthotopic sites on the dorsum of athymic mice. After
allowing 7-10 days for healing of the grafts, the
dressings were removed and nitrocellulose membranes,
which had been dipped into molten paraffin containing a
high concentration of benzo[a]pyrene crystals, were
affixed to the center of the skin grafts with surgical
adhesive tape. Control grafts were treated with membranes dipped in paraffin alone. Occlusive dressings
were then applied. In the first experiment (Table 4),
the carcinogen was kept in direct contact with the
graft for 10 weeks and then it was removed for 8 weeks;
the carcinogen was then applied for an additional 5

weeks. The animals were closely observed for the development of benign and malignant tumors. Tumors appeared beginning at the tenth week and continued to present until the fortieth week. The tumors which first developed were usually near the periphery of the human skin grafts. The lesions first appeared papillomatous (Fig. 1) and subsequently they developed central ulcerations. The mice were then killed and H&E sections prepared. Epidermoid carcinomas infiltrating the subjacent epidermis were the most commonly encountered tumors, although two fibrosarcomas were also found.

**TABLE 4.** Induction of Epidermoid Carcinomas in Human Skin Grafts with Benzo[a]pyrene Treatment

| Treatments | No. Tumors/Total Grafts |
| --- | --- |
| None | 0/24 |
| BP | 71/141(50%) |

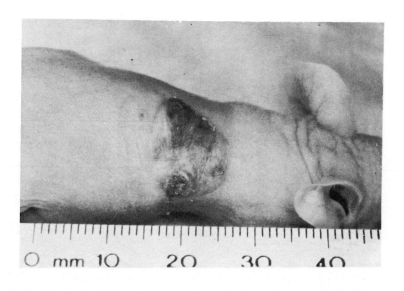

**FIG. 1.** Athymic mouse with human skin graft treated with benzo[a]pyrene- impregnated nitrocellulose membrane. Two epidermoid carcinomas have developed in the skin graft, one at twelve o'clock and the other at 6 o'clock.

It was possible that some of the tumors which developed in the human skin grafts might be of murine rather than of human origin. One method of resolving this issue would be to directly compare the response of human and nude mouse skin grafts to benzo[a]pyrene treatments. Accordingly, nude mice received either human or nude mouse skin grafts and were treated with benzo[a]pyrene applied as previously described, but the duration of the treatment was varied. Groups received carcinogen for 4, 6, 8, or 10 weeks; another group received the previous treatment protocol. The results demonstrated that the tumors which developed in the human and nude mouse grafts were similar in frequency and that each treatment duration was of approximately equal effectiveness in altering human and nude mouse skin grafts (Table 5). This suggested that it was possible that the responding cells were the same in both graft types and that the tumors were of murine rather than human origin. To test this hypothesis, mice with lesions which developed in either human or nude mouse skin grafts were killed with carbon dioxide gas and the skin grafts and attendant cancers were removed, and divided into half. One half was fixed in formalin and H&E sections prepared. The other half was snap-frozed in liquid nitrogen and then smasked with a cold hammer on a cold steel plate. The tissue fragments were then collected and extracted with BPS. Content of human and murine LDH isoenzymes were identified with the use of a commercial kit ("Authentikit", Corning Glass Works, East Walpole, MA 02032). Each assay included known standards of human and mouse skin processed identically to the controls (Fig. 2).

**TABLE 5.** Induction of Epidermoid Carcinomas in Human and Athymic Mouse Skin Grafts Treated with Benzo[a]pyrene

| | | | | Duration of BP Treatment | | | |
|---|---|---|---|---|---|---|---|
| Exp. | Skin | None | 4 | 6 | 8 | 10 | 10-8-5 |
| 1 | Human | 0/18 | 5/15 (33%) | 8/16 (50%) | 12/20 (60%) | 17/28 (61%) | 13/16 (81%) |
| 2 | Human | 0/8 | 0/8 | 4/8 (50%) | 3/9 (33%) | 5/10 (50%) | 7/9 (78%) |
| | Mouse | 0/9 | 3/6 (50%) | 5/7 (71%) | 4/7 (57%) | 10/12 (83%) | 5/6 (83%) |

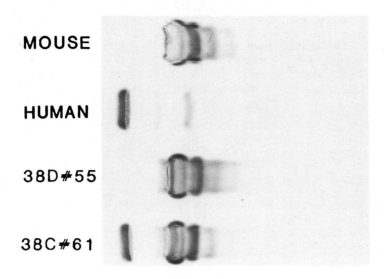

**FIG. 2.** Electrophoresis of LDH enzymes in extract of known standards of skin of mouse and humann, and of two experimental specimens consisting of epidermoid carcinomas which developed in two human skin grafts. Mouse and human known standards differ strikingly in LDH patterns. Experimental specime 38D#55 shows only mouse LDH signal, but specimen 38C#61 reveals strong mouse and human signals both in the same extract.

**TABLE 6.** Frequency of Human LDH Isoenzymes in Epidermoid Carcinomas Developing at the Site of Benzo[a]pyrene-Treated Human Skin Grafts

| Graft Source | No. Human LDH Positive Tumors/ Total Tumors |
|---|---|
| Nude mouse | 0/13 |
| Human | 11/65 |

The results demonstrated that none of 13 carcinomas which developed in nude mouse isografts were human LDH positive (Table 6). By contrast, 11 of 65 tumors which developed from carcinogen-treated human skin grafts were positive for human LDH. These results clearly demonstrated that human cells were present in some of the tumors which developed at the sites of the human skin grafts. However, it was not possible to determine if the human cells were the epidermoid carcinoma cells or whether they were normal human epidermis or stromal cells which had survived in the neoplastic lesions. To resolve this problem we used in situ hybridization of paraffin sections of the carcinomas. The method employed was a modification of that previously described (12). We used a $^{35}$S-labelled riboprobe specific for the human ALU region (M.K. Howett and J.W. Kreider, unpublished observations). When the probe was applied to normal human or mouse skin, there was strong binding to the former and not to the latter. Long-term human skin grafts on an athymic mouse on one occasion showed a curious chimera with interspersion of murine and human epidermis (Fig. 3). We do not know how often this phenomenon occurs. In some of the sections, this probe demonstrated positively-reacting, persisting human hepidermis in association with epidermoid carcinomas (Fig. 4), but in none of a total of 87 carcinomas were the tumor cells positive for human ALU segments. This included the tumors which were positive for human LDH. Therefore, in these experiments, benzo[a]pyrene treatment of human skin grafts did not produce human cancers. Epidermoid carcinomas which resulted were likely of murine origin. The cancers were probably the result of host epidermis peripheral to the slowly contracting human skin graft coming into direct contact with the carcinogen-impregnated disc.

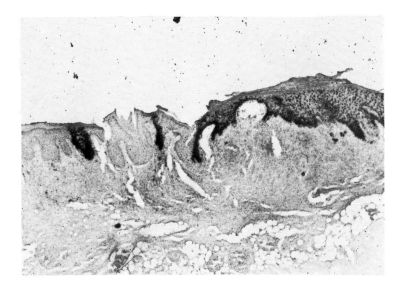

**FIG. 3.** Autoradiograph of microscopic section of benzo[a]-pyrene-treated human skin graft which was on an athymic mouse for 3 months. There are alternating patches of human epidermis which have bound the ALU probe (dark nuclei) and murine epidermis which has not.

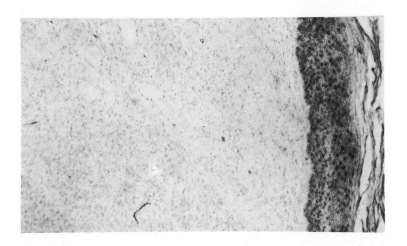

**FIG. 4.** Autoradiograph of microscopic section of human skin graft undermined by epidermoid carcinoma. The normal human epidermis at the right of the photo has virtually all nuclei covered with silver grains exposed in the photographic emulsion by radiolabelled human ALU-specific probe. The subjacent tissues to the left are stroma and epidermoid carcinoma, likely of murine origin, since very few exposed silver grains were present in this region.

In other studies, we are currently evaluating the application of benzo[a]pyrene to established, orthotopic human condylomata induced with HPV-11 in foreskins (Fig. 5). Condylomata at this site have some disadvantages as experimental subjects since they develop with a reduced frequency compared to the subrenal capsule site and are often chewed by the host and its cagemates.

## DISCUSSION

No animal model can precisely replicate the conditions under which cervical carcinogenesis proceeds in the patient. In this disease, neoplastic progression occurs in only a small fraction of patients and may take 2-10 years for the gradual evolution through stages of increasingly severe dysplasia to an invasive malignancy. This process occurs during exposure of the cervical epithelium to a plethora of changes, some of which may contribute as co-factors to the pathogenesis of the tumor. Some of these factors encompass the normal hormonal shifts concomitant to menarche, adolescence, and pregnancy (1). A host of chronic infections may disturb the microenvironment of the cervical epithelium including chlamydia, trichomonas, monilia, herpesviruses, and papillomaviruses (15). Carcinogenic chemicals, including tobacco combustion products, may be secreted in the cervical mucous (9,13,14). Specific and non-specific immunological factors may play a role in inhibiting and possibly stimulating proliferation of neoplastic cells (11).

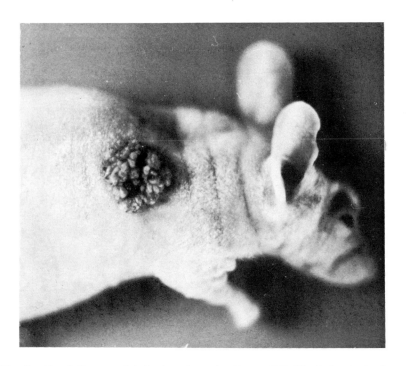

**FIG. 5.** Condyloma which developed from HPV-11 infected human foreskin grafted orthotopically to the dorsolateral thorax of an athymic mouse. Multiple papillae covered with cutaneous horn protrude from the base of the lesion.

For the experimentalist, replication of these complex conditions may not be essential and could be confusing. Since cell transformation in vitro remains an elusive goal, the xenograft system which we have described in this article may be useful in assessing the contribution of isolated co-factors to the pathogenesis of cervical cancer. Some of the advantages of this system are as follows. First, differentiation and maturation of human cervical and cutaneous epithelium is morphologically normal. Lesions which result from infection with HPV-11 or live HSV-2 are identical in morphology and behaviour to those which appear spontaneously in patients. Ethical restrictions do not inhibit interventional studies in this system. It is possible to experimentally vary the normal tissue phenotype, or to study already dysplastic lesions. Donor age, gender, and genotype may also be controlled. Grafts may be exposed to an altered hormonal milieu, secondary virus infections, and chemical and physical carcinogens. The xenograft system might provide answers to some important questions. Are HPVs (especially types 16, 18, 31, 33 and others) necessary and/or sufficient for malignant transformation? Are co-factors required for neoplastic progression?

Our initial studies with xenografts of HPV-11 infected cervix and foreskin have not revealed any alterations in behavior of the transformed cells that could be attributed to superinfection with UV-irradiated HSV-2. However, as with any other negative study, it is possible that an alteration in experimental design may permit detection of neoplastic progression. For example, compared to the time course of the natural disease, our observation period was brief. Studies with the HSV-2 superinfection of Shope papilloma did not reveal an increased frequency of malignant change. In those experiments, the time course was sufficient to detect the spontaneous malignant change, and it may safely be concluded that HSV-2 did not accelerate the course or increase the frequency of cancers. However, since the spontaneous frequency of cancers may be up to two-thirds of the total, an added increment due to herpes may be difficult to detect unless very large numbers of rabbits are studied for very long periods.

We have also described initial attempts to induce epidermoid carcinomas in human skin grafts placed orthotopically on athymic mice. Some problems were encountered. Our first experiments used benzo[a]pyrene or 3-methylcholanthrene dissolved in acetone and applied topically with a fine brush. Carcinogen crystals appeared when the solvent evaporated on the surface of the human skin grafts. The crystals rapidly re-distributed over the integument of the mice due to their custom of huddling together while sleeping. This produced large numbers of cutaneous papillomas and cancers clearly of murine origin. We then switched to the alternative method described previously in which the carcinogen was trapped in paraffin applied to a nitrocellulose disc. The discs were originally smaller than the human skin grafts, but the latter gradually contracted with time and often the discs came into direct contact with the mouse skin. A high frequency of epidermoid carcinomas resulted. In some of the carcinomas human cells could be detected by LDH isoenzyme content. However, we developed a greatly superior method which allowed the precise identification of individual human cells as well as complete preservation of the original histological relationships. With this use of specific human ALU riboprobes, we were able to prove that none of the epidermoid cancers thus far produced were of human origin. These results do not invalidate this experimental approach for inducing malignancy in human tissues, however, they clearly indicate that highly exclusive "targeting" of the carcinogen to the human tissue will be required. Since the experiments also suggest that mouse epidermis may be much more susceptible to benzo[a]pyrene carcinogenesis than human, it will also be extremely important to employ sensitive, histological methods such as human ALU in situ hybridization, to identify the species of origin of the transformed cells.

## ACKNOWLEDGMENTS

This work was supported by the U.S.P.H.S., 5-R01-42011, 2-R01-CA 25305 and P01-CA 27503, and the Jake Gittlen Memorial Golf Tournament. We thank Pat Welch, Janet Weber, Barbara Duncan, Rick Horetsky, Dean Stoesz, and Sue Anne Wolfe for competent technical assistance.

## REFERENCES

1. Allen, E., and Gardner, W.U. (1941): Cancer Res., 1: 359-366.
2. Duff, R., and Rapp, F. (1971): Nature New Biol., 233: 48-50.
3. Howett, M.K., Pegg, A.E., and Rapp, F. (1979): Cancer Res., 39: 1041-1045.
4. Koprowska, I., Bogacz, J., Pentikas, C., and Stypulkowski, W. (1958): Cancer Res., 18: 1186-1190.
5. Kreider, J.W., Howett, M.K., Leure-Dupree, A.E., Zaino, R.J., and Weber, J. (1987): J. Virol., 61: 590-593.
6. Kreider, J.W., Howett, M.K., Lill, N.L., Bartlett, G.L., Zaino, R.J., Sedlacek, T.V., and Mortel, R. (1986): J. Virol., 59: 369-376.
7. Kreider, J.W., Howett, M.K., Stoler, M.H., Zaino, R.J., and Welsh, P. (1987): Int. J. Cancer (in press).
8. Kreider, J.W., Howett, M.K., Wolfe, S.A., Bartlett, G.L., Zaino, R.J., Sedlacek, T.V., and Mortel, R. (1985): Nature, 317: 639-640.
9. Petrakis, N.L., Maack, C.A., Lee, R.E., and Lyon, M. (1980): Cancer Res., 40: 188-189.
10. Rous, P., and Beard, J.W. (1935): J. Exp. Med., 62: 523.
11. Sillman, F., Stanek, A., Sedlis, A., Rosenthal, J.,

Lanks, K.W., Buchhagen, D., Nicastri, A., and Boyce, J. (1984): Am. J. Obstet. Gynecol., 150: 300–308.

12. Stoler, M.H., and Broker, T. (1986): Hum. Pathol., 17: 1250–1258.

13. Trevathan, E., Layde, P., Webster, L.A., Adams, J.B., Benigno, B.B., and Ory, H. (1983): JAMA, 250: 499–502.

14. Winkelstein, W. (1977): Am. J. Epidemiol., 106: 257–259.

15. zur Hausen, H. (1982): Lancet, ii: 1370–1372.

# Sequences Homologous to HSV and HPV Nucleic Acid in Genital Neoplasias

## D. Di Luca, A. Rotola, P. Monini and E. Cassai

*Institute of Microbiology, University of Ferrara, Ferrara, Italy*

Herpes Simplex Virus type 2 (HSV-2) and Human Papillomavirus (HPV) have been the most extensively studied viral agents suspected to be involved as potential carcinogens in genital tumors.

The data regarding the association between HSV and genital neoplasia are sometimes controversial. A greater occurrence of antibodies to HSV-2 in cervical cancer patients than in controls has been found repeatedly (24), even if a recent prospective epidemiologic survey did not detect any association between serological signs of past HSV-2 infections and cervical neoplasia (32). Except for one early report (9), attempts to detect HSV-2 DNA in cervical carcinomas by whole genomic probes provided negative results (4,21, 37). More recently the use of subgenomic fragments of HSV-2 DNA as probes in Southern blot hybridization experiments allowed several laboratories to detect homology to viral DNA in about 14% of all invasive genital carcinomas analysed (11,18,19,22,23,26). Other approaches, such as search for HSV-specific RNA or antigens, also yielded positive results only in some cases (2,8). Since not all the samples are positive when tested for the presence of HSV-2 genetic information and no specific sets of HSV genes are consistently retained or expressed in transformed cells, HSV may act as an initiatior of transformation by mutagenic activity (27,36) via a "hit and run" mechanism (11) or through insertion sequence-like structures (12). These mechanisms would not necessarily require retention or expression of detectable viral DNA sequences for progression. According to these hypotheses, HSV sequences should be more frequent in preinvasive lesions than in invasive carcinomas. However, the few studies available on intraepithelial neoplasias (19,23,26) detected homology to HSV-2 DNA in less than 10% of cases. Such

studies are hindered by the small size of pathological
specimens and by contamination with stromal tissue
producing a decrease in the relative amount of viral
sequences (1).
   A possible role for HPV in the etiology of genital
cancers was proposed initially on the basis of virological considerations (33–35). Afterwards HPV DNA sequences (especially HPV 16 and 18) were detected in up
to 65% of genital neoplasias (7) and, under non stringent hybridization conditions, sequences of yet uncharacterized HPV types can be found in about 90% of all
cervical carcinomas (14). The study of Papillomavirus
malignancies in animal models raised the possibility
that additional agents may cooperate in a multistep
carcinogenic process leading to full malignant conversion. In fact alimentary papillomas of cattle evolve
to carcinomas in animals fed with bracken fern, which
contains a radiomimetic and immunosuppressive toxin
(16). Furthermore clinical follow–up studies in humans
showed that laryngeal papillomas convert to malignancy
after X–ray irradiation (20) and that epidermodysplasia
verruciformis patients develop carcinomas mainly in
sun–exposed areas (13), suggesting that in humans too
HPV may induce neoplastic transformation interacting
synergistically with carcinogens or mutagens. From this
viewpoint HSV, due to its mutagenic potential (27),
could be considered an initiating agent for HPV neoplastic promotion (36); however this interesting hypothesis is still to be verified. Many investigations
analysed the presence of HSV or HPV DNA in genital
tumors, but less attention was payed to the simultaneous search for both viruses in the same pathological
samples, and to the influence of stromal contamination
in searching homology in small pathological samples.


## SEARCH FOR SEQUENCES HOMOLOGOUS TO HSV DNA
## IN GENITAL TUMORS

   DNA from cervical and vulvar intraepithelial neoplasia grade III and invasive carcinoma was examined
for homology to HSV DNA by Southern blot hybridization
(29) in high stringency conditions (Tm – 20°C). The
following HSV DNA cloned restriction fragments were
employed as probes:
- HSV-2 BglII N (m.u. 0.58-0.63) which, upon transfection, alters the growth properties of rodent
  embryo, Balb and NIH 3T3 cells (10,25);
- HSV-2 BglII O (m.u. 0.38-0.42) which contains an
  origin of DNA replication (30) and partially overlaps
  a portion of HSV-1 DNA BglII I fragment with reported
  transforming activity (25);
- HSV-2 BglII C (m.u. 0.42-0.58) which contains two

distinct "in vitro" transforming functions: the left
end of the fragment is able to immortalize normal
diploid hamster cells, while sequences from the right
end convert immortalized cells to tumorigenicity
(15);
- HSV-2 BamHI E (m.u. 0.53-0.58), mostly overlapping to
BglII C and containing the transforming sequences
from the right end of this fragment; it contains
sequences coding for ICP10, one of the HSV-specific
antigens most frequently detected in cervical tumor
cells (15).
- HSV-2 BglII G (m.u. 0.20-0.31), selected to represent
viral DNA sequences with no known transforming
activity;
- HSV-1 BglII I (m.u. 0.31-0.42), able to transform
morphologically rodent cells (3,25). This fragment
was selected since in our geographic area up to 40%
of genital HSV infections are caused by HSV-1 (31).

**TABLE 1.** HSV DNA Fragments Employed as Probes in Analysis
of Genital Tumors

| N° Samples | Diagnosis | Probe | Map Units | Positive Samples |
|---|---|---|---|---|
| 55 | Intr. Neopl. | BglII N HSV-2 | 0.58-0.63 | 5 |
| 121 | Inv. Ca. | | | 17 |
| 10 | Intr. Neopl. | BglII O HSV-2 | 0.38-0.42 | 1 |
| 20 | Inv. Ca. | | | 2 |
| 4 | Intr. Neopl. | BglII C HSV-2 | 0.42-0.58 | 0 |
| 6 | Inv. Ca. | | | 0 |
| 5 | Intr. Neopl. | BglII G HSV-2 | 0.20-0.31 | 0 |
| 10 | Inv. Ca. | | | 0 |
| 19 | Intr. Neopl. | BamHI E HSV-2 | 0.53-0.58 | 0 |
| 24 | Inv. Ca. | | | 3 |
| 11 | Inv. Ca. | BglII I HSV-1 | 0.31-0.41 | 0 |

Intr. Neopl. = Intraepithelial Neoplasia
Inv. Ca.    = Invasive Carcinoma

The results on a large number of pathological samples are shown in Table 1. In each experiment, an
appropriate number of normal genital tissues from the
tumor-bearing patients was included as control, for a
total of samples; in all instances the controls did not
hybridize to any of the viral probes. Hybridization to
HSV-2 BglII N was detected in 5/55 (9.1%) intraepithe-

lial neoplasias and in 17/121 (14%) invasive carcinomas. The hybridization pattern was not the same in all
the positive tumors, one or two bands being detected in
different cases (Fig. 1, lanes B, C and D). The amount

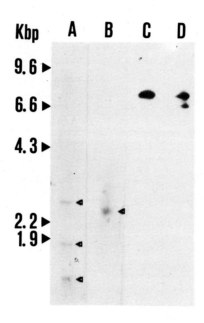

**FIG. 1.** Hybridization in high stringency conditions of DNA from
3 invasive carcinomas (lanes A,B,C) and 1 intraepithelial
neoplasia (lane D). The sample shown in lane A was digested
with BamHI and hybridized to $^{32}$P labelled HSV-2 BamHI E fragment. The other samples, cleaved with EcoRI, were hybridized to
HSV-2 BglII N fragment.

of hybridizing sequences was variable, ranging between
5 and 0.1 copies of a 1.5 kb fragment per diploid
genome, as estimated in reconstruction experiments.
Hybridization to BglII O was detected in 1/10 intraepithelial neoplasias and in 2/20 invasive carcinomas. All
the 3 samples hybridizing to BglII O contained also
sequences homologous to BglII N (Fig. 2). The BglII N
and BglII O probes hybridized to the same size fragments in each of the two invasive carcinomas (respectively 17.7 and 4.2 kb; Fig. 2 lanes A, B), and to two

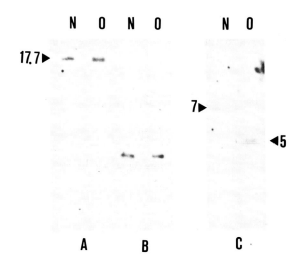

**FIG. 2.** Southern blot hybridization of DNA from 2 invasive carcinomas (lanes A,B) and 1 intraepithelial neoplasia (lane C). After EcoRI/SacI digestion, the sample DNAs were hybridized, in parallel experiments, to $^{32}$P labelled HSV-2 BglII N (lanes N) and BglII O (lanes O) fragments, in high stringency. Molecular weights are given in kilobase paires.

different size fragments in the intraepithelial neoplasia (7 and 5 kb, Fig. 2 lane C). Since in the HSV-2 genome BglII N and O fragments are located more than 26 kb apart, the sequences homologous to the two fragments in the invasive carcinomas may have rearranged and become linked to each other. No hybridization was detected to HSV-2 BglII C and G or HSV-1 BglII I fragments. Three out of 24 (12.5%) invasive carcinomas contained sequences homologous to Bam HI E (Fig. 1, lane A).
These findings suggest the following conclusions:
1) The hybridizations detected do not reflect aspecific crossreactions between human and viral DNA. As already mentioned, all the genital healthy tissues obtained from the tumors bearing patients did not hybridized to any of the HSV-2 probes. Furthermore in a recent work (26) we hybridized 24 labial and 8 cerebral tumors to BglII N, never detecting positive reaction.

2) Several fragments of the HSV-2 genome seem to be
   associated to genital tumors. In addition to the
   fragments described above, other laboratories reported the presence of HSV-2 BglII J fragment (m.u.
   0.31-0.38) in some tumoral tissues (11,23). It is
   clear that the probable association between HSV and
   genital neoplasias is not related to only one specific HSV DNA fragment; therefore screening of pathological tissues with only one HSV-2 DNA fragment
   cannot reveal the real incidence of homology to HSV
   in neoplasias.
3) It is unlikely that the samples hybridizing to HSV-2
   harbored infectious or latent virus; in fact the
   restriction pattern of native HSV-2 DNA yields
   fragments of significantly different size compared
   to the bands detected in tumor samples.

One striking observation is that, contrary to the
"hit and run" model, homology to BglII N is detected
more frequently in invasive carcinomas (14%) than in
intraepithelial neoplasias (9.1%), as shown in Table 1.
This apparent discrepancy could be ascribed to the
different nature of samples: while invasive carcinomas
are relatively large surgical specimens containing
negligible amount of stromal tissue, intraepithelial
neoplasias are much smaller and therefore stromal
contamination could considerably reduce the proportion
of neoplastic cells. To test this possibility, we
examined two groups of genital tumors for homology to
BglII N. One group, consisting of 13 relatively large
intraepithelial neoplasias obtained mostly by conization, was carefully purified from stromal tissue. All
these samples showed histologic features suggestive of
HPV infection (Di Luca et al., manuscript in preparation). Another group, consisting of 19 intraepithelial
neoplasias obtained by colposcopic biopsies, was processed with no specific selection. Homology to BglII N
was detected in 30.8% (4/13) precancerous lesions from
which the stroma had been removed but only in 5.3%
(1/19) intraepithelial neoplasias with stromal contamination (Table 2), suggesting that HSV homologous
sequences are present in more preinvasive lesions than
found up to now.

Our study does not allow to distinguish between two
hypotheses: 1) HSV is preferentially associated to HPV
containing lesions, since 12/13 intraepithelial neoplasias cleaned from stroma contained HPV; 2) alterna-
tively, the abundance of stromal tissue could account
for a decreased sensitivity of the technique in revealing homology to short HSV DNA sequences. In fact
reconstruction experiments showed that sequences
smaller than 1.5 kb present at less than 10 copies per
cell cannot be detected.

**TABLE 2.** Homology to HPV 16 or 18 and HSV-2 BglII N in Genital Tumors

|  |  | N° Positive Samples/N° Examined | |
|---|---|---|---|
| Diagnosis |  | HPV 16-18 | BglII N |
| Intraepithelial Neoplasias | with stroma | 7/14 (50%) | 1/19 (5.3%) |
|  | without stroma | 12/13 (92.3%) | 4/13 (30.8%) |

## PRESENCE OF HPV 16-18 IN GENITAL TUMORS

Since geographical differences were described in the incidence of HPV 16 and 18 infections in human genital cancer (6,7), we studied the prevalence of these two HPV types in cervical and vulvar neoplasias of the Italian population. Southern blot hybridization under high stringency conditions was used throughout our study. The results on the search of HPV 16 and 18 DNA in genital neoplasias show that 27 out of 50 (54%) invasive carcinomas contained sequences homologous to HPV 16 or 18 (data not shown). These results are in agreement with our previous report (6) and do not differ significantly from those reported for USA (56%) (17) or other European countries (64%) (14). More attention was payed to the preinvasive lesions, which were divided in two groups: i) small samples excised by colposcopy which were processed directly were obtained from Dr. S. Costa (St. Orsola Hospital, Bologna) and ii) larger samples were obtained by biopsies and sur- gical specimens from Prof. G. De Palo (Istituto Nazio- nale Tumori, Milano) and cleaned of the stromal tissue. About 50% of colposcopic biopsies contained HPV; the incidence is similar to that already reported by se- veral laboratories (14). All the samples deprived of the stromal tissue showed koilocytosis and 92.3% of them were positive for HPV 16-18 sequences. As already described by Crum (5), the association of HPV 16 with such koilocytic lesions is stronger than that detected in classical intraepithelial neoplasia. No correlation was found between the amount of HPV 16 or 18 DNA and the stage of tumor growth or the location (cervical or vulvar) of neoplasia. We also analysed 20 condylomata: none of them was positive for HPV 18, while 3 of them (all multicentric) contained HPV 16 DNA. None of 20 healthy control tissues was positive to HPV sequences. The autoradiographic pattern of DNA from tumor

samples after cleavage with an endonuclease cutting
once on HPV 16 genome, often showed fragments different
in size from the linear monomeric form (FIII), strongly
suggestive of integrations in the human genome or of
rearrangements in viral DNA, even in some intraepithelial neoplasias (Fig. 3, lane D).

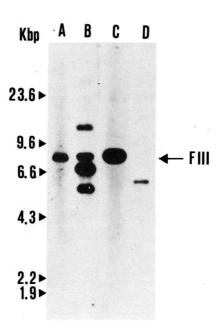

**FIG. 3.** Autoradiography of DNA from 2 invasive carcinomas
(lanes A,B) and 2 intraepithelial neoplasias (lanes C,D) digested with BamHI, cutting once on HPV 16 genome. The samples
were hybridized in high stringency conditions to a $^{32}$P labelled
HPV 16 probe.

### SIMULTANEOUS PRESENCE OF HSV–2, HPV 16 OR 18 DNA

Since "in vitro" systems for HPV are still lacking,
it is difficult to design studies providing experimental support to the suggested cooperation between HSV
and HPV in genital oncogenesis. The problem can be
approached indirectly by searching the two viral agents
in the same tumor tissues. We therefore focused our
attention on the simultaneous presence in genital
tumors of sequences hybridizing to HSV–2 Bgl II N fragment and HPV 16–18 DNA. Eight invasive carcinomas and 5
intraepithelial neoplasias hybridizing to Bgl II N were
probed in high stringency conditions to HPV DNA. The

results, reported in Table 3, show that 12/13 tissues which hybridized to BglII N contained also HPV 16-18 DNA. This simultaneous presence in intraepithelial neoplasias is not surprising, HPV 16-18 being present in most intraepithelial neoplasias (Table 2). Conversely, the data on invasive lesions may offer significant indications: 7/8 samples contained homology to both viruses. Since HPV was found in about 50% of invasive carcinomas, one would expect that only 50% of samples homologous to HSV-2 BglII N contain also HPV DNA, in the case HSV and HPV are not associated. The numbers are still too low to draw any firm conclusion, but could be indicative of a possible cooperation between HSV-2 and HPV.

**TABLE 3.** Presence of HPV 16 or 18 in Samples Positive to HSV-2 BglII N

| Diagnosis | N° Samples | HPV 16-18/BglII N |
|---|---|---|
| CIN III | 3 | 3/3 |
| VIN III | 2 | 2/2 |
| Cervical Inv. Ca. | 7 | 7/7 |
| Vulvar Inv. Ca. | 1 | 0/1 |

CIN III = Cervical intraepithelial neoplasia grade III
VIN III = Vulvar intraepithelial neoplasia grade III

## CONCLUSIONS

Several virus-specific antigens and different sequences of HSV-2 DNA and/or RNA have been detected in genital tumors; however no specific set of HSV-2 footprints was common to all positive cases. Therefore no viral gene could be identified as responsible for in vivo oncogenicity. Also, cells transformed in vitro by HSV-2 maintain their altered phenotype without any detectable expression or permanence of viral sequences. Such observations could be accounted for by the HSV mutagenic potential (27) or by the insertion of small HSV-2 DNA sequences within the host genome; viral functions could be temporarily expressed, transactivating cellular promoters, or could disrupt genic regulation within the host cell genome.

On the other hand, a substantially different situation was shown studying the molecular mechanisms by which HPV could be responsible for in vivo oncogenicity. In fact HPV 16 E6 and E7 Open Reading Frames (ORFs), whose counterparts in the Bovine Papillomavirus

DNA have in vitro transforming potential, are transcribed in some genital tumors (28). Furthermore, interruption of these ORFs was never detected in the neoplastic samples analysed, suggesting that transformation could be due to their persistent expression.

The multistep amd multifactorial theories of the natural history of cancer suggest that HSV and HPV could play a role in transformation by different molecular mechanisms, cooperating synergistically in tumor induction. According to such hypothesis, HSV could act as an initiating agent, through its mutagenic potential; then HPV-specific functions persistently expressed could complete the neoplastic phenotype.

We detected the simultaneous presence of sequences homologous to HSV and HPV in more tumors than expected on the basis of merely casual events; this finding could be indicative of an actual cooperation of the two viral agents in the genesis of cervical cancer.

## ACKNOWLEDGEMENTS

The studies done in our laboratory were supported by grants from the Italian National Research Council (Special Project "ONCOLOGY") and from the Associazione Italiana per la Ricerca sul Cancro (AIRC). P. Monini was recipient of a AIRC fellowship. We thank Prof. De Palo (Istituto Nazionale Tumori, Milano) and Prof. Orlandi (St. Orsola Hospital, Bologna) for providing the neoplastic tissues. We are very grateful to Prof. Rilke and Dr. Pilotti (Istituto Nazionale Tumori, Milano) for their invaluable assistance in processing the specimens.

## REFERENCES

1. Aurelian, L. (1983): In: Viruses associated with human cancer, edited by L.A. Phillips, pp. 79–123. Dekker, New York.
2. Aurelian, L., Kessler, I.I., Rosenshein, N.B., and Barbour, G. (1981): Cancer, 48: 455–471.
3. Camacho, A., and Spear, P.G. (1978): Cell, 15: 993–1002.
4. Cassai, E., Rotola, A., Meneguzzi, G., Milanesi, G., Garsia, S., Remotti, G., and Rizzi, G. (1981): Eur. J. Cancer, 17: 685–693.
5. Crum, C.P., Mitao, M., Levine, R.U., and Silverstein, S. (1985): J. Virol., 54: 675–681.
6. Di Luca, D., Pilotti, S., Stefanon, B., Rotola, A., Monini, P., Tognon, M., De Palo, G., Rilke, F., and Cassai, E. (1986): J. Gen. Virol., 67: 583–589.
7. Durst, M., Gissmann, L., Ikenberg, H., and zur Hausen, H. (1983): Proc. Natl. Acad. Sci. USA,

60: 3812–3815.

8. Eglin, R.P., Kitchener, H.C., McLean, A.B., Denholm, R.B., Coordiner, J.W., and Sharp, F. (1984): Br. J. Obstet. Gynaecol., 91: 265–269.

9. Frenkel, N., Roizman, B., Cassai, E., and Nahmias, A. (1972): Proc. Natl. Acad. Sci. USA, 69: 3784–3789.

10. Galloway, D.A., Goldstein, L.C., and Lewis, J.B. (1982): J. Virol., 45: 530–537.

11. Galloway, D.A., and McDougall, J.K. (1983): Nature, 302: 21–24.

12. Galloway, D.A., Nelson, J.A., and McDougall, J.K. (1984): Proc. Natl. Acad. Sci. USA, 81: 4736–4740.

13. Gissmann, L. (1984): Cancer Surv., 3: 161–181.

14. Gissmann, L., and Schneider, A. (1986): In: Viral etiology of cervical cancer, edited by R. Peto, and H. zur Hausen, pp. 217–224. Banbury Report 21.

15. Hayashi, Y., Iwasaka, T., Smith, C.C., Aurelian, L., Lewis, G.K., and Ts'O, P.O.P. (1985): Proc. Natl. Acad. Sci. USA, 82: 8493–8497.

16. Jarrett, W.F.H., McNeil, P.E., Grimshaw, W.T.R., Selman, I.E., and McIntyre, W.I.M. (1978): Nature, 274: 215–217.

17. Lorincz, A.T., Lancaster, W.D., Kurman, R.J., Bennett Jenson, A., and Temple, G.F. (1986): In: Viral etiology of cervical cancer, edited by R. Peto, and H. zur Hausen, pp. 225–237. Banbury Report 21.

18. MacNab, J.C.M., Walkinshaw, S.A., Coordiner, J.W., and Clements, J.B. (1986): N. Engl. J. Med., 23: 1052–1058.

19. Manservigi, R., Cassai, E., Deiss, L., Di Luca, D., Segala, V., and Frenkel, N. (1986): Virology, 155: 192–201.

20. Mounts, P., and Shah, K.V. (1984): Prog. Med. Virol., 29: 90–114.

21. Pagano, J.S. (1975): J. Infect. Dis., 132: 209–223.

22. Park, M., Kitchener, H.K., and MacNab, J.C.M. (1983): EMBO J., 2: 1029–1034.

23. Prakash, S.S., Reeves, W.C., Sisson, G.R., Brenes, M., Godoy, J., Bacchetti, S., de Britton, R.C., and Rawls, W.E. (1985): Int. J. Cancer, 35: 51–57.

24. Rawls, W.E. (1985): In: The Herpes Viruses, Vol. 3, edited by B. Roizman, pp. 241–255. Plenum Press, New York.

25. Reyes, G.R., LaFemina, R., Hayward, S.D., and Hayward, G.S. (1980): Cold Spring Harbor Symp. Quant. Biol., 44: 629–641.

26. Rotola, A., Di Luca, D., Monini, P., Manservigi, R., Tognon, M., Virgili, A.R., Segala, V.,

Trapella, G., and Cassai, E. (1986): Eur. J. Cancer Clin. Oncol., 10: 1256-1265.

27. Schlehofer, J.R., and zur Hausen, H. (1982): Virology, 122: 471-475.

28. Schwarz, E., Freese, U.K., Gissmann, L., Mayer, W., Roggenbuck, B., and zur Hausen, H. (1985): Nature, 314: 111-114.

29. Southern, E.M. (1975): J. Mol. Biol., 98: 503-517.

30. Spaete, R.R., and Frenkel, N. (1985): Proc. Natl. Acad. Sci. USA, 82: 694-698.

31. Taparelli, F., Squadrini, F., Cassai, E., Tognon, M., and Fornaciari, A. (1985): Med. Malad. Infect., 9: 509-513.

32. Vonka, V., Kanka, J., Hirsch, I., Zavadova, H., Kromar, M., Suchankova, A., Rezakova, D., Broucek, J., Press, M., Domorazkova, E., Svoboda, B., Havrankova, A., and Jelinek, J. (1984): Int. J. Cancer, 33: 61-66.

33. Woodruff, J.D., Julian, C., Puray, T., Mermut, S., and Katayma, P. (1973): Am. J. Obstet. Gynecol., 115: 677-684.

34. zur Hausen, H. (1975): Biochim. Biophys. Acta, 417: 25-33.

35. zur Hausen, H. (1976): Cancer Res., 36: 794.

36. zur Hausen, H. (1982): Lancet, ii: 1370-1372.

37. zur Hausen, H., Schulte-Holthausen, H., Wolf, H., Dorries, K., and Egger, H. (1974): Int. J. Cancer, 13: 657-664.

# The Analysis of Benign and Malignant Ano-Genital Tumors for HPV DNA

R.S. Ostrow[1,5], D.A. Manias[1,5], B.A. Clark[4], S.J. Gustafson[1,5], B.E. Kloster[5], J.L. Slack[5], M.K. Shaver[2], L.F. Carson[4], T. Okagaki[3,4], L.B. Twiggs[4] and A.J. Faras[1,5]

Departments of [1]Microbiology,
[2]Cell Biology and Genetics,
[3]Laboratory Medicine and Pathology,
[4]Obstetrics and Gynecology, and
[5]Institute of Human Genetics,
University of Minnesota, Minneapolis, Minnesota, USA

Many laboratories have shown a strong correlation between the presence of various types of HPV DNAs and benign and premalignant tumors of the genital tract of both sexes (8,12,15,20). In addition, HPV DNAs, particularly HPV 16, 18 and 31 have been found in between 30% to 100% of cervical cancers, depending upon the geographical location of the target study group (2,10, 14,21). In this laboratory, we have used several techniques for the detection of HPV DNAs in malignant tumors of the cervix, vulva, vagina and penis. Techniques such as filter hybridization and in situ hybridization offer complementary means of diagnosing HPV infection (17). The former technique offers high sensitivity and the capability of extensive characterization using both high and low stringency hybridization conditions and restriction endonuclease analysis. The second technique, while being somewhat less sensitive, can detect foci of cells containing 5 or more copies each of an HPV genome in a minute tissue specimen and define those cells in a specific morphological setting (16, 17). In addition, this method offers the possibility of conducting retrospective DNA or RNA studies in fixed tissues which have been kept in storage for several years. Together these methods have revealed the presence of HPV DNA in a significant portion of malignant tumors from various genital organs.

## METHODS

Filter hybridizations under both low and high stringency conditions in conjunction with restriction endonucleases were performed with nicked translated HPV DNA
probes and plasmid probes as described previously (13).
In situ hybridizations on formalin fixed paraffin
embedded tissues or cells grown in tissue culture were
performed as previously reported (17). Cells from
tissue culture or exfoliated cervical cells suspended
in isotonic saline were either centrifuged or smeared
onto microscope slides prior to in situ hybridizations.
In addition, cellular DNA was extracted from formalin
fixed paraffin embedded tissues by a slight modification of our usual extraction methods in conjunction
with previously reported methods (1,4).

## RESULTS

Previously we had detected HPV DNA in approximately
18% to 33% of cervical cancers (6,17). To date we have
now studied a total of 39 cancers of the cervix and
have found 41% to be positive for HPV infection. This
corresponds well with findings from other laboratories.
However, seven of the ten most recently obtained of
these samples were found to be positive for HPV DNA
(Table 1). Whether this represents a change in the

**TABLE 1.** Summary of Findings of HPV DNA in
Invasive Cervical Cancers

| Patients | HPV 16* | HPV 18* | Other HPVs | Total* |
|---|---|---|---|---|
| All | 9/39 (23%) | 3/39 (8%) | 5/39 (13%) | 16/39 (41%) |
| Most Recent | 4/10 (40%) | 2/10 (20%) | 1/10 (10%) | 7/10 (70%) |

* One patient had both HPV 16 and HPV 18 –related DNA.

infection rates of our study population or is simply a
statistical fluctuation is unclear at this time. However, since the conditions of hybridization were virtually identical in all of these analyses, it is clear
that these differences were not due to sensitivity
differences. Studies are currently in progress on new
samples as well as a retrospective study on DNA extracted from decade old fixed tissues in order to further
study this question. In addition, preliminary in situ
hybridization results on over 100 new adenocarcinomas,
adenosquamous carcinomas, and squamous cell carcinomas

show overall about 43% to contain detectable HPV genomes (T. Tase, et al., in preparation). Our studies on
malignant tumors of the vulva and vagina have also
shown a portion of those samples to contain HPV DNA. In
malignant squamous cell tumors of the vulva approximately 19% (5/26) were found to contain HPV DNA. This
number could be slightly higher as 7 of the samples
were studied only by in situ hybridization which may
not have detected samples containing less than 5 copies
per cell of HPV DNA throughout the entire tissue.
Overall, when all malignant tumors of the vulva (including pseudoglandular squamous cell carcinoma and a
basal cell carcinoma) were studied for HPV infections,
only 14% were found to contain HPV DNA (2). This would
seem to indicate either that the role of HPV in pseudoglandular and basal tumors of the vulva is minimal, or
that those specimens (7/16) with which only in situ
hybridization analysis was possible, contained less
than 5 copies per cell of HPV DNA. Similarly, our study
of 14 invasive carcinomas of the vagina revealed 21% to
be associated with HPV DNA (16). Only two of these
samples were studied by filter hybridization. Together,
all of these results show a fairly consistant association of HPV DNA in various tumors of the entire female
genitalia. Interestingly, it is now becoming evident
that HPV 16 is not strictly found in genital or oral
mucosa. On two occasions we have detected HPV DNA in
cutaneous Bowen's diseases. One case was in a patient
who was diagnosed as having epidermodysplasia verruciformis with impared immune functions (19). While we
found only HPV-3, and not HPV-5 in several cutaneous
flat wart and pityrasis like lesions, we found HPV 16
in a Bowen's disease of the thumb. However, in another
subject with no evidence of immune deficiency, a palmar
Bowen's disease was found to contain HPV 16 DNA (Fig.
1) (19).
   The potential for some HPV to be involved in the
transformation from a benign to a malignant lesion in
the genital tract may, in fact, be mirrored in a closely related model system. Some evidence for the possible existence of primate papillomas and the visuali-
zation of putative papillomavirus virions has been
previously reported (22). In addition, genital premalignant and malignant tumors in primates have been
reported (5,9,11). Recently we have studied various
benign and malignant lesions of primates for the presence of papillomavirus genomes. The benign lesion had
previously been found to contain virion-like particles
by electron microscopy (22). Under low stringency
hybridization conditions with a mixed probe of HPV 6,
16 and 18 for genital and malignant lesions or HPV 1
and 2 for cutaneous papillomas, we detected papillomavirus-related bands in both a lymph node metastasis in

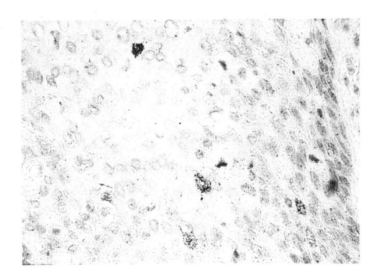

**FIG. 1.** In situ hybridization of a palmar Bowen's Disease  with tritium labeled HPV 16 DNA.

a Rhesus monkey in  which a squamous cell carcinoma  of the penis was observed, and in a foot wart of a Colebus guereza monkey (Fig. 2). This finding would point to an oncogenic potential of a primate papillomavirus in  the genital tract  of  a species  more closely  related  to humans than has  previously been  studied. We are  currently in  the process  of  cloning and  characterizing these papillomavirus  species  in the  hopes  that  the study of genital malignancies induced in primates  with primate or perhaps HPV  may further delineate the  role of various HPVs in human genital malignancies.

It has  been  reported  that  approximately 10% of "normal" PAP  smears actually contain  evidence of  HPV infection (5). In  an effort  to develop more  reliable screening methods  for genital HPV  infections, we  are developing methodologies which  combine in situ  hybridization with  the collection of  exfoliated cells  and PAP smears  for highly  sensitive diagnostic  screening for papillomavirus  infection  in  the  female  genital tract. In a preliminary  study, we have obtained  exfoliated cervical cells from patients diagnosed as having condylomatous or dysplastic genital lesions. Cells were treated as normal or modified PAP smears, or  centrifuged onto microscope slides  for in situ  hybridization. From nine patients studied using mixed tritium labelled HPV DNA probes  of HPV 6,  16 and 18,  we were able  to detect positive  signals  in  one-third of the  samples

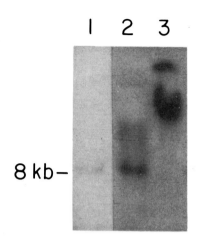

**FIG. 2.** Papillomavirus DNA in primate lesions. DNA extracts from benign (lane 1) or metastatic (lanes 2, 3) primate tumors were treated with (lanes 1, 2) or without (lane 3) BamHI prior to filter hybridization analysis under low stringency condi- tions with a mixed probe of HPV 1 and 2 (lane 1) or HPV 6, 16, and 18 (lanes 2, 3).

indicating the feasibility of this type of analysis (Fig. 3). Further studies with sulphur labelled DNA probes and modified hybridization techniques are in progress to increase the sensitivity of this method. The ability to detect even a single infected cell offers promise for maximal diagnostic sensitivity.

Since HPV is so closely associated with ano-genital neoplasia (70, the question arises as to what possible role HPV may play in neoplasia of other epithelial linings. Our previous studies of over 200 tumors have indicated that HPV can be detected in a few additional tumors including carcinomas of the lung, cecum, tongue and neck (18). To this end we have begun to study various neoplasia of the colon including colon polyps and invasive cancers. Two techniques have been used for this analysis. First, when fresh biopsy material is available, we extracted the tissues for DNA under our normal procedures. We have also selected a series of tissue specimens which had been fixed in formalin and embedded in paraffin. Using a slight variation of a

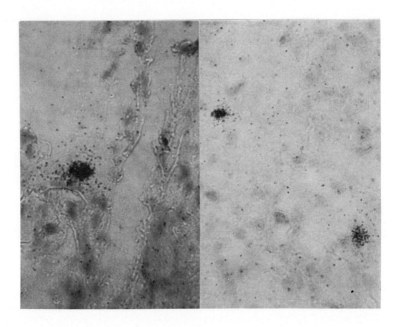

**FIG. 3.** In situ hybridization of exfoliated cervical cells from a patient with genital neoplasia. Exfoliated cervical cells from a patient with clinically diagnosed condyloma were prepared for normal PAP smear (left) or simply centrifuged (right) onto a microscope slide and hybridized in situ with a tritium labelled mixed probe of HPV 6, 16 and 18 and exposed for 30 days.

method previously reported (1,4), we have extracted good quality, high molecular weight cellular DNA which can be cleaved with restriction endonucleases. Extracts were then analyzed by filter hybridization with a mixed DNA probe of HPV 6, 16 and 18 under low stringency conditions. In test tissues known to contain HPV 6 DNA, we were able to detect this viral DNA in formalin fixed tissues. To date we have studied using standard techniques 13 fresh tissues including 5 benign colon polyps, 4 malignant tumors of the colon, and 4 normal control tissues obtained from patients with colon carcinomas at distal sites (Fig. 4). No evidence for HPV DNA was found in any of these tissues. The sensitivity of the experiments would have permitted the detection of less than 0.25 HPV genomic copies per cell. These preliminary results would appear to indicate that HPV is not involved in the etiology of these neoplasias. Further

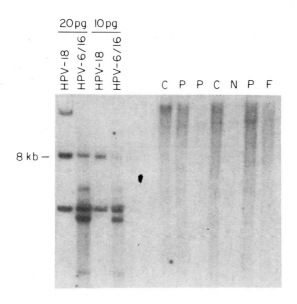

**FIG. 4.** Analysis of neoplasia of the colon for HPV DNA. DNA extracts from polyps (P), carcinomas (C) or normal adjacent tissue (N), or foreskin (F) were treated with BamHI prior to filter hybridization analysis under low stringency conditions with a mixed DNA probe of HPV 6, 16 and 18. Also shown are two sets of standard HPV DNAs (20 and 10 pg).

samples of fresh and fixed tissues are currently being analyzed to obtain a larger and more significant population sampling.

## ACKNOWLEDGEMENTS

This work was supported by grants from the National Institutes of Health (CA 25462) and the Minnesota Leukemia Research Fund.

## REFERENCES

1. Blin, N., and Stafford, D. (1976): Nucleic Acids Res., 3: 2302-2308.
2. Carson, L., Okagaki, T., Fukushima, M., Twiggs, L., Clark, B., Manias, D., Ostrow, R., and Faras, A.

(1987): Int. J. Gynecol. Pathol. (submitted for publication).

3. Choo, K., Pan, C., Liu, M., Ng, H., Chen, C., Lee, Y., Chao, C., Meng, C., Yeh, M., and Han, S. (1987): J. Med. Virol., 21: 101–107.

4. Dubeau, L., Chandler, L., Gralord, J., Nichols, P., and Jones, P. (1986): Cancer Res., 46: 2964–2969.

5. Ferenczy, A., Mitao, M., Nagai, N., Silverstein, S., and Crum, C. (1985): N. Engl. J. Med., 313: 784–788.

6. Fukushima, M., Okagaki, T., Twiggs, L., Clark, B., Zachow, K., Ostrow, R., and Faras, A. (1985): Cancer Res., 45: 3252–3255.

7. Gal, A., Meyer, P., and Taylor, C. (1987): J.A.M.A., 257: 337–340.

8. Gissmann, L., Wolnick, L., Ikenberg, H., Koldovsky, U., Schnurch, H., and zur Hausen, H. (1983): Proc. Natl. Acad. Sci. USA, 80: 560–563.

9. Hertig, A., MacKey, J., Feeley, G., and Kampschmidt, K. (1983): Am. J. Obstet. Gynecol., 145: 968–977.

10. Lorincz, A., Lancaster, W., and Tample, G. (1986): J. Virol., 58: 225–229.

11. Morin, M., Renquist, D., and Allen, A. (1980): Lab. Anim. Sci., 30: 110–112.

12. Okagaki, T., Twiggs, L., Zachow, K., Clark, B., Ostrow, R., and Faras, A. (1983): Int. J. Gynecol. Pathol., 2: 153–159.

13. Ostrow, R., Bender, M., Niimura, M., Seki, T., Kawashima, M., Pass, F., and Faras, A. (1982): Proc. Natl. Acad. Sci. USA, 79: 1634–1638.

14. Ostrow, R., and Faras, A. (1986): Clin. Micro. News., 8: 53–56.

15. Ostrow, R., and Faras, A. (1987): Cancer Metastasis Rev. (in press).

16. Ostrow, R., Manias, D., Clark, B., Fukushima, M., Okagaki, T., Twiggs, L., and Faras, A. (1987): Am. J. Obstet. Gynecol. (submitted for publication).

17. Ostrow, R., Manias, D., Clark, B., Okagaki, T., Twiggs, L., and Faras, A. (1987): Cancer Res., 47: 649–653.

18. Ostrow, R., Manias, D., Fong, W., Zachow, K., and Faras, A. (1987): Cancer, 59: 429–434.

19. Ostrow, R., Manias, D., Mitchell, A., Stawowy, L., and Faras, A.: Arch. Dermatol. (submitted for publication).

20. Ostrow, R., Zachow, K., Weber, D., Okagaki, T., Fukushima, M., Clark, B., Twiggs, L., and Faras, A. (1985): In: Papillomaviruses: Molecular and Clinical Aspects, edited by P. Howley, and T. Broker, pp. 501–511, Alan R. Liss, New York.

21. Pfister, H. (1984): Rev. Physiol. Biochem.

Pharmacol., 99: 112–181.
22. Rangan, R., Gutter, A., Baskin, G., and Anderson, D. (1980): Lab. Anim. Sci., 30: 885–889.

# The In Situ Hybridization Test in the Diagnosis of Human Papillomaviruses

K.V. Shah[1], J.W. Gupta[1] and M.H. Stoler[2]

[1]Department of Immunology and Infectious Diseases,
The Johns Hopkins School of Hygiene and Public Health,
Baltimore, Maryland, USA;
[2]Department of Pathology, University of Rochester,
School of Medicine, Rochester, NY, USA

In situ hybridization tests localize target nucleic acids "in place" usually in histologic sections or on chromosomes. The technique is sensitive enough to detect oncogenes present as single copies on their chromosomal locations. In human papillomavirus (HPV) investigations the in situ test has been utilized in a variety of ways: (i) to diagnose HPV genotypes, retrospectively, in routinely collected pathological tissues which may have been stored for decades in paraffin blocks; (ii) to localize the specific cells containing the HPV genome in complex pathological lesions; (iii) to relate expression of specific genes to the pathogenesis of the lesions; and (iv) to localize the chromosomal sites of HPV integration in cell lines and tissues derived from invasive cancers. In this article, we will concentrate on the use of the in situ test in the diagnosis of HPV in fixed tissue. Wagner et al. (20) have devised a different type of in situ test in which exfoliated cells (freshly collected or fresh-frozen) are placed on filter, denatured in situ and hybridized with radiolabeled probes. After a period of autoradiography, positive signals are seen as discrete spots on the x-ray plate. This test has been used extensively in epidemiologic investigations of HPV. It does not permit localization of the HPV genome to specific cells and will not be discussed in this article.

## VARIABLES IN TISSUE IN SITU HYBRIDIZATION

Many factors affect the intensity of the signal in in situ tests of tissues (1). Some fixatives (e.g., glutaraldehyde, or formalin) cross-link proteins more tightly than others. The prehybridization treatment of tissues is aimed at making the target nucleic acids accessible to the probes and may have to be adapted to the type of fixatives used. Different tissues respond differently with respect to fixation, extent of non-specific binding of probes, etc., so the conditions may have to be standardized separately for each tissue studied. The target nucleic acids may have degrated if the time interval between collection of tissue and fixation has been long; RNA degrades more rapidly than DNA. Shorter probes are better able to penetrate the tissue and rearch the target nucleic acids and so give stronger signals. Highest signals are obtained when the probe concentration is sufficient to saturate the target nucleic acids. Efficiency of hybridization also varies greatly according to the temperature of the hybridization reaction. The most important variables affecting efficiency of hybridization are type of fixative, interval before fixation, probe size and concentration, and temperature of hybridization.

## LABELS AND PROBES UTILIZED IN HPV DIAGNOSIS

Cloned HPV DNAs maintained in plasmid vectors are the starting point for preparation of the probes. Both DNA and RNA probes have been used. For preparation of DNA probes, the label ($^3$H, $^{35}$S or biotin) is most often incorporated by nick translation of the double-stranded viral DNA. $^3$H-labeled probes, because of the short path lenght of the label, give excellent resolution, and can distinguish between cytoplasmic and nuclear localization of the signal. They also have a long half-life. As compared to $^3$H-labeled probes, the $^{35}$S-labeled probes are less stable, but they attain higher levels of specific activity and require shorter time for autoradiography. Non-radioactive labels like biotin have several important advantages (3) (Figs. 1, 2). They do not pose the hazards associated with radioactivity and are stable over long periods of time. Also, because the detection depends on a color change by an enzymatic reaction and not on autoradiography, the test can be completed in a matter of hours rather than of days. Typically, the times required for completion of tests utilizing biotin, $^{35}$S and $^3$H labels are, respectively, one day, 4-6 days, and about 3 weeks. However, the sensitivity of detection by biotin-labeled probes (estimated to be 800 copies/cell) (6) is at present lower than that for radioactive probes (estimated to be 20-100 copies/cell) (10,17).

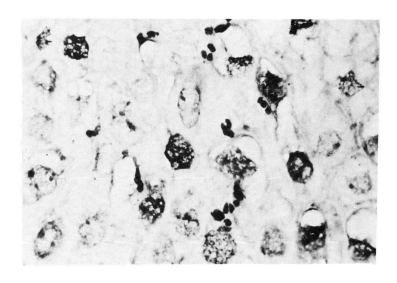

**FIG. 1.** Biotin labeled HPV-6 DNA probe with hematoxylin counterstain and DAB-nickel chloride specific stain. Positive nuclei in biopsy of a cervical condyloma.

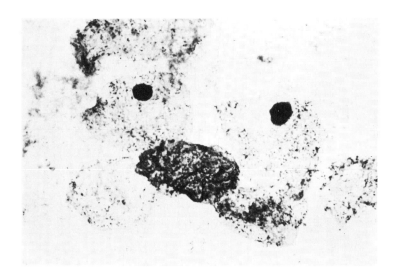

**FIG. 2.** Biotin labeled HPV-6 DNA probe with hematoxylin counterstain. Positive signals localized to nuclei of condylomatous squamous cells in cervical smear.

## ASYMMETRIC SINGLE-STRANDED RNA PROBES

Asymmetric RNA probes are transcribed as single strands from the viral DNA inserted into the polylinker of several new, commercially available transcription vectors (17). The polylinker is flanked by bacterial polymerase promoters (e.g., SP6 and T7) which are activated by appropriate polymerases. Because all of the genetic information of HPVs is located on one strand of the double-stranded DNA molecule, it is possible to transcribe either the coding or the noncoding strand by use of the appropriate polymerase. If the target DNA strands in a tissue are not separated by denaturation, the anti-sense probe (transcribed off the non-coding DNA strand) will detect only viral mRNA whereas the sense probe (transcribed off the coding DNA strand) will not hybridize at all and will serve as a control for non-specific binding. Both probes will detect viral DNA if the tissue is denaturated prior to hybridization. The anti-sense single-stranded RNA probe, which detects viral mRNA, may be the most efficient way for detection of HPV genome in situ (17). In genital tract tissues tested for both viral mRNA and viral DNA by single-stranded RNA probes, the signals for viral mRNA were always stronger, and more extensive, than those for viral DNA (17). The anti-sense probe, being single-stranded, will not hybridize with itself, and will form RNA-RNA hybrids, which are more stable than RNA-DNA or DNA-DNA hybrids. This makes it possible to employ higher post-hybridization wash temperatures (and reduce non-specific binding) after RNA-RNA hybridization than after RNA-DNA hybridization.

## CONDUCT AND INTERPRETATION OF THE IN SITU TEST

The detailed protocols of the tests have been published (3,8,17). Here, an outline is given for tests with $^3$H or $^{35}$S-labeled anti-sense RNA probes. Four to six micron sections are cut and placed on slides which are specially treated (poly-d-lysine treated or more recently by organosilanation (19), to prevent loss of section during the hybridization procedure. A panel of probes are tested on adjacent sections, one probe per section. After deparaffinization and hydration of tissue, the sections are treated with a proteolytic enzyme to make the target nucleic acid accessible to the probe, and with acetic antihydride to reduce non-specific binding of the probe. If the objective is to detect viral DNA in the tissue, the sections are denatured to separate the DNA strands using either heat, formamide, or both. They are not denatured if the purpose is to detect viral mRNA.

Single-stranded RNA probes are transcribed from the

viral DNA in the transcription vector using one or more labeled nucleotide precursors and the appropriate polymerase. The probe is reduced in size to about 200 base pair lenght by alkaline hydrolysis. Hybridization is performed at conditions of high stringency and is followed by dipping the slides in photographic emulsion and autoradiography.

Signals are confined to epithelial cells. Signals of highest intensity are found in areas showing koilocytotic changes and/or mild dysplasia (Fig. 3). The

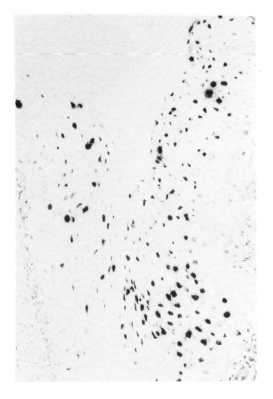

**FIG. 3.** $^{35}$S-labeled HPV-16 DNA probe with hematoxylin counterstain. Strong focal hybridization pattern in an antigen positive cervical condyloma.

hybridization is focal and is not seen uniformly in cells showing similar cytopathological features, even in the same microscopic field. Invasive carcinoma cells may show low level uniform staining which "high-light" them over the surrounding stroma (17) (Fig. 4). A positive hybridization indicates the presence of the

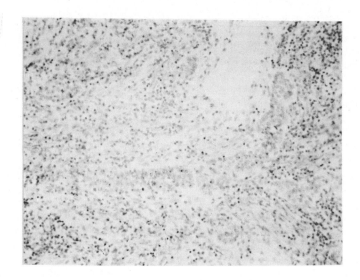

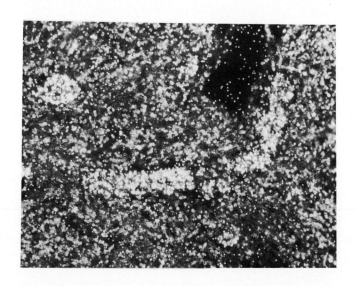

**FIG. 4.** [3]H– labeled HPV–18 anti–sense probe with hematoxylin counterstain. Brightfield illumination (top) demonstrates nests of squamous cell carcinoma invading an inflammatory and fibrous cervical stroma. Under darkfield illumination (bottom) the HPV–18 mRNA signal highlights the tumor cells and outlines them over the negative stroma.

virus used as the probe or a virus closely related to
the probe virus. Closely related viruses (e.g., HPV-6
and HPV-11, HPV-16 and HPV-31) can be distinguished
from one another by relative signal strength if both
viruses are used as probes. Subgenomic monospecific
probes have been devised which show no cross-hybridization even with closely related viruses (4). A negative test does not rule out the presence of HPV. The
amount of HPV in the tissues may be low and beyond the
limit of detection or the tissue may contain an HPV
which does not cross-hybridize with the used probes.

## CONTRIBUTIONS OF THE IN SITU TEST TO HPV RESEARCH

Many aspects of the etiology and pathogenesis of HPV
lesions have been clarified by studies using the ·in
situ hybridization test. For example, HPV-6 and HPV-11
were associated with the conjunctival papilloma of
childhood (13) and with neoplastic progression of
respiratory papillomas (5). In a study of oral warts,
it was shown that HPV-2 was associated frequently with
cutaneous lesions of the lip but rarely with mucosal
lesions inside the oral cavity (7). The genital tract
viruses were found to frequently infect the oral cavity
(18). HPV-16 was detected in the tumor cells themselves
in in situ and invasive carcinomas of the cervix (6,12,
15-17) (Fig. 5). It was demonstrated that the most

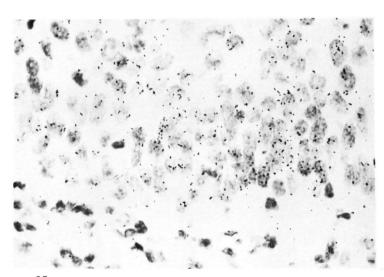

**FIG. 5.** $^{35}$S-labeled HPV-16 DNA probe with hematoxylin counterstain. Bottom half of epithelium of a CIN III lesion. Faint
diffuse hybridization signal is strongest over the basal cells.
The stroma below is negative.

differentiated neoplastic lesions  contain the  highest
amount of  viral DNA  (6). HPV-16  was associated  with
carcinoma of the anal canal (12,14) (Fig. 6) and with
in situ and microinvasive carcinoma of the vulva  (10).
Viral mRNA was found to be more readily detectable than
viral DNA (17). The in situ technique has been  applied
to cervical cytology smears  (2,8,9). It also has  been
utilized to study the molecular basis of the  evolution
of HPV-associated pathology by  use of single gene  RNA
probes (4).

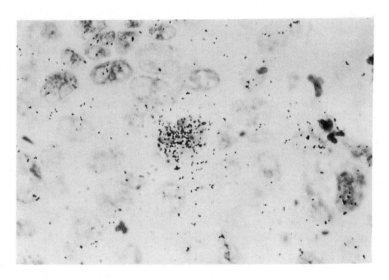

**FIG. 6.** $^{35}$S-labeled HPV-16 DNA probe with hematoxylin  counterstain. High power view of a squamous cell carcinoma of the anus
showing focal signal over a single malignant cell.

## ACKNOWLEDGEMENTS

This work was supported in part by US Public  Health
Services grants  CA-42074, AI-16959  and CA-36200  from
the National Institutes of Health, Bethesda, Maryland.

## REFERENCES

1. Angerer, L.M.,  Stoler,  M.H.,  and Angerer,  R.C.
   (1987): In: In  Situ Hybridization. Applications
   to Neurobiology,  edited by  K. Valentino, J.
   Eberwine, and J. Barchas. Oxford  University
   Press, Oxford (in press).
2. Beckmann, A.,  Chu, J., and McDougall, J.  (1987):
   Sixth International  Papillomavirus  Workshop,
   Washington, DC, June 14-18, Abstract.

3. Beckmann, A., Myerson, D., Daling, J. Kiviat, N., Fenoglio, C., and McDougall, J. (1985): J. Med. Virol., 16: 265–273.
4. Chow, L., Hirochika, H., Nasseri, M., Stoler, M., Wolinski, S., Chin, M., Hirochika, R., Arvan, D., and Broker, T. (1987): In: Cancer Cells, Vol. 5, Papillomaviruses, edited by B. Steinberg, J. Brandsma, and L. Taichman. Cold Spring Harbor Laboratory, New York (in press).
5. Crissmann, J., Kessis, T., Weiss, M., Fu, Y., and Shah, K. (1987): Sixth International Papilloma-virus Workshop, Washington, DC, June 14–18, Abstract.
6. Crum, C., Nagai, N., Levine, R., and Silverstein, S. (1986): Am. J. Pathol., 123: 174–182.
7. Eversole, L., Laipis, P., and Green, T. (1987): J. Cutan. Pathol. (in press).
8. Gupta, J., Gendelman, H., Naghashfar, Z., Gupta, P., Rosenshein, N., Sawada, E., Woodruff, J., and Shah, K. (1985): Int. J. Gynecol. Pathol., 4: 211–218.
9. Gupta, J., Gupta, P., Rosenshein, N., and Shah, K. (1987): Acta Cytol. (in press).
10. Gupta, J., Pilotti, S., Rilke, F., and Shah, K. (1987): Am. J. Pathol., 127: 206–215.
11. Gupta, J., Saito, K., Saito, A., Fu, Y., and Shah, K. (1987): Sixth International Papillomavirus Workshop, Washington, DC, June 14–18, Abstract.
12. Gupta, J., Taxy, J., Gupta, P., and Shah, K. (1987): Lab. Invest., 56: 29A, Abstract.
13. McDonnell, P., McDonnell, J., Kessis, T., Green, W., and Shah, K. (1987): Hum. Pathol. (in press).
14. McDougall, J., Beckmann, A., and Kiviat, N. (1986): In: Papillomaviruses (Ciba Foundation Symposium 120), edited by D. Evered, and S. Clark, pp. 86–103. Wiley, Chichester.
15. Ostrow, R., Manias, D., Clark, B., Okagaki, T., Twiggs, L., and Faras, A. (1987): Cancer Res., 47: 649–653.
16. Schneider, A., Oltersdorf, T., Schneider, V., and Gissmann, L. (1987): Int. J. Cancer (in press).
17. Stoler, M., and Broker, T. (1986): Hum. Pathol., 17: 1250–1258.
18. Syrjanen, S., Syrjanen, K., and Lamberg, M. (1986): Oral Surg., 62: 660–667.
19. Tourtellotte, W.W., Verity, A.N., Schmid, P., Martinez, S., and Shapshak, P. (1987): J. Virol. Methods, 15: 87–99.
20. Wagner, D., Ikenberg, H., Boehm, N., and Gissmann, L. (1984): Obstet. Gynecol., 64: 767–772.

# Human Papillomavirus Types 16 and 18 Present and Expressed in Cervical Cancers and Their Transforming Activity

Y. Tsunokawa[1], Y. Inagaki[1], N. Takebe[1], S. Nozawa[2], M. Terada[1] and T. Sugimura[1]

[1]Genetics Division, National Cancer Center Research Institute, Tokyo, Japan
[2]Department of Obstetrics and Gynecology,
School of Medicine, Keio University, Tokyo, Japan

Human papillomavirus type 16 (HPV 16) and human papillomavirus type 18 (HPV 18) are reported to be frequently associated with cervical cancers in Germany, Brazil, Kenya and England (2,6,23). We and others have previously reported that HPV 16 and HPV 18 DNA sequences and their transcripts are also frequently found in cervical cancer tissues and cell lines of Japanese patients (28,32). Besides this epidemiological evidence of association of HPV 16 and 18 with cervical cancers in various parts of the world, little information is available on the molecular mechanisms underlying the development of such cancer by these viruses. In order to obtain insight into their biological significance, the subgenomic regions of HPV 16 and 18 and their transcripts consistently present in cervical cancers were analyzed, and two types of cDNA clones representing 3.4 kb and 1.6 kb HPV 18 transcripts in HeLa cells were sequenced. We report here that the E6 and E7 regions were consistently present and that at least the E6 region was expressed as mRNA in all the cultured cervical cancer cell lines tested. Sequence analysis of two types of HPV 18 cDNA clones from HeLa cells showed that 3.4 kb transcript contained E6, E7, 5'portion of E1 and human sequence, and 1.6 kb transcript contained spliced and frame-shifted E6 (E6*), E7 and human sequence. We also show here that HPV 16 DNA integrated into genomic DNA of a cervical cancer had transforming activity to NIH3T3 cells upon transfection, and this HPV 16 DNA contained the E6 and E7 regions.

## MATERIALS AND METHODS

SKG–IIIa and SKG–IIIb cells were established from the same cervical cancer (16). SKG–I (15) and SKG–II (10) cells were derived from cervical cancer tissues of two different patients. These cervical cancer cells, HeLa cells and NIH3T3 cells were cultured under humidified atmosphere of 5% $CO_2$ at 37°C as described previously. To obtain surgical specimens, portions of tumors, not including necrotic parts, were removed. The samples were quickly frozen by pressing between precooled metal plates and were kept at −70°C.

Total DNA and RNA were extracted as described previously (3,13). Poly(A)$^+$ RNA was prepared with passing total RNA through an oligo (dT)-cellulose column (1). Southern blot hybridization and Northern blot hybridization analyses were performed as described in details previously (13,26).

The cloned HPV 16 and HPV 18 DNA sequences were generously provided from Drs. zur Hausen and Gissmann.

cDNA library was constructed with Poly(A)$^+$ RNA from HeLa cells using Okayama–Berg's procedure (17) and screened by colony hybridization with HPV 18 genome as a probe (8). Isolated cDNA clones were characterized by restriction enzyme digestions. Sequence analysis of cDNA clones was performed according to the dideoxy chain termination sequencing method using M13 cloning vectors (14,21).

DNA from a cervical cancer tissue obtained from a patient undergoing hysterectomy for stage III cervical cancer was transfected into NIH3T3 cells by the calcium phosphate coprecipitation technique (27,29). The cancer was diagnosed histologically as a moderately differentiated adenocarcinoma. Transformed foci were cloned and tested for tumorigenicity to nude mice as described previously (27).

Cosmid library of genomic DNA of transformed NIH3T3 cells was constructed with Ish–Horowicz and Burke's methods (9,13) using cosmid vector pCV108 (11). Cosmid library was screened and clones were isolated with general procedure described previously (13). To examine tumorigenicity of NIH3T3 transfectants of cosmid clones, tumorigenicity assay described by Fusano et al. (7) was performed.

## RESULTS

### Regions of HPV 16 and HPV 18 Genomes
### Present in Cervical Cancers

The results of our study on the presence of HPV 16 and 18 in surgical specimens and cultured cell lines are summarized in Table 1. By Souther blot analysis,

**TABLE 1.** Presence of the HPV Type 16 or Type 18 Genome and its Transcripts in Cervical Cancer

Surgical Specimens

| Histological Diagnosis | HPV Type | Copy No. x Haploid Genome | Transcript |
|---|---|---|---|
| Adenocarcinoma | 18 | 10 | detected |
| Squamous cell carcinoma | 18 | 2-3 | ND |
| Squamous cell carcinoma | 16 | 20 | detected |
| Squamous cell carcinoma | 16 | 1-2 | ND |
| Squamous cell carcinoma | 16 | 20 | detected |
| Adenocarcinoma | 16 | 100 | ND |
| Squamous cell carcinoma | — | | |
| Squamous cell carcinoma | — | | |
| Adenosquamous cell carcinoma | — | | |
| Adenocarcinoma | — | | |

Cell Lines

| Cell Line | Histological Diagnosis | HPV Type | Copy No. | Transcripts |
|---|---|---|---|---|
| SKG-I | Squamous cell carcinoma | 18 | 2 | 1.5kb, 4.3kb |
| SKG-II | Squamous cell carcinoma | 18 | 3-4 | 2.0kb, 2.6kb, 4.4kb, 6.6kb |
| SKG-IIIa | Squamous cell carcinoma | 16 | 1 | 1.5kb, 5.8kb |
| SKG-IIIb | Squamous cell carcinoma | 16 | 1 | 1.5kb, 5.8kb |

ND: Not determined.

four cervical cancers out of ten were found to have HPV type 16 DNA sequences and two others to have type 18 DNA sequences. The copy numbers of HPV DNA per human haploid genome varied from approximately 1 to more than 100. SKG-I, -II, -IIIa and -IIIb cell lines contained one to a few copies of HPV 16 or HPV 18 DNA sequences.

In order to determine the subgenomic regions of HPV 16 or those of HPV 18 DNA consistently present in cervical cancers, DNAs from cervical cancer cell lines and surgical specimens of cervical cancers were analyzed. SKG-IIIb cellular DNA was first cleaved with HindIII, XbaI and SstI which were non-cutting restriction enzymes for HPV 16 (25), and then hybridized to

HPV 16 DNA as a probe. Hybridization analysis showed one band, indicating that there was one integration site of the HPV 16 DNA in SKG-IIIb DNA. By comparing the sizes of bands detected by Southern blot hybridization analysis of SKG-IIIb DNA after double cleavage with BamHI/AvaII and BamHI/PstI with those of the restriction fragments of HPV 16 prototype DNA, the subgenomic form of HPV 16 DNA on SKG-IIIb cells was determined. It covered the L1, E6 and E7 regions with deletions of entire sequences corresponding to the E4, E5 and E2 regions, and parts of the L2 and E1 regions (Fig. 1). Hybridization analysis of three DNA samples from surgical specimens of cervical cancers indicated that all or most of the HPV 16 genome including E6 and E7 regions were present in these DNA samples.

Hybridization analysis of SKG-I cellular DNA with HPV 18 DNA after digestion with BglII, HindIII or SstI consistently gave two bands, indicating that there were two different integration sites for HPV 18 DNA in SKG-I cells, since these enzymes do not cut HPV 18 DNA (4). Hybridization analysis of SKG-I DNA with total HPV 18 DNA as a probe after double cleavage with Sau3AI/EcoRI and HincII/BamHI showed that the E2 region was one of the integration sites of HPV 18 DNA, and most of the HPV 18 genome including the E6 and E7 regions were present in the cells. By the same analysis, it was found that SKG-II cells contained three to four copies of HPV 18 DNA sequences, which included the E6 and E7 and parts of the L1 and E2 sequences. Hybridization of two DNA samples from surgical specimens of cervical cancers with total HPV 18 DNA as a probe showed that the E6 and E7 regions were present in the integrated HPV 18 DNA.

## Expression of HPV Genomes

Three surgical specimens containing HPV, two of type 16 and the other of type 18 were found to have HPV transcripts by Northern blot hybridization. The presence of HPV transcripts in three other samples of cervical carcinoma tissue containing HPV could not be tested due to the degradation of RNAs. By Northern blot hybridization analysis of Poly (A)$^{+}$ RNA, we found that the HPV transcripts ranged from 1.5 kb to 6.6 kb in all of the cultured cell lines derived from cervical cancers.

The 0.4 kbp AvaII fragment of HPV 16 DNA was subcloned, purified and used as a probe covering a part of the E6 region. Northern blot analysis of RNAs from SKG-IIIb with HPV 16 DNA and 0.4 kbp AvaII fragment as probes showed that the E6 region was transcribed as mRNAs with sizes of 1.5 kb and 5.8 kb.

The 0.2 kbp XbaI-BamHI fragment of HPV 18 DNA was

subcloned, corresponding to a portion of the E6 region.
Northern blot analysis of poly(A)$^+$ RNA from SKG-I cells

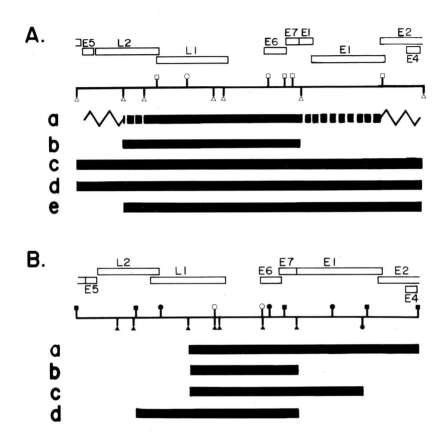

**FIG. 1.** Schema  of the HPV  16 or HPV  18 sequences present  in
cellular DNA.
A. Linear  map of  HPV 16  with cleavage sites  of the  enzymes
BamHI (O),  AvaII  (□) and PstI  (▵), and putative open  reading
frames (▭) are shown in the top (25). The subgenomic sequences
of HPV 16 DNA (▬)  present in the cellular genomes,  cellular
DNA sequences (/\/\/) and virus-cell junctions (▪▪▪▪) are  indicated. (a), SKG-IIIa and SKG-IIIb; (b), T601; (c), (d) and (e),
surgical specimens of cervical cancers.
B. Linear map of HPV  18 with cleavage sites of enzymes,  EcoRI
(∗), XbaI (●), HincII (▪), BamHI ( O ) and Sau3Ai (▲), and putative open reading  frames (▭)  are shown in  the top (4).  The
subgenomic sequences of HPV  18 DNA (▬) present in the  cellular genome are  indicated. (a), SKG-I;  (b), SKG-II; (c)  and
(d), surgical specimens of cervical cancers.

with HPV 18 DNA and its 0.2 kbp XbaI–BamHI fragment showed the E6 region was transcribed as mRNA of 1.5 kb and 4.3 kb. In SKG–II cells, the E6 region was transcribed as mRNA of 2.0 kb, 2.6 kb, 4.4 kb and 6.6 kb.

### Sequence Analysis of cDNAs for HPV 18 Transcripts in HeLa Cells

HeLa cells contained about 10 copied of HPV 18 DNA per haploid genome, and expressed 3.4 kb and 1.6 kb transcripts of HPV 18 genome (24). We isolated two types of cDNA clones representing 3.4 kb and 1.6 kb transcripts. The sequence analysis of these two types of cDNA clones showed that 3.4 kb transcript contained E6, E7, 5'portion of E1 and 3'flanking human sequence, and 1.6 kb transcript contained spliced and frame-shifted E6, designated as E6* by Schneider–Gadicke and Schwarz (22), E7 and 3'flanking human sequence

cDNA clone No. 125 included 3135 nucleotides representing a nearly full-sized cDNA for 3.4 kb transcript. The analysis of clone No. 125 showed that 3.4 kb transcript contained three open reading frames: entire E6 and E7 and the 5'portion of E1 (ΔE1) ( Fig. 2). No

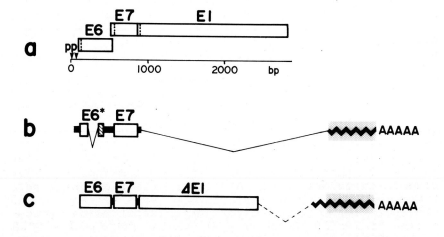

**FIG. 2.** Two types of HPV 18 transcripts in HeLa cells. The 5'portion of the early regions of HPV 18 genome (a), 1.6 kb transcript(b) and 3.4 kb transcript(c) are schematically presented. The open reading frames E6, E6*, E7, E1 and 5'portion of E1 (ΔE1) are indicated by open boxes. Hatched box means frame shifted open reading frame. The first ATG in each open reading frame was shown by a dotted line in the box. Two TATA boxes (p) upstream of the E6 region are indicated by arrows. Zig-zag lines show flanking cellular sequences. Shaded boxes on the zig-zag lines indicate identical sequences.

splicing or frame shift was observed within the E6 and E7 open reading frames, coding 158 and 105 amino acids, respectively. The 3.4 kb transcript contained 742 nucleotides of human flanking sequence with a poly(A)-addition signal, AATAAA.

Analysis of cDNA clone No. 20 revealed that 1.6 kb transcript contained two open reading frames, E6* and E7, coding for 57 and 105 amino acids, respectively. The 1.6 kb transcript contained both of the two viral TATA boxes upstream of E6 in the 5'portion of mRNA, and 571 nucleotides of human sequence was completely identical with that of 3'portion of human flanking sequence of 3.4 kb transcript except that there were 5 more additional nucleotides upstream of the poly(A)-addition site of 1.6 kb transcript. No open reading frame was found in human sequences of 3.4 kb or 1.6 kb transcript.

## Transforming Activity of HPV 16 DNA Integrated into a Cervical Cancer

NIH3T3 transfection assay using calcium phosphate coprecipitation technique has been used successfully to identify transforming genes in various cancers (5,29). We have tested the genomic DNA from a human cervical cancer containing HPV 16 DNA for transforming activity on NIH3T3 cells. Southern blot analysis of BamHI-digested DNA of this sample showed a main band of 5.1 kbp with an additional band of 7.9 kbp, hybridized to HPV 16 DNA. Based on the intensity of the band, the copy number of HPV 16 DNA was estimated to be approximately 100 copies per haploid genome. When this DNA sample was transfected into NIH3T3 cells, a transformed focus composed of crisscrossed and piled up cells was detected (Fig. 3). The DNA obtained from the primary transformant induced transformed foci upon transfection into NIH3T3 cells. The transformed cells were less refractile than those with activated c-Haras from T24 bladder carcinoma (7). All these transformants were tumorigenic to nude mice; tumors were formed in all mice tested within 10 days after subcutaneous inoculation of $1 \times 10^6$ cells of the transformants. Southern blot hybridization with HPV 16 DNA showed that BamHI digested DNAs of the primary and secondary transformants contained 5.1 kbp fragment containing HPV 16 DNA sequence. It was found that DNA from a primary transformant contained conspicuous bands that hybridized with the human specific Alu family sequence (20). BamHI digests of DNAs of the secondary transformants had distinct fragments containing human specific Alu family sequence.

Southern blot analysis showed that an NIH3T3 primary transformant (T601) contained the sequences of the L1,

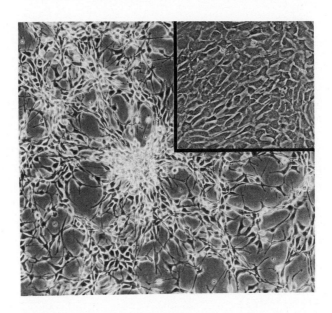

**FIG. 3.**   Morphological   appearance of   a primary   transformant
(T601) and parent NIH3T3 cells (inset).


E6 and E7 regions but the entire regions of the   E4, E5
and E2 and parts of the L2 and E1 regions   were deleted
(shown in Fig. 1). It was found that HPV 16 DNA and its
human flanking   sequences were integrated   at a   single
integration site   into the genomic   sequence of   NIH3T3
cells. Northern blot analysis showed that the E6 region
was transcribed   as mRNAs in   the transformant.   Cosmid
clones containing   HPV 16   DNA were   obtained from   the
cosmid library prepared from   DNA of one of the   NIH3T3
secondary transformants. When two cosmid clones containing HPV 16 DNA with its human flanking sequences  were
transfected into NIH3T3 cells,   the cells became   tumorigenic to nude mice.

## DISCUSSION

The present results   showed that the   E6 and E7   regions of HPV 16 and 18 DNA were consistently present in
all cervical cancer cell lines examined. These   regions
of HPV 16 and   HPV 18 were   also present in the   biopsy
materials. In contrast, the E2, L2 regions and parts of
the E1 and L1 regions of HPV 16 and HPV 18 were deleted
in some cervical cancers. These results are   consistent
with   the   reports   from   other   laboratories   (12,18),

showing the E6 and E7 regions of HPV 16 and HPV 18 to be consistently intact in cervical cancer cell lines; these regions of HPV 16 were present in the surgical specimens of cervical cancers. The E6 regions of HPV 16 and HPV 18 were transcribed as mRNA in all the cell lines tested.

Sequence analysis of HPV 18 cDNA clones obtained from the cDNA library prepared from HeLa cells provides us with more information on HPV 18 transcripts. HeLa cells contained 3.4 kb and 1.6 kb transcripts. The 3.4 kb transcript had E6, E7 and 5'portion of E1, whereas 1.6 kb transcript contained spliced and frame-shifted E6, designated E6*, and E7. It was also found that 1.6 kb transcript contained two viral TATA boxes in the non-coding region upstream of E6, indicating that a human cellular promoter is used for the transcription of viral sequences in HeLa cells. It was not possible to determine whether 3.4 kb transcript utilizes the viral or cellular promoter for its transcription. The other unique finding on HPV 18 transcripts in HeLa cells was that 3.4 kb transcript contained 742 nucleotides of human sequence containing a poly(A) addition signal. The 3'portion of 571 nucleotides was completely identical with that of 1.6 kb transcript, except that there were additional 5 nucleotides upstream of the poly(A)-addition site of 1.6 kb transcript. HPV 18 DNA sequences were reported to be localized on chromosomes 5, 8, 9, and 22 in HeLa cells (19). The present results indicated that both 3.4 kb and 1.6 kb mRNAs were transcribed from the HPV genome at the same integration site with different splicing. The human flanking sequences containing poly(A)-addition signals might play a role in the stabilization of mRNAs. The human flanking sequences did not hybridize to the bands containing HPV 16 or 18 DNA and were not expressed as mRNA in any other cervical cancer cell lines we tested. It is very unlikely that the insertional activation of specific cellular genes occurs in the development of cervical cancers.

We have shown here that HPV 16 DNA sequences in total genomic DNA from a cervical cancer had transforming activity to NIH3T3 cells. Cosmid clones containing HPV 16 DNA and human flanking sequences showed tumorigenic activity to NIH3T3 cells upon transfection. The importance of the E6 and E7 regions of HPV for transformation was further strengthened by showing that the NIH3T3 transformant contained the E6 and E7 regions of HPV 16. The E5 and E6 regions of bovine papillomavirus have transforming activity on C127 cells and NIH3T3 cells upon transfection (30,31). Since the E2, E4 and E5 sequences were not present in the NIH3T3 transformant induced by transfection of HPV 16 DNA integrated into genomic DNA of a cervical cancer, these

regions were not required for the transforming activity. It is likely that the E6 and E7 regions are
important for the transforming activity on NIH3T3
cells, and possibly, since they are consistently present, for the development of cervical cancers. The
biological function of the E6, E6*, and E7 encoded
products of HPV 16 and 18 should be elucidated to
understand their molecular mechanisms involved in the
development of cervical cancers.

## ACKNOWLEDGEMENTS

We express our appreciation to Drs. H. zur Hausen
and L. Gissmann for their generous gift of HPV 16 and
HPV 18 probes. This study was supported in part by a
Grant-in-aid from the Ministry of Health and Welfare
for a Comprehensive 10-year Strategy for Cancer
Control, Japan.

## REFERENCES

1. Aviv, H., and Leder, P. (1972): Proc. Natl. Acad.
   Sci. USA, 69: 1408-1412.
2. Boshart, M., Gissmann, L., Ikenberg, H.,
   Kleinheinz, A., Scheurlen, W., and zur Hausen, H.
   (1984): EMBO J., 3: 1151-1157.
3. Chirgwin, J.M., Prizybyla, A.E., MacDonald, R.J.,
   and Rutter, W.J. (1979): Biochemistry, 18: 5294-
   5299.
4. Cole, S.T., and Danos, O. (1987): J. Mol. Biol.,
   193: 599-608.
5. Cooper, G.M. (1982): Science, 218: 801-806.
6. Durst, M., Gissmann, L., Ikenberg, H., and zur
   Hausen, H. (1983): Proc. Natl. Acad. Sci. USA,
   80: 3812-3815.
7. Fusano, O., Birnbaum, D., Edlund, L., Fogh, J., and
   Wigler, M. (1984): Mol. Cell. Biol., 4: 1695-
   1705.
8. Hanahan, D., and Meselson, M. (1980): Gene, 10:
   63-67.
9. Ish-Horowicz, D., and Burke, J.F. (1981): Nucleic
   Acids Res., 9: 2989-2998.
10. Ishiwata, I., Nozawa, S., Kiguchi, K., Kurihara,
    S., and Okumura, H. (1978): Acta Obst. Gynaec.
    Jpn., 30: 731-738.
11. Law, Y.F., and Kan, Y.W. (1983): Proc. Natl. Acad.
    Sci. USA, 80: 5225-5229.
12. Lehn, H., Krieg, P., and Sauer, G. (1985): Proc.
    Natl. Acad. Sci. USA, 82: 5540-5544.
13. Maniatis, T., Fritsch, E.F., and Sambrook, J.
    (1982): Molecular Cloning: A Laboratory Manual.
    Cold Spring Harbor Laboratory, Cold Spring
    Harbor, New York.

14. Messing, J. (1983): Methods Enzymol., 101: 20–78.
15. Nozawa, S., Tsukazaki, K., Udagawa, Y., Ishiwata, I., Ohta, H., Kurihara, S., and Okumura, H. (1982): In: Carcinoma of the cervix, edited by E.S.E. Hafez, and J.P. Smith, pp. 142–151. Martinus Nijhoff Publishers, Amsterdam.
16. Nozawa, S., Udagawa, Y., Ohta, H., Kurihara, S., and Fishman, W.H. (1983): Cancer Res., 43: 1748–1760.
17. Okayama, H., and Berg, P. (1982): Mol. Cell. Biol., 2: 161–170.
18. Pater, M.M., and Pater, A. (1985): Virology, 145: 313–318.
19. Popescu, N.C., DiPaolo, J.A., and Amsbaugh S.C. (1987): Cytogenet. Cell Genet., 44: 58–62.
20. Rubin, C.M., Houck, C.M., Deininger, P.L., Friedman, T., and Schmid, C.W. (1980): Nature, 284: 373–374.
21. Sanger, F., Nicklen, S., and Coulson, A.R. (1977): Proc. Natl. Acad. Sci. USA, 74: 5463–5467.
22. Schneider-Gadicke, A., and Schwarz, E. (1986): EMBO J., 5: 2285–2292.
23. Scholl, S.M., Pillers, E.M.K., Robinson, R.E., and Farrel, P,J, (1985): Int. J. Cancer, 35: 215–218.
24. Schwarz, E., Freese, U.K., Gissmann, L., Mayer, W., Roggenbuck, B., Stremlau, A., and zur Hausen, H. (1985): Nature, 314: 111–114.
25. Seedorf, K., Krammer, G., Durst, M., Suhai, S., and Rowekamp, W.G. (1985): Virology, 145: 181–185.
26. Southern, E.M. (1975): J. Mol. Biol., 98: 503–517.
27. Tsunokawa, Y., Takebe, N., Kasamatzu, T., Terada, M., and Sugimura, T. (1986): Proc. Natl. Acad. Sci. USA, 83: 2200–2203.
28. Tsunokawa, Y., Takebe, N., Nozawa, S., Kasamatzu, T., Gissmann, L., zur Hausen, H., Terada, M., and Sugimura, T. (1986): Int. J. Cancer, 37: 499–503.
29. Wigler, M., Sweet, R., Sim, G.K., Wold, B., Pellicer, A., Lacy, E., Mantias, T., Silverstein, S., and Axel, R. (1979): Cell, 16: 777–785.
30. Yang, Y.-C., Okayama, H., and Howley, P.M. (1985): Proc. Natl. Acad. Sci. USA, 82: 1030–1034.
31. Yang, Y.-C., Spalholz, B.A., Rabson, M.S., and Howley, P.M. (1985): Nature, 318: 575–577.
32. Yoshikawa, H., Matsukura, T., Yamanoto, E., Kawana, T., Mizuno, M., and Yoshiike, K. (1985): Jpn. J. Cancer Res., 76: 667–671.

# Clinico-Pathologic Correlations of Papillomaviruses-Related Lesions of the Lower Genital Tract

S. Pilotti and F. Rilke

*Division of Pathology and Cytology*
*Istituto Nazionale Tumori, Milan, Italy*

Recent advances in molecular biologic technology, such as in situ hybridization (ISH) and Southern transfer, contributed to the acquisition of new data on the etiology and the clinico-pathologic features of early vulvar neoplasia (EVN). In favor of the existence and the recently increased prevalence of this new clinico-pathologic entity – also named Bowenoid type VIN (1) – and its relatedness to human papillomavirus (HPV) speak two studies of our group, one retrospective and the other prospective.

The retrospective study was based on the re-investigation by ISH of 20 cases of EVN the majority of which had already been shown to be HPV-related on the basis of immunohistochemistry and ultrastructure (15). In these 20 cases the areas of intraepithelial neoplasia (IN) were suitable for ISH with radiolabelled (with 35S) DNA probes for HPV types 6/11, 16 and 18 (11).

The prospective analysis (6) was performed by Southern blot hybridization with HPV types 16 and 18 radiolabelled (with 32P) DNA probes on 21 cases including eight of EVN and 13 of invasive squamous cell carcinoma. The cases were consecutive, without histologic pre-selection for epithelial cytopathic effect (CE) even though a selection of the cases before admission to the Institute can not be ruled out.

## IN SITU HYBRIDIZATION

In ten of 20 lesions HPV DNA could be detected with definite predominance of HPV 16 which was present in nine. One patient was positive for HPV 6/11 and had a giant condyloma of the Buschke-Lowenstein type which, contrary to the findings reported in literature, had already given regional nodal metastases (8). In eight

of 14 cases (57%) with bowenoid type VIN, in situ
hybridization was positive. This figure is significant
because it can be compared with the results of the
prospective investigation which was carried out only on
cases with EVN of bowenoid type. Nonetheless, two cases
which turned out to be HPV 16 DNA-positive, were originally diagnosed as VIN of the basaloid type (1). This
finding is in agreement with the known fact that not
always do HPV 16-related INs show evidence of CE (3,10)
and confirms the usefulness of ISH for the assessment
of HPV-related EVN.

## SOUTHERN BLOT HYBRIDIZATION

HPV type 16 DNA was detected in all eight cases of
EVN and in two of 13 cases (15%) of invasive squamous
cell carcinoma investigated. None of the nine control
healthy tissues contained HPV DNA. The striking difference in positivity between the cases with VIN and
those with invasive carcinomas, in addition to the
different median ages – 45 and 73 years respectively –
suggests that the vulva may be affected by two diverse
diseases in contrast to the uterine cervix. In fact,
the same type of study which was conducted at the same
time on 7 cases of in situ and 16 of invasive squamous
cell carcinoma of the cervix showed positivity for HPV
16 DNA in 100% and 81% respectively. Also the median
ages of the patients with intraepithelial and invasive
cervical lesions were similar, 40 and 43 years, respectively. The findings described showe that as far as the
vulva is concerned our prevalence data on the type of
HPV involved are in agreement with other reports (7,9,
10,12), whereas they are at variance with reference to
the association of HPV with invasive carcinoma (7). The
same holds true for the detection of HPV DNA in healthy
controls (13) none of whom was positive in our series.
We are unable to offer any explanation in this respect
at the present time. It should, however, be noted that
some of the results reported in the literature were
obtained on material deriving from heterogeneous sources, as it appears from the acknowledgments (13), and
that apparently normal tissues of the genital tract of
healthy women may contain biologically inactive HPV DNA
(16). We underscore that the tissues for DNA extraction
have to be properly selected and treated in order to
avoid under – as well as overestimations. Therefore,
tissue samples have to be taken by the pathologist and
checked on frozen sections in order to (i) select
uniform lesions and (ii) discard non-representative
epithelial components and most of the stroma. These two
points are very important for the study of intraepithelial lesions. The same procedure should be applied to
healthy controls which should comprise the same type(s)

of tissue(s) and organ(s).

Finally, our data suggest that the majority of cases of VIN are HPV-related and that the predictive significance of the CE in hematoxylin and eosin-stained histologic sections is high. If we consider only the cases of both series which showed CE (Table 1), the percentage of HPV-related cases was the same, even though the methods applied were different in terms of sensitivity.

**TABLE 1.** PV-associated VIN*: Results by Methods (No. 22)

|  | No. of Cases | Evidence of HPV DNA** | | Age (mean) yrs |
|---|---|---|---|---|
|  |  | No. | % |  |
| In situ Hybridization | 14 | 8 | 5/ | 4/ |
| Southern blot Hybridization | 8 | 8 | 100 | 45 |

\* VIN: vulvar intraepithelial neoplasia
\*\* HPV 16 in all but one case

Crum et al. (4) recently found that among 18 cases of CIN, only 60% of those which were positive with Southern blot for HPV 16 DNA were also positive by ISH. It should also be mentioned that in some HPV-16 related cases the CE may be minimal as was in 2 cases of the retrospective series. Finally, the young age of the patients with VIN of bowenoid type was confirmed as was the prevalence of HPV 16.

A peculiar feature of EVN of bowenoid type is the not uncommon co-existence, with the clinically dominant vulvar lesion, of other HPV-related lesions at other sites of the lower genital tract (LGT) and/or adjacent cutaneous areas. We observed this event in the course of both retrospective histopathologic studies (in about 50% of the cases) (15) and the ongoing colposcopic examinations of outpatients. This phenomenon has been known as "field effect" of neoplasia (5) or, more recently, as "genital neoplasm papilloma syndrome" (14). One of its main features is the similar clinical presentation irrespective of the presence or absence of coexistant IN which can be ascertained only histologically. We selected from our files and those of the outpatients' clinic, 2 series of consecutive patients with synchronous multicentric presentation of the disease, one with and the other without associated early neoplasia. Our aim was to verify whether the type

of HPV associated with the lesion was correlated merely
with histology or also with the clinical findings and
had possible prognostic implications as well.

**TABLE 2.** Multiple Condylomatous Lesions: Characteristics
of Patients

| | PV-associated Early Neoplasia (No=12) | PVI (No=14) |
|---|---|---|
| Diagnosis of Vulvar Lesions | 4 VIN 8 Microinvasive Carcinoma | all PVI |
| **Organs Involved:** | | |
| Vulva | 12 | 14 |
| Cervix | 6 | 14 |
| Perianal skin | 6 | 4 |
| Vagina | 1 | 8 |
| **No. of Sites Involved:** | | |
| 2 | 11 | 4 |
| 3 | 1 | 7 |
| 4 | – | 3 |
| **No. of Cases with recurrences** in | | |
| Lower Genital Tract | 8 | 14 |
| Adjacent Sites | 5 | 5 |
| **Age** (years) | | |
| mean | 42.5 | 30 |
| median | 40 | 25.5 |

Table 2 summarizes the clinico-pathologic features
cf both groups of patients: 12 showed histologically
more or less advanced early neoplasia and 14 only
evidence of HPV infection (PVI). Extravulvar sites,
often synchronously involved, were the cervix and the
perianal skin in the first group and the vagina in the
second. The number of involved sites varied from a
minimum of two to a maximum of four; more than two
sites were often involved by PVI. The incidence of
recurrences was high and similar in the two series,
both by percentage of incidence and type of site involved. The recurrences involved not only the LGT but
also adjacent sites, such as the crural and gluteal
skin, the urethra and the anal canal. A preliminary
immunohistochemical investigation had already confirmed
the light microscopic evidence of PV-relatedness by

proving the presence of PV-antigen in the vulvar lesions in similar percentages in both series, with and
without neoplasia, - 67% and 43% respectively, - as
well as in the extravulvar sites, - 50% and 57% respectively.

In situ hybridization with probes for HPV 6/11, 16
and 18 reconfirmed both at the DNA level and percenta-
gewise, the immunohistochemical data for both groups,
with and without neoplasia: for the vulvar lesions 58%
and 43% respectively, and the extravulvar sites, 50%
and 57% respectively. However, the most significant
finding of the ISH test was related to the distribution
of HPV types. Having proven that the same types of HPV
were present in the various sites of each single case,
it appears from Table 3 that HPV 16 was not only
strongly associated with early neoplasia, but also with
50% of the PVI cases. Therefore, five cases with PVI
were at risk for progression because of the presence of
HPV 16 and also of HPV 18 in one of them.

**TABLE 3.** Multiple Condylomatous Lesions:
HPV-DNA in Situ Hybridization*

|  | HPV by Cases | |
|  | PV-associated Early Neoplasia (No=12) | PVI (No=14) |
| --- | --- | --- |
| HPV-16 | 6** | 5*** |
| HPV-6/11 | 1 | 5 |
|  | 7 (58%) | 10 (71.5%) |

\*     Retrospective study
\*\*    One case with mixed infection HPV 6/11 and 16
\*\*\*   One case with mixed infection HPV 16 and 18

It has been reported that in a high percentage of
recurring acuminated condymolas HPV-16 was detected
(2). The natural history of our series of 14 cases of
PVI is for many aspects similar to that recently reported for male patients with HPV infection with reference to relapses, spontaneous regressions and response to therapy. The multicentricity of the lesions
in this series, in which the disease featured a genital
neoplasm-papilloma syndrome is most likely linked to
the anatomical complexity of the female LGT.

The correlation of the incidence data of HPV 16, and
the mean ages of the patients with respectively PV-

associated early neoplasia and with PVI only is highly suggestive of a progression of the disease from infection to neoplasia. This event may correlate on the hand with the hypothesis that a carcinoma with bowenoid features may arise in condylomas harboring HPV 16, with or without the association of other types of HPV (9), and on the other hand with the hypothesis of the significance of the mechanism of intracellular surveillance in viral carcinogenesis (16).

## REFERENCES

1. Buckley, C.H., Butler, E.B., and Fox, H. (1984): J. Clin. Pathol., 37: 1201–1211.
2. Campion, M.J., Singer, A., Clarkson, P.K., and McCance, D.J. (1985): Lancet, i: 943–945.
3. Crum, C.P., Mitao, M., Levine, R.U., and Silverstein, S. (1985): J. Virol., 54: 675–681.
4. Crum, C.P., Nagai, N., Levine, R.U., and Silverstein, S. (1986): Am. J. Pathol., 123: 174–182.
5. Deligdisch, L., and Szulman, A.E. (1975): Gynecol. Oncol., 3: 181–190.
6. Di Luca, D., Pilotti, S., Stefanon, B., Rotola, A., Monini, P., Tognon, M., De Palo, G., Rilke, F., and Cassai, E. (1986): J. Gen. Virol., 67: 583–589.
7. Durst, M., Gissmann, L., Ikenberg, H., and zur Hausen, H. (1983): Proc. Natl. Acad. Sci. USA, 80: 3812–3815.
8. Gissmann, L., Wolnik, L., Ikenberg, H., Koldovsky, U., Schnurch, H.G., and zur Hausen, H. (1983): Proc. Natl. Acad. Sci. USA, 80: 560–563.
9. Gross, G., Hagedorn, M., Ikenberg, H., Rufli, T., Dahlet, C., Grosshans, E., and Gissmann, L. (1985): Arch. Dermatol., 121: 858–863.
10. Gross, G., Ikenberg, H., Gissmann, L., and Hagedorn, M. (1985): J. Invest. Dermatol., 85: 147–152.
11. Gupta, J., Pilotti, S., Shah, K.V., De Palo, G., and Rilke, F. (1987): Am. J. Surg. Pathol., 11: 430–434.
12. Ikenberg, H., Gissmann, L., Gross, G., and Grussendorf-Conen, E.I. (1983): Int. J. Cancer, 32: 563–565.
13. MacNab, J.C.M., Walkinshaw, S.A., Cordiner, J.W., and Clements, J.B. (1986): N. Engl. J. Med., 315: 1052–1058.
14. Okagaki, T. (1984): Pathol. Ann., 2: 31–62.
15. Pilotti, S., Della Torre, G., Rilke, F., De Palo, G., and Shah, K.V. (1984): Am. J. Surg. Pathol., 8: 751–761.
16. zur Hausen, H. (1986): Lancet, ii: 489–490.

# Morphological Relationship of Papillomavirus Infections to Cervical, Vulvar and Penile Cancer

K. Syrjanen[1] and S. Syrjanen[2]

[1]*Laboratory of Pathology & Cancer Research,*
*Finnish Cancer Society, Kuopio, Finland*
[2]*Department of Oral Pathology,*
*University of Kuopio, Kuopio, Finland*

Until the mid 1970's, it was believed that all different types of human warts, e.g., cutaneous, anal, and genital warts, would be caused by one and a single Human Papillomavirus (HPV) type, the variable morphology of the lesions being ascribed to their different anatomical location (104). This issue has been completely revised during the past ten years, however, following the discovery of many different types and subtypes of HPV each shown to possess a remarkable specificity in their site of infection (47,60,76,104). The previous concept on Condylomata acuminata as a sole and innocuous manifestation of HPV has been subjected to complete reappraisal since 1976, when lesions morphologically distinct from the classical exophytic condyloma, i.e., the flat and inverted (endophytic) condylomas were attributed to HPV (50,68).

During the past 7-8 years, ample morphological documentation has been generated, indicating that HPV lesions in the genital tract are frequently associated with intraepithelial neoplasia (CIN), carcinoma in situ (CIS) and invasive squamous cell carcinomas as well (17,21,24,29,30,42,46, 51–53,55,63,64,71, 75–81,83,91, 104–107).

When immunohistochemistry was applied to genital lesions, HPV structural proteins were readily disclosed in benign as well as in all grades of precancer lesions. Subsequently, DNA sequences of certain HPV types have been detected by DNA hybridization technology in genital precancer lesions and in genital squamous cell cancer, including that of the uterine cervix, vagina, vulva, and penis. Recent prospective follow-up data also indicate that cervical HPV infections (like CIN) possess a definite potential to progress into CIS and to invasive cancer, if left untreated (82,84-86,91-93).

Reports on malignant transformation of HPV lesions like laryngeal papillomas and cutaneous lesions of epidermodysplasia verruciformis (EV)(104), as well as epidemiological data on cervical cancer as a sexually transmitted disease (STD) (40,72), suggest that HPV infections are true precancer lesions in the genital tract. Recent progress made in the field of molecular biology of papillomaviruses also strongly implicates HPV as the most probable etiological agent of genital squamous cell carcinomas in both sexes (21,24,29,30,42, 46,51-53,55,63,64,71,76-81,83,104-107).

In the present chapter, the morphological relationships of HPV infections to premalignant and malignant lesions in the cervix, vulva and penis are shortly reviewed. Summary is given on the applicability of the morphological techniques (histopathology, cytology, immunohistochemistry, and in situ DNA-hybridization) in assessment of the malignant potential associated with HPV-infections at these sites.

## HPV-INFECTIONS IN THE GENITAL TRACT

The incidence of genital warts is being steadily increasing since the 1970's, as recently demonstrated in an epidemiologic study, where the mean annual incidence from 1950 to 1978 reached the peak of 106.5 per 100,000 population (7). Reliable incidence and prevalence data of cervical HPV infections in an unselected population have been elucidated only recently by an ongoing study utilizing the cytological mass-screening programme for detection of CIN in Finland (86,92); the prevalence of cervical HPV infections in 22-year-old women (a cohort of 2,000) proved to be 2.7% and the annual incidence as high as 4.5% (86). So far, no such figures are available on HPV infections in the male genital tract.

### Penile HPV-Infections

In 1930, Buschke and shortly afterwards Lowenstein described condylomas in the penis, which were of huge size and closely resembled an invasive squamous cell cancer both in gross appearance and on light microscopy. Since then, these Buschke-Lowenstein (B-L) tumors have been regarded as a variant of verrucous carcinoma, characterized by slow growth, fungus-like appearance and ulceration (97,101). The tumor is bulging rather than invading into the connective tissue (5,97,101). The HPV etiology of the tumor has been confirmed by an extensive literature describing HPV particles, HPV antigens and HPV DNA in the tumor cells

(4,104). By 1977, 65 cases had been reported, where a B-L tumor had transformed into an invasive squamous cell carcinoma (summarized in 5). Even ultrastructurally, these two entities resemble each other, thus further emphasizing the neoplastic character of the B-L tumor (35).

Recently, a squamous cell lesion distinct from the penile warts was described, and known as Bowenoid papulosis (2,99). Morphologically this lesion closely resembles Bowen's disease, which by definition is an in situ squamous cell carcinoma (2,99). Typical HPV particles and HPV antigens have been repeatedly discovered in Bowenoid papulosis lesions speaking for their viral etiology (41,74). Although the biological behaviour of the majority of cases reported so far has been entirely benign, many of them undergoing spontaneous regression, Bowenoid papulosis should be recognized as a distinct entity due to its frequent association with HPV 16 and HPV 18 (2,27,28,41,74,99).

The importance of examination of the male sexual partners of HPV-infected women should be emphasized, because of the increasing evidence on the link between penile and cervical cancer, pertinent to the high risk HPV types 16 and 18 (8,40,45,56,72,95). These types have been also discovered in the majority of penile Bowenoid papulosis lesions studied so far (27,28,37). In a recent study of 114 men with penile warts, the anatomical distribution of condyloma acuminatum, papular and flat condylomata was practically identical, and the gross appearance of the warts did not bear any correlation with their morphology on light microscopy or, more importantly, with the type of HPV DNA disclosed (95). The detection rate of dysplasia was markedly different in the flat, acuminatum, and papular warts, 25%, 50% and 75%, respectively. HPV antigen expression was inversely related to the grade of dysplasia (95).

A definite association of HPV 16 and HPV 18 with the dysplastic lesions was found, as shown in Table 1. In that series, none of the HPV 16- and 25% of the HPV 18-positive cases were devoid of concomitant dysplasia, the corresponding figures for HPV 6 and HPV 11 being 59.2% and 68.8%, respectively.

## Urethral HPV Infections

Condyloma acuminatum confined to adult male urethra has been a well recognized entity since its first description in 1891. It has been estimated that in urological practice, condylomas involve urethra in some 5% of cases, and the bladder only exceptionally (13). Owing to their luxuriant growth, frequently huge size, ulceration, and extension into the deeper structures, the gross similarities between urethral condylomas   and malignancy have been emphasized, and not   infrequently, these lesions   pose   serious   problems   in   eradication (13).

TABLE 1. HPV DNA in Penile Lesions Related to Grade
of Dysplasia

| Grade of Dys- plasia | No.of Cases | HPV No. | DNA % | Per cent of HPV DNA-Positive Lesions | | | |
|---|---|---|---|---|---|---|---|
| | | | | HPV 6 | HPV 11 | HPV 16 | HPV 18 |
| None | 62 | 10 | 14.5 | 55.8 | 42.3 | 0.0 | 1.9 |
| Mild | 36 | 6 | 16.7 | 56.6 | 26.7 | 10.0 | 6.7 |
| Moderate | 8 | 1 | 12.5 | 42.9 | 28.5 | 14.3 | 14.3 |
| Severe | 2 | 0 | 0.0 | 0.0 | 0.0 | 100.0 | 0.0 |
| Total Series | 108 | 17* | 15.8 | 53.8 | 35.2 | 6.6 | 4.4 |

* Includes 9 cases with double infections: HPV 6 & 11, 7 cases; HPV 6 & 18, one case; HPV 11 & 16, one case.

Although the   majority   of urethral   condylomas   de- scribed so   far   presented with   papillary   morphology, flat warts also exist as shown by recent   demonstration of HPV   structural proteins   in   such   lesions   (54,88). More studies with the DNA-hybridization techniques   are urgently needed .especially   on   the   subclinical   HPV infections in   the   male urethra.   Such   lesions   could represent a potential reservoir for reinfections to   be transmitted to   the   sexual   partners   (45). Of   special interest in this respect is the recent discovery of HPV DNA in human semen (61).

## Vulvar Infections

Ample documentation is currently available to   indi- cate that   HPV infections   have morphological   associa- tions with   precancer lesions   of the   vulva, shown   to undergo malignant transformation (70). A strong   epide- miologic association was   recently described   between condyloma acuminatum   and vulvar squamous cell   carci- noma, suggesting a causal relationship (12). An   entity known as   verrucous   carcinoma   (97,101)   was   recently reviewed with   special   emphasis   on   the   differential diagnostic problems   with   condylomas   and   B-L tumors morphologically (97).   Quite lately, HPV   DNA was   dis- closed in a verrucous carcinoma of the vulva (69).

The interest in vulvar intraepithelial neoplasia (VIN) has increased in parallel with the emerging morphological data on the associations of HPV infections with CIN (9,11,17,21,24,29,52,55,63,64,71,77-81, 83,89). Both the cytopathic effects of HPV (koilocytotic atypia) (43) and HPV particles have been found in substantial (70%) percentage of VIN lesions (11). When stained for HPV structural proteins, 50% to 64% of VIN lesions proved to be positive (9,65). DNA hybridization analysis have disclosed HPV DNA of the known genital types, (e.g. HPV 6, 11, 16, 18, 31, 33, 35) in lesions of VIN. In the majority of vulvar carcinomas studied in our laboratory, the high risk HPV types 16 and 18 DNA have been encountered (unpublished observation).

Bowenoid papulosis lesions have also been reported in the vulva (2), which should be distinguished from usual condyloma, because of the frequent association with the high risk HPV types 16 and 18 as pointed out before (2,27,28,41,74,99).

## Infections in the Uterine Cervix

The classical condyloma acuminatum in the uterine cervix has been described in detail by a number of case reports (66,103); a total of 254 such lesions being reported in the literature until 1974 (reviewed in 76). As pointed out, the concepts of cervical HPV lesions have been subjected to complete reapprisal since 1976, since when the flat, inverted and papillary condylomas in the uterine cervix have been shown to frequently accompany CIN, CIS and cancer (14,17,21,23,24,29,30,42, 46, 51-53,55,63,64,71,75-81,83,89).

These reports, based on morphology and cytology, were the first to suggest that HPV might be involved in cervical carcinogenesis (50,68,75). There is little doubt at the moment that cervical HPV infections are a sexually transmitted disease (STD), found in young age groups (peak 20-24 years), associated with early sexual activity and promiscuity (59,90). Less well elucidated is the natural history of the disease, i.e., why some of the HPV lesions disappear spontaneously, and why some progress into more severe grades of CIN, and eventually into a squamous cell carcinoma even within a short period of follow-up.

According to our experience based on a long-term prospective follow-up of over 500 women, cervical HPV infections frequently involve the vagina, either concomitantly with the primary lesion, after a period of follow-up, or following the eradication of cervical infection by conization, cryotherapy or laser (84-86, 92,93). This is consonant with the number of case histories and larger series indicating that HPV infections in the female genital tract are frequently multifocal, i.e., both the external genitalia, vagina and cervix are simultaneously or sequentially affected (66,73,100). Accordingly, vaginal in situ squamous cell carcinoma seems to be associated with identical lesions elsewhere in the genitalia in 88% of cases (36). In fact, such a multicentricity was emphasized in the earlier literature on invasive carcinomas of the genital tract (39).

In an analysis of vaginal intraepithelial neoplasia (VAIN) by DNA hybridization techniques, 15/19 (79%) lesions studied contained HPV 6 DNA, and the rest, DNA of at that time unidentified HPV type (HPV 16?) (57). These authors also found HPV 6 DNA in two lesions of vaginal verrucous carcinoma (57). A double infection by HPV 16 and 18 was disclosed in a vaginal carcinoma developing in the lateral fornices in less than three years of prospective follow-up (82).

## MORPHOLOGICAL LINK BETWEEN HPV-INFECTIONS AND GENITAL CANCER

The gross morphology of the classical genital wart is familiar to anyone engaged in diagnosis of genito-urinary diseases, and will not be surveyed in detail here. Most authors agree that no reliable criteria exist to differentiate the flat and endophytic HPV lesions from those of the classical CIN and CIS on visual inspection only (15,42,51,52). This is because in the majority of cases, the flat and inverted condylomas are indiscernible by the naked eye, making necessary the use of other means to settle the proper diagnosis.

### Colposcopic Patterns

HPV lesions of the vulva, vagina and uterine cervix are readily accessible to colposcopic examination, and a number of excellent descriptions on their colposcopic appearance are available (15,42,98). Colposcopic examination in experienced hands has proved to be a reliable means to carry out the prospective follow-up of the cervical HPV infections, as evidenced by the good correlation between the colposcopic patterns and the findings in cervical PAP smears and directed punch biopsy (85,86,98). Despite such a good correlation, however, it is to be emphasized that a few HPV lesions exist that escape detection by colposcopy (15,68,98), thus necessitating the inclusion of cervical PAP smears and directed punch biopsy in diagnostic procedures of these lesions. Quite lately, the importance of colposcopic examination of the male external genitalia to disclose the subclinical HPV-infections has been emphasized (45,98).

## Cytologic Changes

Although the term "koilocytotic atypia" was introduced thirty years ago in 1956 (43), it took two decades until its significance as the cytopathic effect of HPV was fully established (50,68). The discovery of the new HPV lesions in cervical biopsy has resulted in a series of reports and reviews on the cytological patterns of cervical HPV lesions (6,42,46,51–53,64,83).

According to the experience of our laboratory, the diagnosis of cervical HPV infection can be established in routine PAP smears with a high degree of reliability, provided that the smear is adequate (78–81,83). Cervical HPV lesions characteristically and almost constantly shed cells (either singly or in clusters) classifiable as dyskeratotic superficial cells (Table 2). Such cells exhibit an intensely orangeophilic cytoplasm, and an enlarged, hyperchromatic (frequently pyknotic) nucleus. This hyperchromasia (karyopyknosis) is due to the fact that replication of HPV particles usually takes place in these superficial dyskeratotic cells, as established by detection of the complete viral particles. Not infrequently, single dyskeratotic cells are found deeper in the epithelium admixed with the intermediate cells. The nuclei of the superficial dyskeratotic cells may or may not present with dyskaryotic changes, depending on whether concomitant CIN is present or not (53,83). Thus, the importance of evaluating the nuclear/cytoplasmic ratio in these cells is emphasized, because of diagnostic value to assess the grade of HPV lesions, e.g. whether HPV–NCIN (HPV infection without CIN) or HPV–CIN. This in turn, is of prognostic significance for the subsequent clinical course of the cervical HPV infections, as established by our prospective follow–up study (85,86) (Table 2).

**TABLE 2.** PAP Smear Changes Related to Natural History of HPV Infections

| Smears Consistent with | No. of Cases | Regressed No. | % | Persistent No. | % | Progressed No. | % | Recurred No. | % |
|---|---|---|---|---|---|---|---|---|---|
| Normal | 66 | 24 | 36.4 | 39 | 59.1 | 3 | 4.5 | 0 | 0.0 |
| HPV–NCIN* | 160 | 35 | 21.9 | 107 | 66.9 | 18 | 11.2 | 0 | 0.0 |
| HPV–CIN | 158 | 24 | 15.2 | 95 | 60.1 | 33 | 20.9 | 6 | 3.8 |
| Total Series | 384 | 83 | 21.6 | 241 | 62.8 | 54 | 14.1 | 6 | 1.6 |

* HPV–NCIN = HPV infection without CIN

The cell currently regarded as the most reliable sign of HPV infection is known as a koilocyte or a ballon cell (43,50,68). Albeit not invariably detectable in the PAP smears derived from cervical HPV lesions, koilocytotic change is considered as the cytopathic effect of HPV in the cells infected by this virus (6,42,46,51–53,64,83). The most characteristic koilocyte is an intermediate cell with an enlarged, hyperchromatic nucleus, surrounded by a distinct cytoplasmic clear zone called halo. At the margins of the halo, cytoplasm is condensed and usually exhibit an ambophilic staining pattern. Also the superficial dyskeratotic cells (and infrequently parabasal cells) may undergo koilocytotic change. Both the koilocytes and the superficial dyskeratotic cells may present with bi- or multinucleated forms. In addition, cells known as condylomatous intermediate cells are encountered in a few per cent of PAP smears from HPV lesions (68,83). Equally important as with the superficial dyskeratotic cells, is the evaluation on the nuclear/cytoplasmic ratio also in koilocytotic cells, to assess the grade of lesions, i.e. whether HPV-NCIN or HPV-CIN.

To conclude, the routine PAP smear is reliable means to establish the diagnosis of cervical HPV infection. It is also a technique providing evidence on the association of HPV infections with severe precancer lesions and cervical cancer. This is shown by the discovery of HPV-induced cytopathic changes in PAP smears derived from 272 consecutive lesions of severe dysplasia, in situ carcinoma and invasive cancer, as summarized in Table 3. In cases, where the lesions fail to shed the characteristic cells, however, directed punch biopsy remains the next step in the diagnostic process.

**TABLE 3.** HPV-suggestive Cells in Cervical Smears Derived from Severe Dysplasia (SD), Carcinoma In Situ (CIS) and Cervical Cancer

| HPV-suggestive Cells | Source of Cervical Smear | | | |
| --- | --- | --- | --- | --- |
| | SD | CIS | Cancer | Total |
| Dyskeratotic Cells, single | 8.4% | 6.2% | 12.5% | 8.1% |
| Dyskeratotic Cells, in sheets | 11.3% | 10.0% | 11.1% | 11.0% |
| Koilocytotic Cells | 11.3% | 5.4% | 1.4% | 5.8% |
| Strongly Degenerative Nuclear Forms | 4.2% | 3.9% | 8.3% | 5.1% |
| Binucleated Cells (large nuclei) | 9.8% | 2.3% | 9.7% | 5.5% |
| Binucleated Cells (small nuclei) | 0.0% | 0.0% | 1.4% | 0.4% |
| Multinucleated Cells | 9.9% | 6.9% | 9.7% | 8.4% |
| Condylomatous Intermediate Cells | 4.2% | 0.8% | 1.4% | 1.8% |
| Total Series | 71 | 129 | 72 | 272 |

## Histological Evidence

On light microscopy, the exophytic genital wart is characterized by papillomatosis, acanthosis, elongation and thickening of the rete pegs, parakeratosis, and cytoplasmic vacuolization or koilocytosis (66,103). In practice, this lesion is indistinguishable from the squamous cell papilloma, the latter name being practically never used in HPV lesions of the uterine cervix and longer (76).

Meisels et al. in 1976 (50) in Canada, and Purola and Savia in 1977 (68) in Finland, independent of each other, described in the uterine cervix epithelial changes devoid of the papillary contour of condylomata acuminata, but still exhibiting their characteristic cytological features. These new lesions were named flat and inverted (endophytic) condylomas, and since then their HPV etiology has been unequivocally confirmed by electron microscopic demonstration of HPV particles (6,33), by immunohistochemical techniques disclosing HPV antigens both in punch biopsy and in PAP smears (32,38,67,87,102), and by DNA hybridization experiments with HPV DNA probes (24,26,105,106).

Extensive series of descriptions on the light microscopic appearance of the flat and inverted condylomas have been published during the last 7 – 8 years. A flat condyloma is a flat focus of acanthotic squamous epithelium with accentuated rete pegs and elongated dermal papillae. In many cases, there is a striking contrast between the deep and the superficial layers in the epithelium, the latter crowded by koilocytotic cells. The lesion is usually covered with layers (varying in thickness) of superficial dyskeratotic cells. As pointed out before, single dyskeratotic cells may be present in the intermediate cell layers as well. Another characteristic feature, not detectable in all lesions, however, are the tiny epithelial projections called spikes or asperities (51,53,68,76,79–81).

When changes consistent with CIN are encountered in association with the flat condyloma, the lesions have been called by various names, including: atypical condylomas, condylomatous atypias, condyloma with CIN, or condylomatous dysplasias (17,21,24,29,30,42,46, 51–53,55,63,64,71,75–81,83,89). Although the nomenclature is far from being unified yet, there is a general agreement that HPV lesions are frequently accompanied by CIN and CIS, and less frequently by an invasive squamous cell carcinoma as well. This is also shown in Table 4, where a retrospective series of 620 cervical CIN lesions and cancer was scrutinized for morphological evidence of HPV infection.

**TABLE 4.** Morphological Association of HPV Infections with CIN Lesions and Cervical Cancer

| Grade of CIN | Number of Cases | No Signs of HPV (%) | HPV Infection (%) |
|---|---|---|---|
| CIN I | 194 | 53.1 | 46.9 |
| CIN II | 121 | 28.1 | 71.9 |
| CIN III | 262 | 39.3 | 60.7 |
| Cancer | 43 | 83.7 | 16.3 |
| Total Series | 620 | 44.4 | 55.6 |

In practice, the concomitant CIN lesion can be encountered either admixed with the HPV lesion proper, or situated adjacent to characteristic flat condyloma. In the former case, dyskaryotic (transformed) basal cells invade the varying depth of the epithelium, subjacent to the layers of characteristic koilocytes and dyskeratotic superficial cells. In such cases, it may be sometimes difficult to assess the grade of HPV-CIN even for an experienced pathologist. If, however, the CIN lesion is located adjacent to the HPV lesion, the correct grading of the former is usually readily obtainable, using the criteria outlined for the classical CIN. As emphasized above, this grading is important, because of prognostic value for the clinical outcome of the HPV infection (84-86).

The third type of cervical HPV lesion, the inverted or endophytic condyloma is in most respects identical to the flat one, except that it shows as additional features, pseudoinvasive penetration into the underlying stroma and/or endocervical gland openings. Thus, it shares many of the growth characteristics of the in situ carcinoma, which it actually seems to be frequently connected with morphologically (75,77,78,89). Because of these evident similarities, difficulties are sometimes encountered in differentiating the flat and endophytic condyloma from each other. In doubtful cases, however, more important than attempt to make morphological distinction between these two entities, is from the biological point of view, to complete an accurate grading of the concomitant CIN, as it is of predictive value for the clinical course of these lesions (84-86) (see also Table 5).

The most recently described cervical lesion attributed to HPV is called atypical immature metaplasia (AIM) (10). According to the original report, AIM was found associated with cervical condylomas in 34 per cent, and with CIN II or III in 16 per cent of cases (10), and 16 per cent of the lesions contained HPV structural proteins. Further work is still needed to fully elucidate the relationship of this entity to the other HPV lesions in the uterine cervix.

**TABLE 5.** Clinical Course Related to Grade of HPV Lesions

| HPV Lesion Grade | No.of Cases | Regressed No. | % | Persistent No. | % | Progressed No. | % | Recurred No. | % |
|---|---|---|---|---|---|---|---|---|---|
| HPV-NCIN* | 232 | 70 | 30.2 | 144 | 62.1 | 18 | 7.8 | 0 | 0.0 |
| HPV-CIN I | 104 | 15 | 14.4 | 72 | 69.2 | 15 | 14.4 | 2 | 2.0 |
| HPV-CIN II | 69 | 8 | 11.6 | 50 | 72.5 | 11 | 15.9 | 0 | 0.0 |
| HPV-CIN III | 40 | 5 | 12.5 | 4 | 10.0 | 26 | 65.0 | 5 | 12.5 |
| HPV-CIN | 213 | 28 | 13.1 | 126 | 59.2 | 52 | 24.4 | 7 | 3.3 |

* HPV-NCIN = HPV infection without CIN

## Immunohistochemistry

In early 1980's, an indirect immunoperoxidase (IP-PAP) method was introduced to disclose HPV antigens (structural proteins) in paraffin sections of cervical lesions (38,102). SDS-disrupted virions of papillomaviruses were shown to possess common group-specific antigens giving rise to antisera capable of reacting with all the known papillomavirus types (38,102). Such widely cross-reacting antisera have proved applicable tools in assessing a variety of squamous cell lesions for the presence of HPV antigens.

With the IP-PAP technique, the presence of HPV antigens is confined exclusively to the nuclei of the koilocytes and/or superficial dyskeratotic cells (32, 38,67,87,102). In most series stained with the IP-PAP technique, some 50 per cent of the lesions have been shown to contain HPV antigens. The same technique was recently applied to PAP smears derived from cervical condylomas, and 67% of the smears were positive for HPV antigens (32). There are differences in HPV antigen expression related to lesion morphology in that the papillary warts usually show the highest and flat lesions of the lowest frequency of positive results. It also seems that the positive staining is inversely related to the degree of concomitant CIN in HPV lesions

(78,89). Invasive carcinomas stain positive only exceptionally.

At present, IP-PAP technique is used by many laboratories as a screening method to assess the suggested HPV etiology of genital (and other) squamous cell tumors, especially when the commercial kits became available. Albeit of definite diagnostic value in positive cases, the applicability of IP-PAP staining in HPV tumor research is limited by the fact that it can only disclose the productive HPV infection, where viral structural proteins are expressed. In lesions with nonpermissive infection leading to cell transformation and progression to CIN, CIS and cancer, structural proteins are not likely to be expressed (24,34,62). Recent results showed only insignificant differences in structural protein expression between the lesions infected by different HPV types (84,85). As disclosed in prospectively followed-up cervical HPV lesions, no correlation exists between HPV antigen expression in the first biopsy and the subsequent clinical course, thus invalidating the use of IP-PAP test as a prognostic predictor in this disease (85,86).

## MALIGNANT POTENTIAL OF GENITAL HPV-INFECTIONS

The molecular cloning technology with aid of the restriction endonucleases has significantly increased our knowledge on molecular biology and biochemistry of papillomaviruses in a few years (16,24,25,34,48,62, 107). The first genital HPV type found was HPV 6, preferentially disclosed in benign cervical lesions and in CIN (26), whereas HPV 11 DNA was also present in a few cases of cervical carcinomas. In all these lesions, HPV DNA was found exclusively as non-integrated episomal form outside the host cell genome (26).

In 1983, however, significant new data were obtained following the discovery of two new HPV types 16 and 18 in invasive cervical carcinomas (19). It soon became apparent from blot hybridization and restriction enzyme cleavage studies that the DNA patterns in these carcinomas did not follow those found in the HPV lesions previously studied. Albeit the majority of the HPV DNA still seemed to persist episomally (3,20), many of the carcinomas analysed contained HPV 16 or 18 DNA exclusively linked to the host cell genome (3,20,24). When analysed with HPV 16 and HPV 18 DNA probes, it was shown that these DNAs were present in 5.1% of condylomata acuminata, in 16.7% of flat condylomas, and in 53.8% of CIS and in 57.4% of invasive cervical cancers (25). Thus, integration in the host cell genome seems to be the special feature of the high risk HPV types 16 and 18, and most probably has implications in tumorigenicity of these viruses.

These findings have been confirmed by a number of other authors by now (16,18,44,49,96). In these studies, usually a single biopsy of each HPV lesion has been analysed, however, with no follow-up data available on the previous clinical course of the lesion. Recently, we reported the first documented case progressing from CIN I to an invasive cancer in less than three years, and which on DNA hybridization disclosed a double infection by HPV 16 and HPV 18 (86).

The prospective follow-up project conducted in our clinic was actually the first study to provide firm evidence that HPV 16 and (less dramatically) HPV 18 are clearly the HPV types predisposing the cervical lesions to clinical progression (84-86,92,93). There was in general, a close association between HPV type and grade of the lesion in that HPV 16 and 18 DNA (analysed using the in situ hybridization) was mostly confined to higher grades of CIN, in contrast to HPV 6 and 11 found predominantly in HPV-NCIN lesions (85,86). Thus, morphology alone (as evaluated in the first diagnostic punch biopsy) proved to be of significance in predicting the subsequent clinical behavior of the cervical HPV infections, as depicted in Table 5.

The highest progression rate seems to be associated with HPV 16 lesions (33.3%), which also are the least frequent to undergo spontaneous regression (5.6%). All the lesions recurred after a radical cone treatment also contained HPV 16 DNA (86). This is in sharp contrast to the lesions induced by HPV 6 or 11, which do regress in 25.6% of cases. Noteworthy, however, was the relatively high progression rate established for HPV 6/11 lesions as well (25.6%). Although these data clearly substantiate the concept on HPV 16 and HPV 18 as the high risk HPV types in cervical carcinogenesis, it is to be emphasized that also these "low risk" types HPV 6 and 11 represent a potential risk to a woman for subsequent development of more severe precancer lesions (81,85,86).

Prospective follow-up of a large series of patients also permits evaluation of the eventual latent infections in cervical epithelium. This concept of latent HPV infections was first substantiated by the discovery of HPV particles (91), structural proteins (93), and HPV DNA sequences (22) in spontaneously regressed or laser-eradicated genital HPV lesions. These data are in full agreement with our recent observations confirming the occurrence of HPV 6, 11, 16, 18 and 31 in lesions with no morphological evidence of HPV infection on light microscopy (86). Indeed, HPV 16 and 18 comprised 40% of the HPV types, and HPV 6/11 represented a minority of only 30% in such biopsies. Thus, latency seems to be an established feature of the infectious cycle of these and probably other HPV types as well. Such HPV genomes present in apparently normal epithelium have been recently shown to be responsible for new lesions after a seemingly successful removal of an adjacent lesion (22), a fact that should be taken into account in therapeutic considerations.

## CONCLUSIONS

In routine diagnosis as well as in research of HPV infections, light microscopical methods (histology, cytology, and immunohistochemistry) currently have a central role. These were the first techniques to provide evidence that HPV might be involved in the development of genital squamous cell carcinomas, subsequently supported by the data obtained by other means. The morphological methods are supplemented by the DNA-hybridization techniques, including Southern blot, dot blot, and filter in situ hybridization, which, however, are not suitable for routine diagnosis at the moment.

In the future, the role of light microscopy will be further accentuated by the development of the DNA-hybridization technology applicable to routine diagnosis. As a sign of that, in situ DNA hybridization methods have been recently introduced (31), which are applied to paraffin sections. Evidently, these promising recent developments leading to replacement of the isotope-labelled HPV DNA probes with the non-radioactive (e.g. biotin) probes (1,94), will render the in situ DNA hybridization technology into more general availability in the near future. Combined with the data provided by the molecular biological methods and careful follow-up of the patients, these techniques will undoubtedly provide powerful means to obtain further evidence of the suggested causal relationship between HPV and human cancer.

## ACKNOWLEDGEMENTS

The original investigations included in this review were supported by PHS grant number 1 R01 CA 42010-01 awarded by the National Cancer Institute, DHHS, and in part by a research grants from the Finnish Cancer Society and from the Medical Research Council of the Academy of Finland (SA 07/014). The skillful technical assistance of Mrs. Heli Eskelinen, Miss Soili Finska, Miss Helena Kemilainen, Mrs. Maritta Lipponen and Miss Ritva Savolainen is gratefully acknowledged.

## REFERENCES

1. Beckmann, A.M., Myerson, D., Daling, J.R., Kiviat, N.B., Fenoglio, C.M., and McDougall, J.K. (1985):

J. Med. Virol., 16: 265–272.

2. Berger, B.W., and Hori, Y. (1978): Arch. Dermatol., 114: 1698–1699.

3. Boshart, M., Gissmann, L., Ikenberg,H., Kleinheinz, A., Scheurlen, W., and zur Hausen, H. (1984): EMBO J., 3: 1151–1157.

4. Boshart, M., and zur Hausen, H. (1986): J. Virol., 58: 963–966.

5. Boxer, R.J., and Skinner, D.G. (1977): Urology, 9: 72–78.

6. Casas-Cordero, M., Morin, C., Roy, M., Fortier, M., and Meisels, A. (1981): Acta Cytol., 25: 383–392.

7. Chuang, T-Y., Perry, H.O., Kurland, L.T., and Ilstrup, D.M. (1984): Arch. Dermatol., 120: 469–475.

8. Cocks, P.S., Peel, K.R., Cartwright, R.A., and Adib, R. (1980): Lancet, ii: 855–856.

9. Crum, C.P., Braun, L.A., Shah, K.V., Fu, Y.S., Levine, R.U., Fenoglio, C.M., Richart, R.M., and Townsend, D.E. (1982): Cancer, 49: 468–471.

10. Crum, C.P., Egawa, K., Fu, Y.S., Lancaster, W.D., Barron, B., Levine, R.U., Fenoglio, C.M., and Richart, R.M. (1983): Cancer, 51: 2214–2219.

11. Crum, C.P., Fu, Y.S., Levine, R.U., Richart, R.M., Townsend, D.E., and Fenoglio, C.M. (1982): Am. J. Obstet. Gynecol., 144: 77–83.

12. Daling, J.R., Chu, J., Weiss, N.S., Emel, L., and Tamini, H.K. (1984): Br. J. Cancer, 50: 533–535.

13. Debenedictis, T.J., Marmar, J.L., and Praiss, D.E. (1977): J. Urol., 118: 767–769.

14. De Brux, J., Orth, G., Croissant, O., Cochard, B., and Ionesco, M. (1983): Bull. Cancer, 70: 410–422.

15. De Palo, G., and Stefanon D. (1983): The Cervix, 1: 17–22.

16. De Villiers, E-M., Schneider, A., Gross, G., and zur Hausen, H. (1986): Med. Microbiol. Immunol., 174: 281–286.

17. De Virgiliis, G., Mauri, L., Masserini, M., Le Grazie, C., Beolchi, S., Sideri, M., Rainoldi, R., Maggi, R., and Remotti, G. (1982): Tumori, 68: 465–468.

18. Di Luca, D., Pilotti, S., Stefanon, B., Rotola, A., Monini, P., Tognon, M., De Palo, G., Rilke, F., and Cassai, E. (1986): J. Gen. Virol., 67: 583–589.

19. Durst, M., Gissmann, L., Ikenberg, H., and zur Hausen, H. (1983): Proc. Natl. Acad. Sci. USA, 80: 3812–3814.

20. Durst, M., Hotz, M., Kleinheinz, A., and Gissmann, L. (1985): J. Gen. Virol., 66: 1515–1522.

21. Fenoglio, C.M., and Ferenczy, A. (1982): Semin. Oncol., 9: 349–372.

22. Ferenczy, A., Mitao, M., Nagai, N., Silverstein, S.J., and Crum, C.P. (1985): N. Engl. J. Med., 313: 784-788.
23. Franceschi, S., Doll, R., Gallowey, J., La Vecchia, C., Peto, R., and Spriggs, A.I. (1983): Br. J. Cancer, 48: 621-628.
24. Gissmann, L. (1984): Cancer Surv., 3: 161-181.
25. Gissmann, L., Boshart, M., Durst, M., Ikenberg, H., Wagner, D., and zur Hausen, H. (1984): J. Invest. Dermatol., 83: 26s-28s.
26. Gissmann, L., Wolnick, L., Ikenberg, H., Koldovsky, U., Schnurch, H.G., and zur Hausen, H. (1983): Proc. Natl. Acad. Sci. USA, 80: 560-563.
27. Gross, G., Hagedorn, M., Ikenberg, H., Rufli, T., Dahlet, C., Grosshans, E., and Gissmann, L. (1985): Arch. Dermatol., 121: 858-863.
28. Gross, G., Ikenberg, H., Gissmann, L., and Hagedorn, M. (1985): J. Invest. Dermatol., 85: 147-152.
29. Grunebaum, A.N., Sedlis, A., Sillman, F., Fruchter, R., Stanek, S., and Boyce, J. (1983): Obstet. Gynecol., 62: 448-455.
30. Guillet, G., Breun, L., Shah, K., and Ferenczy, A. (1983): Ann. Dermatol. Venereol., 110: 43-51.
31. Gupta, J.W., Gendelman, H.E., Naghashfar, Z., Gupta, P., Rosenshein, N., Sawada, E., Woodrufff, J.D., and Shah, K.V. (1985): Int. J. Gynecol. Pathol., 4: 211-218.
32. Gupta, J.W., Gupta, P.K., Shah, K.V., and Kelly, D.P. (1983): Int. J. Gynecol. Pathol., 2: 160-170.
33. Hills, E., and Laverty, C.R. (1979): Acta Cytol., 23: 53-56.
34. Howley, P. (1982): Arch. Pathol. Lab. Med., 106: 429-432.
35. Hull, M.T., Eble, J.N., Priest, J.B., and Mulcahy, J.J. (1981): J. Urol., 126: 485-489.
36. Hummer, W.K., Mussey, E., Decker, D.G., and Dockerty, M.B. (1970): Am. J. Obstet. Gynecol., 108: 1109-1116.
37. Ikenberg, H., Gissmann, L., Gross, G., Grussendorf-Conen, E.I., and zur Hausen, H. (1983): Int. J. Cancer, 32: 563-565.
38. Jenson, A.B., Rosenthal, J.D., Olson, C., Pass, F., Lancaster, W.D., and Shah, K. (1980): JNCI, 64: 495-500.
39. Jemerson, G.K., and Merril, J.A. (1970): Cancer, 26: 150-153.
40. Kessler, I.I. (1976): Cancer Res., 36: 783-791.
41. Kimura, S., Hirai, A., Harada, R., and Nagashima, M. (1978): Dermatologica, 157: 229-237.
42. Kirkup, W., Evans, A.S., Brough, A.K., Davis, J.A., O'Loughlin, T., Wilkinson, G., and Monaghan, J.M.

(1982): Br. J. Obstet. Gynaecol., 89:571-577.
43. Koss, L.G., and Durfee, G.R. (1956): Ann. NY Acad. Sci., 63: 1245-1261.
44. Lancaster, W.D., Castellano, C., Santos, C., Delgado, G., Kurman, R.J., and Jenson, A.B. (1986): Am. J. Obstet. Gynecol., 154: 115-119.
45. Levine, R.U., Crum, C.P., Herman, E., Silvers, D., Ferenczy, A., and Richart, R.M. (1984): Obstet. Gynecol., 64: 16-20.
46. Ludwig, M.E., Lowell., D.M., and Livolsi, V.A. (1981): Am. J. Clin. Pathol., 76: 255-262.
47. Lutzner, M.A. (1983): Arch. Dermatol., 119: 631-635.
48. McCance, D.J. (1986): Biochim. Biophys. Acta 823: 195-205.
49. McCance, D.J., Clarkson, P.K., Dyson, J.L., Walker, P.G., and Singer, A. (1985): Br. J. Obstet. Gynaecol., 92: 1093-1100.
50. Meisels, A., Fortin, R., and Roy, M. (1976): Acta Cytol., 20: 505-509.
51. Meisels, A., and Morin, C. (1981): Gynecol. Oncol., 12: 111-123.
52. Meisels, A., Morin, C., and Casas-Cordero, M. (1982): Int. J. Gynecol. Pathol., 1: 75-94.
53. Meisels, A., Roy, M., Fortier, M., and Morin, C. (1979): Am. J. Diagn. Gynecol. Obstet., 1: 109-116.
54. Murphy, W.M., Fu, Y.S., Lancaster, W.D., and Jenson, A.B. (1983): J. Urol., 130: 84-85.
55. Nyeem, R., Wilkinson, E.J., and Grover, L.J. (1982): Int. J., Gynecol. Pathol., 1: 246-257.
56. Obalek, S., Jablonska, S., Beaudenon, S., Walczak, L., and Orth, G. (1986): J. Am. Acad. Dermatol., 14: 433-444.
57. Okagaki, T., Clark, B., Zachow, K.R., Twiggs, L.B., Ostrow, R.S., Pass, F., and Faras, A.J. (1984): Arch. Pathol. Lab. Med., 108: 567-570.
58. Okagaki, T., Twiggs, L.B., Zachow, K.R., Clark, B.A., Ostrow, R.S., and Faras, A.J. (1983): Int. J. Gynecol., Pathol., 2: 153-159.
59. Oriel, J.D. (1981): Sex. Transm. Dis., 8: 326-329.
60. Orth, G., Jablonska, S., Breitburd, F., Favre, M., and Croissant, O. (1978): Bull. Cancer, 65: 151-164.
61. Ostrow, R.S., Zachow, K.R., Niimura, M., Okagaki, T., Muller, S., Bender, M., and Faras, A.J. (1986): Science, 231: 731-733.
62. Pfister, H. (1984): Rev. Physiol. Biochem. Pharmacol., 99: 112-181.
63. Pilotti, S., Alasio, L., Rilke, F., and Fontanelli, R. (1982): Diagn. Gynecol. Obstet., 4: 357-362.
64. Pilotti, S., Rilke, De Palo, G., Della Torre, G., and Alasio, L. (1981): J. Clin. Pathol., 34:

532-541.

65. Pilotti, S., Rilke, F., Shah, K.V., Della Torre, G., and De Palo, G. (1984): Am. J. Surg. Pathol., 8: 751-761.

66. Pitkin, R.M., and Kent, T.H. (1963): Am. J. Obstet. Gynecol., 85: 440-446.

67. Portolani, M., Borgatti, M.A., Bartoletti, A.M., Mariuzzi, M.G., Beltrami, C.A., Di Loreto, C., De Nictolis, M., and Stramazzotti, D. (1983): Microbiologica, 6: 115-120.

68. Purola, E., and Savia, E. (1977): Acta Cytol., 21: 26-31.

69. Rando, R.F., Sedlacek, T.V., Hunt, J., Jenson, A.B., Kurman, R.J., and Lancaster, W.D. (1986): Obstet. Gynecol., 78: 70S-75S.

70. Rhatigan, R.M., and Safflos, R.O. (1977): South Med. J., 70: 591-594.

71. Roy, M., Morin, C., Casas-Cordero, M., and Meisels, A. (1983): Clin. Obstet. Gynaecol., 26: 949-967.

72. Singer, A., Reid, B.L., and Coppleson, M. (1976): Am. J. Obstet. Gynecol., 126: 110-115.

73. Stanbridge, C.M., and Butler, E.B. (1983): Int. J. Gynecol. Pathol., 2: 264-274.

74. Steffen, C. (1982): Am. J. Dermatopathol., 4: 5-8.

75. Syrjanen, K.J. (1979): Arch. Gynecol., 227: 153-161.

76. Syrjanen, K.J. (1980): Obstet. Gynecol. Surv., 35: 685-694.

77. Syrjanen, K.J. (1980): Surg. Gynecol. Obstet., 150: 372-376.

78. Syrjanen, K.J. (1983): Obstet. Gynecol., 62: 617-622.

79. Syrjanen, K.J. (1984): Obstet. Gynecol. Surv., 39: 252-265.

80. Syrjanen, K.J. (1984): The Cervix, 2: 103-126.

81. Syrjanen, K.J. (1986): Pathol. Annu., 21: 53-89.

82. Syrjanen, K.J., de Villiers, E-M., Vayrynen, M., Mantyjarvi, R., Parkkinen, S., Saarikoski, S., and Castren, O. (1985): Lancet, i: 510-511.

83. Syrjanen, K.J., Heinonen, U.M., and Kauraniemi, T. (1981): Acta Cytol., 25: 17-22.

84. Syrjanen, K.J., Mantyjarvi, R., Parkkinen, S., Vayrynen, M., Saarikoski, S., Syrjanen, S., and Castren, O. (1986): Banbury Report, 21: 167-177.

85. Syrjanen, K.J., Mantyjarvi, R., Vayrynen, M., Syrjanen, S., Parkkinen, S., Yliskoski, M., Saarikoski, S., and Castren, O, (1986): Eur. J. Gynaecol. Oncol., 8: 5-16.

86. Syrjanen, K.J., Mantyjarvi, R., Vayrynen, M., Syrjanen, S., Parkkinen, S., Yliskoski, M., Saarikoski, S., Sarkkinen, H., Nurmi, T., and Castren, O. (1987): Cancer Cells 5. Papillomaviruses (in press).

87. Syrjanen, K.J., and Pyrhonen, S. (1982): Arch. Gynecol., 233: 53–61.
88. Syrjanen, K.J., and Pyrhonen, S. (1983): Scand. J. Urol., Nephrol., 17: 267–270.
89. Syrjanen, K.J., Vayrynen, M., Castren, O., Mantyjarvi, R., Pyrhonen, S., and Yliskoski, M. (1983): Int. J. Gynaecol. Obstet., 21: 261–269.
90. Syrjanen, K.J., Vayrynen, M., Castren, O., Yliskoski, M., Mantyjarvi, R., Pyrhonen, S., and Saarikoski, S. (1984): Br. J. Vener. Dis., 60: 243–248.
91. Syrjanen, K.J., Vayrynen, M., Hippelainen, M., Castren, O., Saarikoski, S., and Mantyjarvi, R. (1985): Arch. Geschwulstforsch., 55: 131–138.
92. Syrjanen, K.J., Vayrynen, M., Mantyjarvi, R., Parkkinen, S., Saarikoski, S., Syrjanen, S., and Castren, O. (1985): In: Papilloma Viruses: Molecular and Clinical Aspects, edited by P.M. Howley, and T.R. Broker, Vol. 32, pp. 31–45. UCLA Symposia on Molecular and Cellular Biology, New Series, Alan R. Liss, Inc., New York.
93. Syrjanen, K.J., Vayrynen, M., Saarikoski, S., Mantyjarvi, R., Parkkinen, S., Hippelainen, M., and Castren, O. (1985): Br. J. Obstet. Gynaecol., 92: 1086–1092.
94. Syrjanen, S., Partanen, P., and Syrjanen, K. (1987): Cancer Cells 5. Papillomaviruses (in press).
95. Syrjanen, S., von Krogh, G., and Syrjanen, K. (1987): Genitourin. Med., 63: 32–39.
96. Tomita, Y., Kubota, K., Kasai, T., Sekiya, S., Takamizawa, H., and Simizu, B. (1986): Intervirology, 25: 151–157.
97. Vayrynen, M., Romppanen, T., Koskela, E., Castren, O., and Syrjanen, K. (1981): Int. J. Gynaecol. Obstet., 19: 351–356.
98. Vayrynen, M., Syrjanen, K., Castren, O., Saarikoski, S., and Mantyjarvi, R. (1985): Obstet. Gynecol., 65: 409–415.
99. Wade, T.R., Kopf, A.W., and Ackerman, A.B. (1979): Arch. Dermatol., 115: 306–308.
100. Walker, P.G., Singer, A., Dyson, J.L., and Oriel, J.D. (1983): Br. J. Vener. Dis., 59: 327–329.
101. Weed, J.C., Lozier, C., and Daniel, S.J. (1983): Obstet. Gynecol., 62: 83S–87S.
102. Woodruff, J.D., Braun, L., Cavalieri, R., Gupta, P., Pass, F., and Shah, K.V. (1980): Obstet. Gynecol., 56: 727–732.
103. Woodruff, J.D., and Peterson, W.F. (1958): Am. J. Obstet. Gynecol., 75: 1354–1362.
104. zur Hausen, H. (1977): Curr. Top. Microbiol. Immunol., 78: 1–30.
105. zur Hausen, H. (1980): Adv. Cancer Res., 33:

77–107.
106. zur Hausen, H., and Gissmann, L. (1980): In: Viral
     Oncology, edited by G. Klein, pp. 433–445. Raven
     Press, New York.
107. zur Hausen, H., Gissmann, L., and Schlehofer, J.R.
     (1984): Prog. Med. Virol., 30: 170–186.

# Natural History of Genital Papilloma Virus Lesions

G. De Palo[1], B. Stefanon[1], M. Del Vecchio[2] and F. Falcetta[2]

[1]Division of Diagnostic Oncology and Out-patient Clinic,
[2]Division of Medical Statistic,
Istituto Nazionale Tumori, Milan, Italy

Human papilloma virus (HPV) infection is a sexually transmitted disease. The disease is mainly recorded in the age group 20–35 years, in subjects who are sexually promiscuous (multiple partners or only a partner if that partner has had another or several partners).

The incidence of HPV infection as a clinically recognisable condylomata acuminata markedly increased comparing the years '70 and '80 (6,27). A tremendous increase in subclinical cervical HPV infection visible only by colposcopy was also reported. Although subclinical HPV infection could be in part the result of a reinterpretation of cytologic, pathologic and colposcopic findings, in the past misdiagnosed as cervical intraepithelial neoplasia (CIN) grade I (12), HPV infection seems to have in many countries an epidemic outbreak, attributable to an increased sexual promiscuity, to a decrease in the age of the first sexual experience, and to the use of oral contraceptives rather than a condom, especially in young people, in the years of free love.

Over the same period of time, the incidence of cervical premalignant and malignant lesions of the uterine cervix has also increased in women under 40 years, in the UK and Australia (3,48) and CIN has been found in teenagers (37). Since many of these lesions are associated with HPV infection, it has been supposed that sexual activity, HPV infection, and premalignant lesions of the uterine cervix, are strictly related.

## PATHOGENESIS

HPV comes into contact with the basal cells of the squamous epithelium of the cervix, one of the most active of human tissues in which cells are continually generated and replaced, by direct or indirect sexual contact (Fig. 1). Transmission by fomites, commonly occurring with non-genital strains of HPV, is possible.

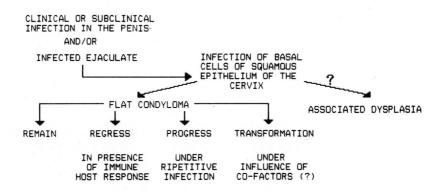

**FIG. 1.** Pathogenesis of HPV infection in the uterine cervix.

The basal cells are transformed; these transformed cells replicate to a flat condyloma, which colposcopically appears as white patches condylomatosis. The incubation period is calculated between 4 weeks-8 months. The flat condyloma may remain flat, may regress in the presence of a good immune host response, or may progress under ripetitive infection derived from the same route of primary and/or by viral particles shed from exfoliated koilocytes, to lesions that colposcopically appear as mixed, mosaic-like and finally florid or leucoplakia-like condylomatosis (Fig. 2). Finally under the influence of cofactors, it may undergo a premalignant transformation resulting in CIN I, which progresses to CIN II and to CIN III.

Although there is a consensus that a co-factor, genetic or environmental, is necessary to act together with HPV to produce the malignant transformation, such as ultraviolet and ionizing radiation for epidermodysplasia verruciformis (7), these co-factors are still unknown. Herpes virus type 2, Chlamydia, smoking, and

oral contraceptives have been considered. Although no
correlation with the clinical course of the HPV lesions
could be established for Chlamydia (45) and there are
no data on oral contraceptive steroids, epidemiological
studies (4) have shown that infected women who smoke
cigarettes (and smoking is increasing among women) have
a higher risk of developing cervical cancer than do
non-smoking infected women. It could be that primary
and secondary smoke constituents that are excreted in
the urine and can appear in cervical fluid (38) might
interact with HPV in the cervix as a co-factor for
malignant transformation in an unknown way.

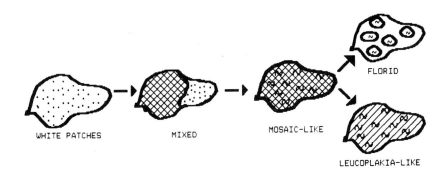

FLORID

WHITE PATCHES          MIXED

MOSAIC-LIKE

LEUCOPLAKIA-LIKE

**FIG. 2.** Colposcopic evolution of HPV infection in the uterine
cervix.

Furthermore, the lesion may recur after treatment.
The reasons may be reinfection or persistence of HPV.
HPV DNAs may be present in clinically and histologically normal tissues near to HPV infection alone or
associated to intraepithelial neoplasia or invasive
carcinoma as demonstrated by Ferenczy et al. (13), by
MacNab et al. (22) in the lower female genital tract,
and by Steinberg et al. (43) in laryngeal epithelium.
It serves as a source of infection to the sexual partner and to the woman herself.

## HPV AND CERVICAL CANCERS

Findings which favor the hypothesis of a relationship between HPV infection and genital cancer are the following: a) coexistence of HPV infection with CIN, such as HPV-associated intraepithelial neoplasia, HPV infection adjacent to intraepithelial neoplasia or both (9) (the different types explain the difficulty in the colposcopic diagnosis); b) coexistence of HPV infection with VIN III and early vulvar carcinoma (30); c) coexistence of HPV-associated VIN and CIN (30) with or without concomitant HPV infection in both sites; d) coexistence or preexistence of HPV infection with in situ or invasive carcinoma of the penis (18,31); e) demonstration of HPV 16 DNA sequences in a large percentage of genital cancer (10,22); f) detection of HPV 18 DNA sequences in cell lines derived from cervical cancer (2); g) detection of HPV 18 DNA integrated into the cellular genome in cell lines (HeLa, C4-1 and 756) derived from human cervical cancer (39); h) malignant transformation of NIH 3T3 cells by HPV 16 DNA from a cervical cancer (47).

These observations are in favor of the hypothesis that patients exposed to HPV infection should be considered at a higher relative risk for malignant transformation than non-exposed patients, and that a lesion containing HPV16/18 has a higher risk of progressing to cancer than a lesion harboring HPV 6/11.

Five longitudinal studies have evaluated the natural history of virus-induced epithelial lesions in the uterine cervix. In the study of De Brux et al. (8), 764 women with untreated HPV-associated CIN I-II-III were followed by cytology. During 18 months of follow-up, 205 patients (26.8%) regressed, 404 (52.9%) had persistent disease, and 90 (11.8%) progressed. Sixty-five (8.5%) patients (10 HPV-CIN II and 55 HPV-CIN III) had relapse after cone biopsy or $CO_2$ laser surgery.

In the study of Mitchell et al. (24), 846 women aged 15-69 years, with cytological evidence of HPV infection alone on Papanicolaou cervical smears in the year 1979, were followed to establish the biological potential of HPV in cervical carcinogenesis. To be eligible for the study the women had to have had either a repeat smear or histology of the cervix during 1980-1985. Histologically proven carcinoma in situ developed in 30 (3.5%) and dysplasia in 33 (3.9%) women over the 6-year period. Another 50 women had cytological evidence of dysplasia but had not undergone cervical biopsy. Therefore, histologically, dysplasia or carcinoma in situ developed in 7.4%, and overall (histology plus cytology) in 13.4% of the exposed cohort of 846 women over the 6-year period.

In the study of Evan-Jones et al. (11), 29 patients

with HPV infection alone of the uterine cervix were followed for 1 year with colposcopy, cytology and biopsy every four months. Six patients had regression (20.7%), 8 persistent disease (27.6%), 15 developed CIN (51.7%), and all but 1 of these patients had CIN II or III.

In the study of Syrjanen et al. (45,46), 513 women with cervical HPV infection were followed by colposcopy, cytology and eventually punch biopsy. The study was started in 1981, and the mean duration of follow-up was 25.6 months (range, < 6 - > 60). Patients were examined at 6-month intervals with colposcopy and cytology. If cytological changes consistent with HPV-CIN were disclosed, a punch biopsy was performed, in contrast to the patients with HPV without CIN lesions, who were followed by Papanicolaou smear only. When progression to carcinoma in situ was established, lesions were eradicated by conization. About 25% of lesions regressed, 60% persisted and about 15% progressed. The clinical course was influenced by the HPV DNA type. The lesions caused by HPV 6/11 had a significant tendency to spontaneous regression (~ 60%), whereas the HPV 16/18-induced lesions showed a high rate of progression (~ 36%). Nevertheless, from these data also HPV 6/11-induced lesions had progression in about 12% of the cases, whereas HPV 16/18-induced lesions had regression in 18% of the cases. It is noteworthy that there was a higher rate of progression for HPV-CIN (HPV-CIN I, 13.4%; HPV-CIN III, 31.2%) than for HPV non-CIN (6.9%) (46).

In the study of Campion et al. (5), 100 informed and consenting women, under 30 years of age, who presented cytological (three consecutive cervical smears obtained within a 16-week period) and colposcopic (atypical transformation zone) evidence of CIN grade I with or without cytopathic effects of HPV, were selected. All patients had detection of HPV 6 and 16. Patients were followed by cytology and colposcopy every 4 months. If there was cytological evidence of severe dysplasia and colposcopic evidence of CIN III, a biopsy was carried out and $CO_2$ laser treatment was given. The follow-up period ranged from 19 to 30 months. Of 100 women, 67 had persistent disease, 7 had regression to normal, and 26 had histologically proven evidence of progression to CIN III not before 10 months. Of the 26 women who had progression to CIN III, 22 (85%) were positive for HPV 16. Of the 9 progressive lesions positive for HPV 6, 8 were also positive for HPV 16.

Our study group comprised 416 women consecutively observed in the colposcopic clinic at the Istituto Nazionale Tumori of Milan, from February 1, 1978 to December 31, 1984. All patients underwent colposcopy, cytology and guided biopsy during colposcopy. Cyto-

logical specimens were taken for Papanicolaou staining
by means of both Ayre spatula and endocervical cotton
applicator before application of acetic acid to the
cervix. Colposcopic examination was performed by a
Zeiss colposcope without and with acetic acid (3%
solution). The colpophotographies were obtained with
Ektachrome film (200 ASA, 24 DIN).

The selection criteria for the study group was the
presence of histologically proven HPV infection, without or with associated CIN of advanced grades (grade II
and III). Histology of the biopsy samples showed cervical HPV infection alone in 277 cases and HPV infection associated with CIN or invasive carcinoma in 139
cases. The characteristics of these women, the histologic and colposcopic patterns, and the treatment have
been discussed elsewhere (9). Out of 277 patients with
HPV infection alone, 91 were lost to follow-up. Out of
139 patients with HPV-associated CIN, 28 were lost to
follow-up. The patients were followed by colposcopy and
cytology every 4-6 months. In the presence of colposcopic abnormalities, a directed biopsy was obtained
from the most abnormal area. Not all cases were systematically followed at this time interval; however, in
all cases, cytologic, colposcopic and histologic information was obtained by August 1986. All the data of the
patients were analyzed by use of a computer. The analysis was carried out by the statisticians (M. Del V.
and F.F.) in August 1986. The follow-up period from
recruitment ranged from 6 to 102 months (Table 1).

**TABLE 1.** Duration of Follow-up of Patients
with Cervical HPV Infection

| DURATION OF FOLLOW-UP (months) | TOTAL | HPV ALONE | HPV + CIN or Inv. Ca. |
|---|---|---|---|
| 6-12 | 25 | 14 | 11 |
| 13-24 | 46 | 32 | 14 |
| 25-36 | 70 | 46 | 24 |
| 37-48 | 25 | 15 | 10 |
| 49-60 | 31 | 17 | 14 |
| 61-72 | 59 | 37 | 22 |
| 73-84 | 21 | 14 | 7 |
| 85-96 | 18 | 9 | 9 |
| 97-102 | 2 | 2 | - |
| | 297 | 186 | 111 |

The criteria employed for evaluation of the follow-up data were the following: persistence was defined as the presence of a lesion (histologic diagnosis) in untreated patients or the presence of a lesion within 3 months in treated patients; no evidence of disease was defined as the absence of a lesion; recurrence was defined as the presence of a lesion 3 months after treatment, and progression was defined as the appearance of CIN, the transition to a higher grade of CIN, or the appearance of invasive carcinoma (Inv. Ca.) in treated or untreated patients.

Out of 186 patients with HPV infection alone, 37 were untreated for 12 months after the diagnosis. No evidence of disease was found in 28, persistence in 7, and progression to CIN in 2 patients (HPV-associated CIN II and HPV-associated CIN III, respectively). Of 149 treated patients, 133 had no evidence of disease; persistence (within 3 months) was ascertained in 5, recurrence in 26 and progression in 5 (4 treated with cautery and 1 treated with human fibroblast interferon (HFI) plus cautery). One of these patients progressed to microinvasive carcinoma 13 months after the histologic diagnosis; the other patients progressed to HPV-associated CIN II (2 patients) and HPV-associated CIN III (2 patients). Therefore, progression from HPV infection was ascertained in a total number of 7/186 patients with a median follow-up of 36 months. The median time to progression was 17 months (range, 4–36 months).

Of 108 patients with HPV-associated CIN II–III, 7 were untreated and 101 were treated (plus the 3 patients treated for invasive carcinoma). Of 7 untreated patients (young, intelligent patients assuring a regular follow-up), 4 had no evidence of disease and 3 regression of CIN and persistence of HPV infection. One of the latter was a pregnant woman with HPV-associated CIN III + HPV infection who was submitted to several biopsies during pregnancy. No patient had progression. The median follow-up period in these untreated patients was 35 months. Of 101 treated patients, 88 were treated with cautery, $CO_2$ laser, or HFI ± cautery, 10 with conization, and 3 with hysterectomy. Of the first 88 patients, 63 had no evidence of disease, 2 had persistence as HPV infection and 1 as HPV-associated CIN, 12 relapsed as HPV infection and 4 as HPV-associated CIN. One patient of 10 treated with conization relapsed with HPV-associated CIN. Progression was observed in 6 of 88 cases. Two of these patients progressed from HPV-associated CIN II to invasive carcinoma and from HPV-associated CIN III to microinvasive carcinoma, 21 months and 35 months from histologic diagnosis, respectively. The other patients progressed from HPV-associated CIN II to HPV-associated CIN III. Therefore,

6/88 treated patients with a median follow-up of 45 months progressed to a higher grade of CIN or to invasive carcinoma. The median time to progression was 28 months (range, 17-53).

Although the follow-ups are similar if no longer in this series than those of the other studies, the progression rate is lower than that reported by other authors. However, there are two major differences: most cases were treated, and punch biopsy was systematically used. Both these factors modify the natural history of exposure to HPV. Furthermore, progression from CIN II to CIN III is problematic because it is possible that at first diagnosis the patient may have CIN III near to the biopsied CIN II.

The estimation of the progression distribution function computed by the Kaplan-Meier method (20) with a confidence interval calculated at $\alpha$ = 0.05 showed that as regards HPV infection alone, on 186 patients the percentage of progressed patients at 5 years was 5.6% in untreated cases and 4.8% in treated cases (Fig. 3), whereas this percentage was 10.5% in 88 treated cases with HPV-associated CIN (Fig. 4).

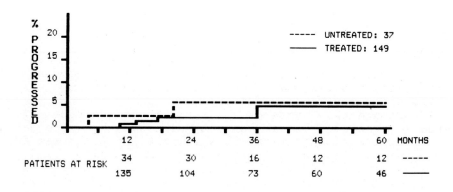

**FIG. 3.** Estimation of the progression distribution function in 186 patients with HPV infection alone of the uterine cervix.

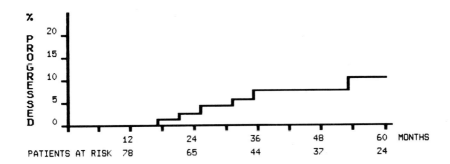

**FIG. 4.** Estimation of the progression distribution function in 88 treated patients with HPV-associated CIN.

## DISCUSSION

The prospective follow-up studies conducted for CIN lesions have reported extremely variable results for progression and regression. Different selection criteria, different methods of conducting the follow-up, and possibly differences in morphologic evaluation are responsible for these discrepancies.

There are two types of studies. The first type of studies report cases of dysplasia as judged by cytological examination only and in which the end-point was a cytological picture suggesting carcinoma in situ. This type of study had the defect that the cytological diagnosis based on a single cervical smear may not exclude the existence of more severe disease at the onset (15,42). The second type of studies report cases of dysplasia as judged by histological examination. This type of study has one defect: the cervical biopsy may alter the natural history of the disease and may induce apparent spontaneous regression (21,26,33,40). In fact, in prospective studies of mild and moderate dysplasia based on cytology alone (15,23,26,34,36) the

progression rate was high (mean percentage of progression: 32%; range, 13-60%) whereas in studies in which
the diagnostic procedure included biopsy (14,17,19,25,
28,32,44) a high regression rate was found with a low
risk of progression (mean percentage of progression:
12%; range, 6-17%).

Although there are some differences, for example
between the data of Campion et al. (5) and those of
Richart and Barron (34), if the progression rate in the
past studies are examined in comparison to those of the
new studies implicating HPV (Table 2), no important
differences appear. Nevertheless, there is a difference
between the two groups: HPV-associated CIN occurred in
women younger than those in the older series. The
absence of a difference in progression rate between the
studies of the past years and the recent studies implicating HPV suggests that there has been an improvement
in the techniques for identification of HPV infection.

**TABLE 2.** Prospective Studies of Cervical HPV Infection
± HPV-associated CIN

|  | Progression |
| --- | --- |
| De Brux et al. (8) | 11.8% |
| Mitchell et al. (24) | 13.4% |
| Syrjanen et al. (45) | 15.0% |
| Campion et al. (5) | 26.0% |
| Evan-Jones et al. (11) | 51.7% |
| | 4.8% |
| De Palo et al. (present series)* | 5.6% |
| | 10.5% |

* by Kaplan-Meier method

This fact is clearly emphasized by the study of
Singer et al. (41). These authors compared two groups
of patients, the first examined in the early 1970s and
the second in the early 1980s, and found no significant
difference in the prevalence of HPV antigen in CIN or
in the category of metaplasia or native squamous epithelium. In this study, the overall prevalence of HPV
antigen was 16% in the 1970s group and 20% in the 1980s
group. In CIN I-II-III, HPV antigen was found in 30% of
lesions studies in the 1970s and 23% of lesions studied
in the 1980s.

The fact that in morphological studies such as those
of Rubinstein (35) and Pilotti et al. (29) there are
two types of CIN, pure and HPV-associated, is of little

significance, since molecular hybridization techniques have evidenced the presence of HPV also in cases in which morphology, immunohistochemistry and electron microscopy were HPV negative. This was clearly shown by the study of our Institute in collaboration with the Department of Immunology and Infectious Diseases of Johns Hopkins University School of Hygiene and Public Health of Baltimore, in which 33% of early vulvar neoplasia without cytopathic effect by histology, was HPV-DNA positive by in situ hybridization (16).

There is no doubt that a change has occurred over the past decade in the natural history of cervical neoplasia. The changing patterns of the disease are the increased number of carcinomas in situ reported in England, Wales, USA, and Canada in the last decade, the increased number of invasive carcinomas in young women rapidly developing after a short premalignant period (1), and the existence of CIN in teen-agers (37).

Nevertheless, it is hard to believe that HPV is responsible for such a situation. In conclusion and in accord to Singer et al. (41), it could instead be possible that although the role of HPV has not changed, the co-factors required by the virus for neoplastic transformation have changed.

## ACKNOWLEDGEMENTS

The authors are grateful to Mrs. Patrizia Di Donato for typing the manuscript and to Ms. Betty Johnston for the editing. This study was supported by a grant (n° 86.00657.44) from Special Project "Oncology" of the Italian National Research Council.

## REFERENCES

1. Bamford, P.N., Beilly, J.O., Steele, S.J., and Vlies, R. (1983): Acta Cytol., 27: 482-484.
2. Boshart, M., Gissmann, L., Ikenberg,H., Kleinheinz, A., Scheurlen, W., and zur Hausen, H. (1984): EMBO J., 3: 1151-1157.
3. Bourne, R.G., and Grove W.D. (1983): Med. J. Aust., 1: 156-158.
4. Brinton, L.A., Schairer, C., Haenszel, W., Stolley, P., Lehman, H.F., Levine, R., and Savitz, D.A. (1986): JAMA, 255: 3265-3269.
5. Campion, M.J., McCance, D.J., Cuzick, J., and Singer, A. (1986): Lancet, ii: 237-240.
6. Chuang, T.Y., Perry, H.O., Kurland, C.T., and Ilstrup, D.M. (1984): Arch. Dermatol., 120: 469-475.
7. Crawford, L. (1984): Nature, 310: 16.
8. De Brux, J., Orth, G., Croissant, O., Cochard, B., and Ionesco, M. (1983): Bull. Cancer, 70: 410-

422.

9. De Palo, G., Stefanon, B., and Del Vecchio, M. (1986): In: Herpes and Papilloma Viruses, edited by G. De Palo, F. Rilke, and H. zur Hausen, pp. 305–327, Raven Press, New York.
10. Durst, M., Gissmann, L., Ikenberg, H., and zur Hausen, H. (1983): Proc. Natl. Acad. Sci. USA, 50: 3812–3815.
11. Evans-Jones, J.C., Forbes-Smith, P.A., and Hirschowitz, L. (1985): Lancet, i: 1445.
12. Ferenczy, A., Braun, L., and Shah, K.V. (1981): Am. J. Surg. Pathol., 5: 661–670.
13. Ferenczy, A., Mitao, M., Nagai, N., Silverstein, S.J., and Crum, C.P. (1985): N. Engl. J. Med., 313: 784–788.
14. Figge, D.P., de Alvarez, R.R., Brown, D.V., and Fullington, W.R. (1962): Am. J. Obstet. Gynecol., 84: 638–647.
15. Fox, C.H. (1967): Am. J. Obstet. Gynecol., 99: 960–974.
16. Gupta, J., Pilotti, S., Shah, K.V., De Palo, G., and Rilke, F. (1987): Am. J. Surg. Pathol., 11: 430–434.
17. Hall, J.A., and Walton, L. (1968): Am. J. Obstet. Gynecol., 100: 662–671.
18. Hanash, K.A., Furlow, W.L., Utz, D.C., and Harrison, E.G. Jr. (1970): J. Urol., 104: 291–297.
19. Johnson, L.D., Nickerson, R.J., Easterday, C.L., Stuart, R.S., and Hertig, A.T. (1968): Cancer, 22: 901–914.
20. Kaplan, E.L., and Meier, P. (1958): J. Am. Statist. Ass., 53: 457–481.
21. Koss, L.G., Stewart, F.W., Foote, F.W., Jordan, M.J., Bader, G.M., and Day, E. (1963): Cancer, 16: 1160–1211.
22. MacNab, J.C.M., Walkinshaw, S.A., Cordiner, J.A., and Clements, B.J. (1986): N. Engl. J. Med., 315: 1052–1058.
23. McGregor, J.E., and Lupen, S. (1978): Lancet, i: 1029–1031.
24. Mitchell, H., Drake, M., and Medley, G. (1986): Lancet, i: 573–575.
25. Nasiell, K., Nasiell, M., Vaclavinkova, V. et al. (1976): In: Health Control in Detection of Cancer, Skandia International Symposia, pp. 244–252, Almkvist & Wiksell, Stockholm.
26. Nasiell, K., Nasiell, M., and Vaclavinkova, V. (1983): Obstet. Gynecol., 61: 609–614.
27. Oriel, J.D. (1986): In: Herpes and Papilloma Viruses, edited by G. De Palo, F. Rilke, and H. zur Hausen, pp. 55–61, Raven Press, New York.
28. Peckham, B., and Greene, R. (1957): Am. J. Obstet.

Gynecol., 74: 804–815.
29. Pilotti, S., Rilke, F., Alasio, L., and Fontanelli, R. (1982): Diagn. Gynecol. Obstet., 4: 357–362.
30. Pilotti, S., Rilke, F., Shah, K.V., Della Torre, G., and De Palo, G. (1984): Am. J. Surg. Pathol., 8: 751–761.
31. Piva, L., Pizzocaro, G., Stefanon, B., and De Palo, G. (1982): In: Prophylaxis and Prevention on Gynaecologic Oncology. Proc. II International Meeting of Gynaecologic Oncology. Venice Lido, April 22-24th, pp. 225–226.
32. Rawson, A.J., and Knoblich, R. (1957): Am. J. Obstet. Gynecol., 73: 120–126.
33. Richart, R.M. (1966): Cancer, 19: 1635–1638.
34. Richart, R.M., and Barron, B.A. (1969): Am. J. Obstet. Gynecol., 105: 386–393.
35. Rubinstein, E. (1980): Acta Obstet. Gynecol. Scand., 59: 529–534.
36. Rummel, H.H., Fick, R., and Heberling, D. (1977): Geburt. Frauenheilh, 37: 521–526.
37. Sadeghi, S.B., Hsieh, E.W., and Gunn, S.W. (1984): Am. J. Obstet. Gynecol., 148: 726–729.
38. Sasson, I.M., Haley, N.J., Hoffmann, D., Wynder, E.L., Hellberg, D.H., and Nilsson, S. (1985): N. Engl. J. Med., 312: 315–316.
39. Schwarz, E., Freese, U.K., Gissmann, L., Mayer, W., Roggenbuck, B., Stremlau, A., and zur Hausen, H. (1985): Nature, 314: 111–114.
40. Sedlis, A., Cohen, A., and Sali, S. (1970): Am. J. Obstet. Gynecol., 170: 1065–1070.
41. Singer, A., Wilkers, J., Walker, P., Jenkins, D., Slavin, G., Cowdell, H., To, A., and Husain, O. (1985): J. Clin. Pathol., 39: 855–857.
42. Spriggs, A.I. (1981): Clin. Obstet. Gynecol., 8: 65–79.
43. Steinberg, B.M., Topp, W.C., Schneider, P.S., and Abramson, A.L. (1983): N. Engl. J. Med., 308: 1261–1264.
44. Stern, E., and Neely, P.M. (1964): Cancer, 17: 508–512.
45. Syrjanen, K., Mantyjarvi, R., Vayrynen, M., Syrjanen, S., Parkkinen, S., Yliskoski, M., Saarikoski, S., and Castren, O. (1987): Eur. J. Gynaecol. Oncol., 8: 5–16.
46. Syrjanen, K., Vayrynen, M., Saarikoski,S., Mantyjarvi, R., Parkkinen, S., Hippelainen, M., , and Castren, O. (1985): Br. J. Obstet. Gynaecol., 92: 1086–1092.
47. Tsunokawa, Y., Takebe, N., Kasamatsu, T., Terada, M., and Sugimura, T. (1986): Proc. Natl. Acad. Sci. USA, 83: 2200–2203.
48. Wolfendale, M.R., King, S., and Usherwood, M. (1983): Br. Med. J., 287: 526–528.

# The Aetiological Factors of Cancer of the Lower Genital Tract. A Different View

B.L. Reid

*Queen Elizabeth II Research Institute for Mothers and Infants*
*The University of Sydney, Sydney, Australia*

Evidence is collected to support a different view on two groups of observations emerging in the literature on lower genital tract neoplasia: the involvement of several viral species in its initiation and an altered epidemiological pattern. The view is based on an electrical approach through an aspect of field theory. In the first group, the field is seen as derived from a novel, very ordered electrical structure induced by the carcinogen. The field can theoretically provide for persistence and amplification of this order by inducing particles of different viral species in appropriate target cells. The ordered field structure produces in the tissue, a relaxation behaviour following a prior stimulation which decays exponentially with interruptions or steps. The relaxation curve for normal tissue also decays exponentially but smoothly without steps. A step relaxation curve is also exhibited by bovine wart virus and by human spermatozoa.

The second group is approached by demonstration of the ability of the permeating field to transmit, in energy form as virtual images through space, the structure and certain properties of living systems such as those of microorganisms and of spermatozoa. The image appears to act as a template to produce a real image on contact with matter of an appropriate form. Thin films of polystyrene drying on glass from a solvent solution were used. The evidence shows that this template or virtual image can be altered in space so that on its subsequent reaction with the film to form an image, novel, structurally simpler real images are produced.

It is possible that this modified template may induce changes in biomatter, just as it does on the plastic film. Modifications to the tissue forming on such template may become the basis of alterations to the incidence, pathological picture, and virulence reported by the epidemiologists to be recently occuring in virus infection patterns of several diseases.

## A Surfeit of Virus as Initiators of Precancer

In the persisting absence of a satisfactory concept for the nature of the neoplastic process, it is scarcely necessary to justify any novel or different approach of the type represented in this paper. The nature and cause of growth, or its abnormal counterpart newgrowth, seem as elusive as ever since the origins of cancer research last century.

In our research on the aetiology of cervical cancer over recent years, we have tended to seek a process caused by an agent as responsible, rather than the agent exclusively. We viewed such a process as being common to the catalogue of miscellaneous agents which have been proposed as initiators of the process. Such an attitude was encouraged by the presence of similarities in competing claims for the role of different virus species as agents in cervical cancer when these are arranged in tabular form for the purpose (14). Since publication of one of the earliest proposals for the complicity of microorganisms in the process (13) at least five agents have attracted sufficient research effort as to make such a comparison quite valid. For this reason we attempted recently to unify the action of various agents by showing that a protein of rather homogeneous amino acid composition found in the sperm head, a protamine, could enhance the amount of wart virus protein found normally in cervical cells (1).

## Is There a Factor Common to Several Viruses?

The conceptual basis of work of this sort derived from Temin's ideas on vironeogenesis (17). Temin sought to modify the well recognised viral latency concept by proposing that the virus was assembled de novo from intracellular precursor molecules. If it could be shown that the cancer inducing process also initiated the virus afresh each time it operated, we would have introduced some desirable parsimony into an obviously complicated story. For the purposes of this sort of thinking, the structure of the induced virus (and thereby its species) is then not as important as the process inducing it, dependent as such a species variable structure would be on presently unknown factors existing in the induced tissue at the time. None of these considerations run counter to the idea that the virus particle, once induced, is perfectly capable of lateral and perhaps vertical transmission thence to act vicariously in place of the original inducer. In this consideration it becomes an infectious amplifier of the process, and will thus be expected to exhibit proper-ties possessed by the process itself.

## ELECTRICAL STRUCTURE OF BIOSYSTEMS:
## A PROPOSED COMMON MECHANISM

### Tissue Dielectrics

Our emphasis in researches on the process relies more on physical than on chemical techniques since it is based on the concept of a relationship of electrical fields with the growth process. This relationship is well known in embryology, in nerve physiology and in bone growth. The branch of electrical theory which interests us is concerned with the penetration and other behaviour of fields within matter and is termed dielectrics. The term was coined by Faraday himself who first studied the topic in relation to the evaluation of insulators. A study of the dielectric properties of biomatter reveals some outstanding differences to those of non-living matter, and within biomatter, neoplastic tissue shows striking differences from non-neoplastic tissue. The unit of comparison used is the dielectric constant often called permittivity by electrical en-gineers. In brief, it measures the capacity of the substance to store the energy of a field of given strength as compared with the capacity of air to store the same field.

### Stimulus-Relaxation as a Probe
### of Dielectric Structure

When an electric stimulus is applied to biomatter in the form of direct current, it conducts the current by means of the movement of charges. These charges can move by the familiar process of the movement of ions or by the less familiar process of the movement of fields associated with charged groups within molecules and macromolecules. Such fields, present beforehand as a result of the disposition of chemical groups in the structure, rearrange under the influence of the sti-mulus (so called polarisation) to create an electrical structure, termed a dipole about the electrical centre of the molecule. When the stimulus is terminated, the formed or induced dipole recovers (or relaxes in elec-trical language). During recovery a relaxation or depolarisation current appears. The relaxational field movement is thus in fact a form of conductivity, just as is that due to ion movement, and can be shown to be an important conduit for field movement under experi-mental arrangements where ion conductivity is absent for any reason (4,18).

We have found that the relaxation conductivity (that is, conductivity in the absence of ion movement) behaviour of tissue responds to a carcinogen. In the case of normal tissue, the decay of the effects of the stimulus over time (the relaxation curve) is a smooth exponential function. In the presence of a chemical carcinogen exposed to the tissue for a few minutes only, the curve assumes a novel shape which includes several steps or interruptions to the decay (2,4).

We interpret these steps as indicating the recruitment by polarisation of polymers by the carcinogen so as to form domains with their own characteristic dielectric constant (2,4,18). Where sufficient matter is recruited to such a domain, the discreteness of the specific dielectric constant appears as a step on the otherwise exponential decay curve. This discrete domain means, in our interpretation, that the carcinogen has electrically induced the polymers into a more aligned or symmetrical pattern. The pattern is very reminiscent of a crystal structure in contrast to a probable, more disordered structure of normal differentiated tissue. The high dielectric constant of cancer tissue at low frequencies shown by our own studies (2-4,18), together with those of others (16) means that its capacity for energy storage is high so that in a particular area, given the energy circulation through the organism as a result of its metabolism, it becomes an energy sink or drain.

The use of a sink analogy presupposes that the effluent energy is released to the system in which the sink is placed so that its quality becomes an important property. The order inherent in the polymer structure of the sink tissue as we have discussed is imposed on the energy flow which itself becomes ordered, or, in more physical terms, coherent. It is known from quantum physical considerations of the passage of coherent energy through a biosystem that such structural energy has the capacity in turn to structurate aggregating macromolecules, such as those in the process of forming a tissue, with which it shares resonance (7). We take up this important point in connection with the ordered electrical structure of human sperm and bovine wart virus in the next section.

## Assimilation of the Electrical Structure of Virus and Sperm with that of Carcinogen-Induced Tissue

These findings have a bearing on the problem of cervical carcinogenesis. We have found, in contrast to normal tissue such as yeast cells and bovine thymus gland, normal human sperm and bovine wart virus show step curves in their relaxation behaviour. This indica-

tes that, at the frequencies we used (~ 1500HZ), they
are highly ordered in the electrical sense and so, by
the tenets of electrical field theory, in a position to
accomodate and emit coherent energy fields at high
density. Expressed in other terms, given a target with
which they can resonate, they can induce corresponding
electrical order in those fields within its elements
(7). The induction process could occur across the
intact cell membrane. This amounts to a restatement of
an older theory of viral carcinogenesis recently re-
vived (10) which was said to be "hit-run" in operation.

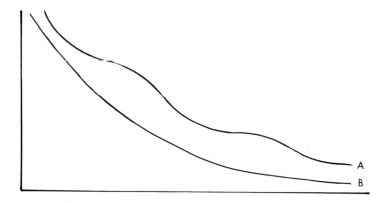

**FIG. 1.** Idealised sketch of relaxation curves following dc
stimulation of biomatter prepared as to expose polarisation
conductivity. Curve B derives from normal differentiated tissue. Curve A, where the current decay is interrupted by steps,
derives from tissue exposed to a carcinogen. Curve B is also
found in preparations of bovine wart virus and of human sperm.
For discussion see 2,4. Ordinate: Current. Abscissa: time.

### The Fate of the Target Tissue upon Successful Induction

The electrical induction process is well understood
by physicists and certain new properties emerge as a
result. These properties can now be described because
they are important in our attempts to understand the
basic nature of the oncogenic process, in particular
how the electrical structure of an inducer including
virus could achieve this state.
First the enhanced energy flow nay interfere with
valency electrons in the component atoms and molecules
of the induced area and so disrupt the cell by an
effect on atomic cohesion. The structural counterpart

is the familiar cytopathogenic effect. In the second case an energy density and flow short of causing disruption can result in varying degrees of induction of electrical order, inducing target tissues to enter the energy sink state. This state we believe to be a key feature of the oncogenic process. Most importantly, the induction process can be intermittent in time with successive induction events summating from energy of any source so long as resonance parameters are in conformity. Successive polymer groups within the target cell or tissue can be recruited over time to produce the observed domain structure so that the process begun by energy of one source can be continued by that from another, procuring throughout, a vicious cycle through an amplification of the energy being passaged. This sequential nature of the induction process can accomodate the documented long latency of the carcinogenic process as well as the evidence for collusion of carcinogens of several sources, such as several viral species or combinations of chemical and viral agents. Cocarcinogenesis is an established phenomenon including the specific instance of carcinogenesis due to the wart virus in animals and man (22).

## THE SECOND THEME: AN ALTERED EPIDEMIOLOGICAL PICTURE

Many authorities are agreed that there have been changes in the epidemiological pattern of lower genital tract carcinogenesis in recent years. These changes have taken the form of increased mortality rates in younger women as well as changes in the age incidence of first recognition of the disease state (5-7,9). Less formally documented but nevertheless widely discussed internationally when gynaecologists meet is an alteration to a property which might be termed aggressiveness of the lesion, in terms of its proclivity for earlier lymph node involvement, earlier metastasis, and earlier display of more serious histological stigmata (6,7,19), all of which may be causally connected with the overall change in the age incidence and mortality.

Authors report a close association between preneoplastic stage and the presence of virus. This has been coupled with prospects for an epidemic of lower genital tract cancer in the same way as might occur with other forms of sexually transmitted disease (21).

These considerations render attractive a simple cause and effect view that something may have happened quantitatively or qualitatively to the virus as to produce a change in its virulence. Precisely the same reasoning has been entered by veterinary practitioners in discussing a recent world-wide epizootic of enteritis in dogs due to the parovirus (15)). The disease spread rapidly between continents in so many months in the presence of means for its control including stringent quarantine. So strange was the epidemiological picture that veterinary virologists incriminated laboratory accidents as may have occurred in the preparation of vaccines, to cope with the unusual features of the spread.

Reports on the changed epidemiology of lower genital tract cancer have ascribed the new patterns to a changed epidemiology of sexually transmitted disease including that due to human wart virus. If we allow that this change includes an increased frequency of sexual contact, then this factor may provide background for a different view on the origin of alterations in viral virulence.

A third viral disease, that of acquired immune deficiency in humans with its own sexual more connotations, has made sudden and dramatic geographic appearances particularly in Africa where it has rapidly assumed epidemic proportions.

Alterations in virulence are often thought of in material terms such as viral mutation. In the vein of the action of fields discussed in connection with the first theme earlier in this paper, our approach has been to watch for a mechanism which involves an alteration in the field that the virus is proposedly using as an inducer. The mechanism discovered hinges on the fact that during their action, sperm (in the case of sexual contact) or virus (during transformation of normal cells) reside in space. Our studies refer to this spatial phase of the operation of these forms of biomatter.

## Physical Background to the Space-Phase Studies

Underlying the dielectric properties of biomatter outlined above, we referred to the chemistry of the molecules concerned, more particularly to charge distribution on their side groups. We return to the chemical bonding of these same molecules as a basis for further discussion. It is accepted that each chemical bond is in a state of vibration so that interaction of these vibrations during normal metabolism produces oscillations over a spectrum of modes. It has been known for many years that cells produce a demonstrable radiation (11). This radiation, which can be conveniently seen as derived from bond vibration has become the object of intense study by biophysicists in the last decade (20).

We have already indicated that the male gamete has an electrical structure prospectively favouring a function of powerfult inducer of a corresponding state in the target tissue. We have also briefly referred to demonstration of transmission properties of the oscil-

latory modes of metabolising tissue (20). We therefore
carried out experiments to demonstrate just how complex
or integrated were these modes in the sense that the
signal propagated may be as elaborate as to amount to
an energetic replica or scaffold of all of the integrated metabolic chemistry of the source. The remainder of
this paper is a description of the results of early
attempts to make such virtual energy replicas real.

### Space-Phase Studies of Biomatter Fields: Methods

A growing culture of living microorganisms is placed
on the laboratory bench at room temperature. At a
distance of 1 to 10m away a thin film of polystyrene
sulphate (Monsanto Chemicals) is prepared by plunging a
clean microscope slide into a 0.25% (w/v) solution of
the polymer in benzol, and allowing it to evaporate.
When dry, the preparation is stained by a suitable dye,
(we use either haematoxylin or gram stain procedure)
and subsequently examined under the oil immersion objective or a light microscope. The growing culture can
be removed from laboratory space after 5 minutes exposure. Films are prepared at desired intervals up to
weeks from the initial exposure. We have used the following microorganisms: E. coli, B. subtilis Rhodospirillum sp., Penicillium sp. As well we have used
fresh ejaculates of human sperm from volunteer healthy
donors.

Examples of the results are shown in Figs. 2 and 3
as illustrative of the real images obtained. The images
stain with the dyestuff but the adjacent film does not
so that good definition is realised. It is a striking
property of the image that the fidelity of structural
copy of the real organism extends to its reaction to
gram staining. E. coli images on polystyrene stained
gram negative, B.subtilis images stained gram negative.

Aside from the many questions raised by observing
the propagation of such images through laboratory
space, which will be the object of further publications, one aspect of their behaviour seems relevant to
the problem of abrupt changes in epidemiological pattern. It was noted that, where preparations of the film
image were carried out during the passage of a meteoro-
logical cold front through the laboratory space and
involving overnight temperature gradients from 15°C to
0°C, the recovered image changed in an abrupt and
striking way. The illustration chosen (Fig. 4) is of a
segment of the image of a Penicillium sp. mycelium. The
mycelium is seen to have enlarged and broken up with a
collection of remarkably geometrical structures. We
have been able to identify at least four such figures
including cube, sphere, tetrahedron and icosahedron.
The latter is shown in Fig. 5.

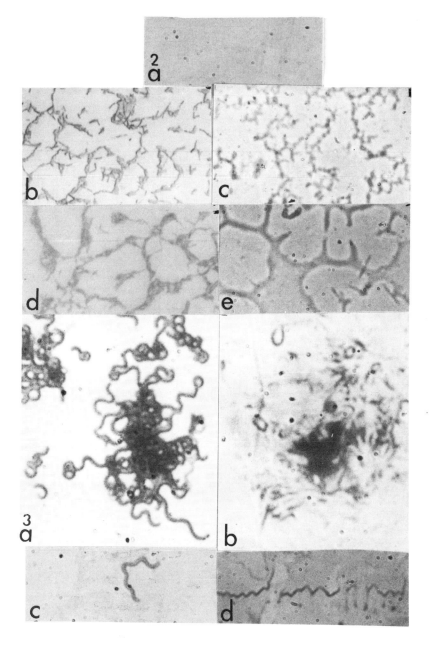

**FIGS. 2 & 3.** Photomicrographs of real microorganisms (Figs. 2 b, 2d E. coli, 3a, 3c Rhodospirillum sp.) for comparison with their respective images (Figs. 2c, 2e, 3b, 3d) recovered from a film of polystyrene solution drying on glass. Fig. 2a is a control slide made prior to exposure. Hematoxylin stain. x1000.

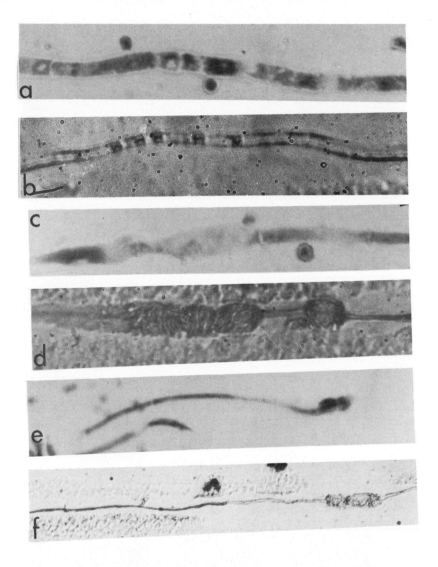

**FIG. 4.** Photomicrographs of real Penicillium sp. (Figs. 4a mycelium 4 c,e fruiting body) for comparison with their respective images (Fig. 4b,d,f) recovered from polystyrene film as in Figs. 2 & 3. Figs. 4 g,h,i,j,k (overleaf) represent mycelium recovered after passage of cold front through laboratory space to show its break up into geometrical figures which include cubes, tetrahedra and (Fig. 4l), a hexagon which could be a section of an icosahedron. x1000 except e,f 400 and 1 2000.

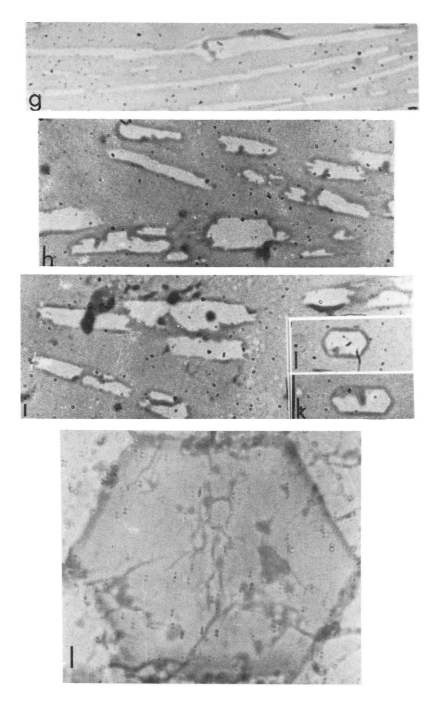

**FIG. 4 cont'd.** For caption see previous page.

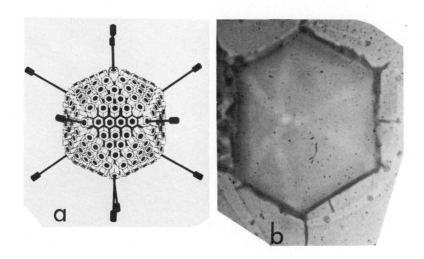

**FIG. 5A.** Model of an adenovirus reconstructed from ultrastructural data to show the overall icosahedral shape x 100,000.
**B.** Image on polystyrene film, history as in **Fig.** 4 g,1 from Penicillium sp. suggesting an icosahedral structure. x 2000. Fig. 5A is reproduced from Horne R.W. et al., J. Ultrastruct. Res., (1975): 51, 233.

It has thus been possible to visualise in Penicillium sp. mycelial images under the microscope, four of the five platonic solids. It is possible that latent geometrical forms underly the apparently complex structure of other biomatter examples as was taught over twenty centuries ago in classical times. However, our interest is focussed on the icosahedron because the ultramicroscopic plan of many animal viruses including those causing the diseases already referred to is formed upon that of an icosahedron. The idea that the formation and growth of all matter including pure crystals and biomatter occurs on a pre-existing energetic scaffold is gaining increasing credance this last decade or so (12). Geometrical pattern is a feature of the ultrastructure of all viruses; animal and many plant viruses are icosahedral (Fig. 5).

An icosahedral image would be an appropriate scaffold for the de novo formation of virus in an appropriate target cell from cellular building blocks of the type proposed by Temin (17). It remains to be seen whether the energetic image of the spermatozoon, which can be transmitted under the same conditions as

obtains in the transmission of microbial forms, contains incipient icosahedral shapes as does Penicillium
sp. The presence of real virus in the sperm head, which
has been recognised for many years, suggests that this
is possible.

There is a uniqueness concerning the complicity of
the male gamete and viruses as inducers. A demonstrable
electrical structure of high order means that its
radiated energy will be more coherent and therefore of
highly competitive signal strength. As a radiated
oscillation, the energy image obeys the laws of elec-
trodynamics so that the theoretical limit to its propagation distance is infinity. Such a trasmission mode
may underlie the surprisingly rapid spread of certain
viral diseases already noted. It is also possible that
the history of the proposed energetic template in space
may admit of mutation – like changes to account for
alteration in the clinical response to the new particle
forming as the cell avails itself of the template.

## ACKNOWLEDGEMENTS

The bovine wart virus sample was the generous gift
of Dr. Spadbarrow, Department of Veterinary Pathology,
University of Queensland. The various microbial species
were generously provided by Mrs. I. Dalins, Department
of Microbiology, The University of Sidney.

## REFERENCES

1. Anderson, H., Reid, B.L., and Coppleson, M. (1984):
   The Cervix, 2: 219–228.
2. Barsamian, S., Reid, B.L., and Thornton, B.S.
   (1985): IRCS Med. Sci., 13: 1103–1104.
3. Barsamian, S.T., Greenoak, G., Barsamian, S., and
   Reid, B.L. (1986): In: Proc. Aust. Soc. Exper.
   Path., 18th Annual Meeting.
4. Barsamian, S.T., and Thornton, B.S. (1984): Phys.
   Lett., 107: 414–418.
5. Carmichael, J.A., Clarke, D.H., Moher, D., Ohlke,
   I.D., and Karchmar, E.J. (1986): Am. J. Obstet.
   Gynecol., 154: 264–269.
6. Coppleson, M., and Reid, B.L. (1987): Med. J.
   Aust. (in press).
7. Del Giudice, E., Doglia, S., and Milani, M. (1985):
   In: The Living State II, edited by R.K. Mishra,
   pp. 437–447. World Scientific, Singapore.
8. Draper, G.J., and Cook, G.A. (1983): Br. Med. J.,
   287: 510–513.
9. Elliott, P.M. (1985): J. Obstet. Gynecol., 6: 145.
10. Galloway, D.A., and McDougall, J.K. (1983): Nature,
    302: 21–24.
11. Gurwitsch, A. (1929): Protoplasma, 6: 449–493.

12. Hagan, B., and Reid, B.L. (1980): Med. Hypotheses, 6: 559-609.
13. Reid, B.L. (1962): In: Proc. 1st. Intern. Congress Exfol. Cytol., Lippincot, Philadelphia, pp. 62-72.
14. Reid, B.L. (1985): In: Clinics in Obstetrics and Gynaecology, 12, edited by A. Singer, pp. 1-17. Saunders, London.
15. Siegl, G. (1984): The Parvoviruses, edited by K. Berns, pp. 363-387. Plenum Press, New York.
16. Singh, B., Smith, C.W., and Hughes, R. (1979): Med. Biol. Eng. Comput., 17: 45-60.
17. Temin, H. (1970): Perspect. Biol. Med., 14: 11-26.
18. Thornton, B.S., Reid, B.L., and Webb, S.J. (1986): In: Modern Bioelectrochemistry, edited by F. Gutmann and H. Keyzer, pp. 315-327. Plenum Press, New York.
19. Ward, B., Monaghan, J., and Sheppard, J. (1985): Br. Med. J., 290: 1301-1303.
20. Webb, S.J. (1985): In: The Living State II, edited by R.K. Mishra, pp. 367-403. World Scientific, Singapore.
21. Wolfendale, M.R., King, S., and Usherwood, M. (1983): Br. Med. J., 287: 526-528.
22. zur Hausen, H. (1982): Lancet, ii: 1370-1372.

# Treatment of Genital Herpes

## G.D. Wilbanks[1] and C.A. Benson[2]

[1]*Department of Obstetrics & Gynecology,*
[2]*Section of Infectious Disease, Department of Medicine*
*Rush Medical College*
*Rush Presbyterian St. Luke's Medical Center*
*Chicago, Illinois, USA*

Physicians have been engaged in the diagnosis and treatment of herpes since ancient Greece. The treatment of herpes has had a long and interesting history (60, 61). Like most subjects in medicine and science, there has been unequal advancement. Gradual inroads have been made, with some peaks and valleys, as knowledge about the disease has increased. However, in the last decade, the growth of basic molecular pathophysiology, antiviral pharmacology and controlled clinical studies have increased geometrically (5). Several excellent reviews (2,15,34,53,79) present the state of the art. Unfortunately, there is still no ideal medication, for either local or systemic treatment of common, genital infections. A preventive vaccine has been proposed and is to be tested. This discussion will attempt to summarize the treatment of genital herpes in 1987.

## History

McNair Scott's recent Samuel J. Zakon Prize lecture (60,61) summarizes the interesting history of herpetic infections. The word "herpes" has been used in medicine from the time of Hippocrates. The term is derived from the Greek word , "Erpein" (to creep), which was originally used to describe a variety of spreading skin lesions. Morton is reported to be the first to use the term herpes to describe oral lesions associated with fever, although a good clinical description was given by Heroditus (100 A.D.). John Astruc described penile and labial lesions in 1736, thought to be due to the same etiology, but the venereal nature was not suggested until the 1830's. Classic illustrations were made by Unna in 1883. It was in the second decade of the

20th century that Gruter and Lowenstein isolated a transmissible agent from vesicles.

Treatment recommended in 1877 by the "great" Philadelphia dermatologist, Duhrning, was a bland ointment. For recurrences, he recommended that "the bowels should be carefully regulated". In 1910 Hyde recommended alcohol or a zinc-containing ointment to abort the attack. Tincture of benzoin was suggested after rupture of vesicles. Zinc was used with some apparent success in reducing recurrences even in 1985 (20). In the 1940's and early 1950's smallpox vaccination was a popular treatment modality until proven ineffectual in 1959 (37). Attempts to develop effective vaccines continues to the present (7,40,45). The modern era of specific antivirals began with the synthesis of idoxuridine in 1959 (56). It is interesting to speculate what such a historical review would contain in the next century.

## Pathogenesis of the Disease

The virus penetrates mucosal surfaces, where it replicates locally in mucosal epithelial cells. At the same time, HSV enters peripheral sensory nerves and is transported to the nerve cell body in the dorsal root ganglion via the nerve axon. The virus then replicates in the neuron. Following replication, virions are again transported to the mucosal surface via the neuronal axon. These virions then cause primary or recurrent infection with its characteristic lesions (34).

The discovery of the ability of HSV to induce viral latency and the neuronal involvement in herpes simplex infections has assisted in the understanding of the chronic, recurrent nature of the disease. However, the nature of the humoral and cell mediated response to the infection and the impact of these immunologic responses to the prevention and treatment of the disease still remain an enigma. The method by which a vaccine would be effective in prevention and possible treatment of the disease remains to be tested. The problems of asymptomatic shedding, neonatal (and intrauterine) infection, possible ascending genital tract infections and the continued spectre of cervical carcinogenesis stress the need for effective treatment and prevention.

## Pregnancy: Special Emphasis on the Need for Effective Treatment and Prevention

Pregnancy complicates the problem of herpes infection, because of the potential involvement of both mother and fetus and stresses the important of prevention and treatment (8,25). Although rare, disseminated disease during pregnancy results in significant material and fetal morbidity and mortality rates approaching 40% even with treatment (55). Grover et al. (28) recently reported treatment of disseminated herpes in a woman at 32 weeks gestation with intravenous acyclovir. The mother and infant survived without problem.

Vaginal delivery in a woman with active genital herpetic infection has been shown logically to result in neonatal herpes infection (8,25). The exact incidence of such infection is still debated, but active infections are indications for cesarean section delivery in most centers. Most studies have shown that vaginal delivery is safe if clinical surveillance and serial cultures indicate no active vaginal infection at the time of delivery.

Despite such active surveillance however, transplacental infection by HSV has been demonstrated in early pregnancy (8,25). The teratogenic and abortive effects of the virus are debated. Monif et al. (49) reported a patient who had primary vulvar herpes diagnosed at 19 weeks gestation. She delivered at 25 weeks a 520 g fetus that was severely affected with cutaneous and systemic HSV-2 infection. The infant died shortly after birth. A recent report by Growdon et al. (29) suggested strongly the transplacental infection of a term twin fetus following negative surveillance for active vaginal involvement. The second twin developed systemic HSV-II infection at 16 days. The first twin had negative cultures and did not develop any signs of infection. If indeed further evidence of late transplacental infection by herpes can be documented, a whole new schema for management of pregnant women with genital herpes will have to be developed (51).

## TREATMENT

### General

The development of treatment modalities for genital herpes has progressed utilizing two main approaches in the past i.e., local treatment and systemic drug therapy (Table 1). Recently, attempts have been made to alter the immune response to the infection with biologic response modifiers (BRMs) such as interferon or prostaglandin inhibitors. Overall (53) reviewed in detail 52 papers published from 1962-1983 describing various treatment regimens. He concluded there was no really effective treatment to that date. Corey and Spear (15) summary of data generated through 1986 suggested that acyclovir was the only current method of treatment effective in reducing the duration and severity of common genital lesions (Table 2). There was little definitive data on effective treatment of other

**TABLE 1.** Agents Used in the Treatment of Genital Herpes

---

**Specific Antivirals**

     Acyclovir
     Deoxy acyclovir
     Ademine arabinoside
     Ademine arabinoside monophosphate
     Amatadine
     Aryl Diketones (avilones)
     Bromovinyl Deoxyuridine (BVDU)
                cytidine
     Carboxyclic bromovinyldeoxylividine
     Cyclaradine
     Cytosine arabinoside
     Digydroxypropoxymethyl guanine (DHPG)
     Ethyldeoxyuridine
     Fluoroiodoaracyticlus
     Iododeoxyuridine
     Phosphonoformate
     Phosphonoformic acid (fosarnet)
     Rimantadine
     Trifluro thymidine
     Vidarabine

**Other Systemic Agents**

     Inosine
     Interferon
     Levamisole
     Lithium
     Lysine
     Photodynamic inactivation
     Prostaglandin inhibitors
     Trimethoprim-Sulfamethoxazole
     Vitamins (bioflavinoids and ascorbid
      acid)

**Topical Agents**

| | |
|---|---|
| Acyclovir | Idoxuridine |
| Adenosine Monophosphate | Interferon |
| Alcohol | Kethoxal |
| Gurrows Solution |    (3-ethoxy-2-oxobutyraldehyde) |
| Gutylated hydroxytolerene | Laser |
| Chloroform | Neutral red photoactivation |
| Epinephrine | Nonoxynol-9 |
| Ether | Povidone codine |
| Gossypol | Semio-semicarbozone |
| Heavy metals (Zinc, borate) | Tinctive of benzoin |
| Heparin | Zinc |
| Hydrogen peroxide | |

---

**TABLE 2.** Current Status of Antiviral Chemotherapy
of HSV Infections

| TYPE OF INFECTION | TREATMENT AND BENEFITS |
| --- | --- |
| **Mucocutaneous HSV Infections** Immunosuppressed Patients | |
| Acute Symptomatic First or Recurrent Episodes | IV or oral acyclovir relieves pain and speeds healing: with localized external lesions, topical acyclovir may be beneficial |
| Suppression of Reactivation of Disease | IV or acyclovir taken daily prevents recurrences during high-risk period (e.g. immediately after transplantation). |
| Immunocompetent Patients First Episodes of Genital Herpes | Oral acyclovir is the treatment of choice. IV acyclovir may be used if severe disease of neurologic complications are present: topical acyclovir may be beneficial in patients without cervical, urethral, or pharyngeal involvement. |
| Symptomatic Recurrent Genital Herpes | Oral acyclovir has some benefits in shortening lesions and viral excretion time: routine use for all episodes is not recommended. |
| Suppression of Recurrent Genital Herpes | Daily oral acyclovir prevents reactivation of symptomatic recurrences; use is at present limited to a 6-month course in patients with frequent recurrences. |
| First Episodes of Oral-Labial HSV | Oral acyclovir has not yet been studied. |
| Recurrent Episodes of Oral-Labial HSV | Topical acyclovir of no clinical benefit; oral acyclovir has not been studied. |
| Herpeticwhitlow | Studies of antiviral chemotherapy have not been performed. |
| HSV Proctitis | IV acyclovir appears to be beneficial in immunosuppressed patients; oral acyclovir is under investigation. |

./.

./. TABLE 2

| | |
|---|---|
| Herpetic Eye Infections (acute keratitis) | Topical trifluorothymidine, vidarabine, idoxuridine, acyclovir, and interferon are all beneficial; debridement may be required; topicalsteroids may worsen disease. |

**HSV Infections of the Central Nervous System**

| | |
|---|---|
| HSV Encephalitis | IV acyclovir or vidarabine descreases mortality: acyclovir is the preferred agent. |
| HSV Aseptic Meningitis | No studies of systemic antiviral chemotherapy have been performed. |
| Autonomic Radiculopathy | No studies are available. |
| Neonatal HSV Infections | IV vidarabine or acyclovir decreases mortality: a comparative trial is in progress. |

**Visceral HSV Infections**

| | |
|---|---|
| HSV Esophagitis | No controlled studies have been performed; systemic acyclovir or vidarabine should be considered. |
| HSV Pneumonitis | No controlled studies have been performed; systemic acyclovir or vidarabine should be considered. |
| Disseminated HSV Infections | No controlled studies have been performed; systemic acyclovir or vidarabine should be tried; there is no definite evidence that therapy will decrease mortality. |
| HSV-associated Erythema Multiforme | Controlled studies are under way; only anecdotal observations are available regarding the use of topical or oral acyclovir. |

Modified from Corey and Spear (15)

manifestations of the disease. Spruance and Freeman
(66) devised an interesting list of medications used
topically or systemically in herpes treatment. A number
of new compounds suggest possible efficacy in in vitro
and animal studies or preliminary human trials (Table
1). Hirsch and Kaplan (34) give a nice review the
development of new drugs, their mechanisms of action
and prospects for the future.

### Local Treatments

Almost every known class of therapeutic agent has
been utilized as a local treatment for mucocutaneous
oral and genital herpes (Table 1).

In recent years a number of compounds have raised
considerable interest initially only to decline with
time and analysis of data generated in controlled
studies. Alcohol, ether (30) and chloroform (72) followed by silver nitrate and tincture of benzoin as
local caustics, which perhaps eliminated local bacterial secondary infections and anesthetized nerve
endings, have been used, but did not affect the natural
course of the disease. These agents caused considerable
local discomfort.

Various soaking or cleansing solutions, such as
Borrow's solution and hydrogen peroxide, had no effect
and were supplanted by Betadine (23). This may have had
practical use associated with its antibacterial and
cleansing properties, however, its efficacy was probably little better than saline solution.

Heparin solution was tried by Grossman and Thornard-
-Neumann (27) based on a suggested in vitro effect. In
a well controlled clinical study, topical heparin in
polyethylene glycol showed no therapeutic benefit.

Incidental observations suggested that vaginal
contraceptives containing gossypol (80) and the topical
spermicidal, surfactant, nonoxynol 9, had apparent
favorable outcome on symptoms of herpetic infections.
Vontver et al. (73) found no beneficial effect in a
study of topical nonoxynols in 37 men and 32 women with
genital herpes. No controlled clinical study of local
gossypol has been reported.

In 1965, Wallis and Melnick (75) studied the dyna-
mics of photooxidation of the virus and suggested that
this mode of clinical therapy might be feasible. Clinical trials were tried with some success in 1973 (22,
35) but the concern over potential carcinogenic effects
of photoactive dyes (42,57) and local skin reactions
associated with its use (26) have prevented further
development of this modality.

Newer antiviral agents, locally applied, such as
idoxuridine (30% in DMSO) (58) and acyclovir in poly-
ethelene glycol (14), have resulted in slight clinical

benefit in reduction of symptoms and virus shedding. However, they showed no effect on the time to healing of lesions and the rate and number of recurrences.

A number of other locally applied drugs that looked promising in vitro or in animal studies have been thus far ineffective in controlled clinical trials. These include trisodium phosphonoformate (fosarnet) (4,74), butylated hydroxytolerene (24) and arildone (an aryl diketone) (18). DeClercq and Cassiman (17) urged careful testing of antiviral drugs regarding mutagenicity as they demonstrated that two new drugs, fluoroiodo-aracytidine and dihydroxypropoxymethylguanine were mutagenic in their investigational system at concentrations achieved therapeutically in humans.

Local Laser (CO2) destruction has been used in the treatment of genital herpes (1). Baggish treated 30 patients with primary lesions and reported a "cure rate" of 83% (25/30). Most successes were treated within 48 hours of onset of lesions. Of the 48 women with recurrent lesions, 16 (33%) had no further infections and 12 had some increase in recurrence intervals. If this effect in primary lesions can be confirmed in repeated studies, it may warrant serious consideration as a form of local treatment.

Even human interferon β (IFNβ) cream has been used as local treatment for genital herpes (50). Using human IFN-β from poly (rI):(rC) induced foreskin diploid fibroblasts in a polyethylene glycol base, an increase in interval between recurrences was observed in 6/6 women and 8/13 men with recurrent genital herpes. This is interesting but a double blind study is currently underway to provide more definitive information.

At this time, there seems to be no truly effective local therapy for genital herpes, although those involved with clinical practice will note occasional amelioration of symptoms with judiciously used topical acyclovir or other local remedies. If topical treatment is to be effective, new agents or new delivery vehicles must be identified and tested (66). Semi-carbozones have been suggested by in vitro and animal studies as a new possibility.

## SPECIFIC SYSTEMIC DRUGS FOR HERPES TREATMENT

The era of specific antiviral therapy begins in the late 1950's when Prusoff (56) synthesized idoxuridine. However, it was not until the 1970's that the increased frequency of occurrence of herpes infections and the development of less toxic second generation antivirals, stimulated biochemists, pharmacologists, virologists and other related specialists to elevate this field to its current intense level of activity. As noted above in Tables 1 and 2, and extensive reviews (2,15,34,53,

79), of all the compounds previously devised and tested, acyclovir is the only drug to be proved effective
and practical in treating genital herpes. [Vidarabine
(ARA-A) is effective in severe systemic infections,
especially in the newborn.] Even systemic therapy with
acyclovir is palliative, as the drug does not reach the
latent virus in the neuron, is not virocidal, and thus
does not cure the disease. Although not as major a
concern as was initially expressed, the development of
resistant strains as a result of chronic use of the
drug remains a possibility (3,44). Also, the effects of
prolonged administration of the drug are unknown. Corey
and Spear (15) list the specific uses of the drug for
various forms of herpes infections (Table 2).

As Corey notes and as shown in several studies (48),
acyclovir seems to be standing the test of time in the
treatment of both primary and recurrent disease in both
immunocompetent and immunosuppressed patients (Table
2). The drug may be given intravenously in severe
infections, with significant but reasonable toxicity.
Prompt oral treatment suppresses symptoms, accelerates
healing and decreases virus shedding, for both primary
and recurrent lesions. Such intermittant oral therapy
is not recommended for routine use as the possibility
of the development of resistant strains persists and
there is no effect on development of recurrences.
Continuous oral therapy will suppress recurrences but
recurrences continue when the drug is stopped. The
toxic effects of long term therapy are not known. It is
anticipated that a new generation of antiviral agents
will be effective in inactivating the latent virus, but
there are no such agents ready for clinical use at this
time.

A number of old and new compounds are in various
phases of development or testing. These have recently
been reviewed by Whitley (79) and Spruance and Freeman
(66). Some of these new compounds and other medications
are listed in Table 1.

Obviously, there is as yet no ideal, specific agent
for the simple curative treatment or prevention of
genital herpes. Perhaps one of the new generation of
compounds either alone or combined with a vaccine or
BRM will be effective for this frustrating disease.

## IMMUNOLOGIC THERAPY

### Immunopotentiating and Immunomodulating Agents

Werner and Zerial (78) who recently summarized the
effects of immunopotentiating and immunomodulating
agents agreed with these conclusions. BCG, C. parvum
and glucan show protective effect in exposed animals,
but are perhaps to pleiotropic to be used in humans.

Levamisole and inosiplex have been used anecdotally  in
humans but show   only modest  activity in treatment   of
experimental HSV infection.   Interleukin-2 (rIL-2)   has
been shown to modify HSV-2 infection in guinee pigs but
no specific clinical studies   have been reported  (76).
The possible  activities  of monokines  or  lymphokines
remains speculative. Perhaps the  most likely role  for
these compounds will be  in combination with  acyclovir
or  similar   drugs  to   potentiate  the   therapeutic
response.
    The interferons have both antiviral and  immunoregu-
latory properties which may  play a role in the  treatment of herpes. The use of interferon-alpha 2  (IFN-2a)
has been  disappointing  in  clinical   studies  (21,41)
altough it appeared  effective  in  animal and in  vitro
models. Mendelson et  al. (46) did   note a decrease  in
healing time and viral  shedding during recurrences  in
men, but not in women. Side effects, both systemic  and
hematolic, are major  problems, especially  with  prolonged usage in high doses.
    Werner and Zerial (78)  speculate that if a  vaccine
is perfected, perhaps compounds such as muramylpeptides
or lipopeptides  could be useful  as immune  adjuvants.
Kawana (36) utilized PS-K,  a protein bound  polysacha-
ride used  in  Japan for  immunotherapy of  cancer, to
treat recurrent  genital herpes in  a preliminary  clinical trial. He treated 19 females and 5 males who  had
recurrent genital  herpes with  3-5  mg/day orally.  He
noted a decrease  in duration  and frequency of  recurrences during  treatment with  the drug and  no  side
effects were observed. Further studies are in progress.

### Prostaglandin

    Host resistance  to HSV infection  bears some  rela-
tionship with  natural  killer  cell  activity.  Since
prostaglandins are known  inhibitors of natural  killer
cytotoxicity, prostaglandin  inhibitors seemed  logical
potential therapeutic agents  for genital herpes.  This
concept was supported by the in vitro studies of  Baker
and Milch (2) showing prostaglandin F2a and E2 enhanced
cell-to-cell spread of HSV-2 and no effect. of ibuprofen
on prostaglandin altered T-cell mitogen response.  This
was confirmed  by the  lack of effect  of ibuprofen  on
recurrent genital herpes in  clinical studies by  Milch
et al (47)  and our own  group (unpublished data);  despite initial  encouraging results  in the  preliminary
trial by Chang (12).
    Although it would seem that several aspects of  cell
mediated immunity are related to herpes infections  and
recurrences, interferon (at least a2) and prostaglandin
inhibitors are not active in treating recurrent  herpes
in the clinical formats tested. Combinations of  active

drugs or an effective vaccine with immunotherapeutic compounds may be effective in treatment programs and should be studied.

## VACCINES

Since the difficulties of neural involvement, latency and recurrences pose major obstacles to treatment of genital herpes, obviously a vaccine or other method to prevent the infection is the treatment of choice. The immunology of herpes is also unusual with recurrences occurring in spite of circulating antibodies. Until recent years this disease was not common and did not carry a high mortality, so the stimulus for vaccine development was small. The apparent rapid increase in the incidence of herpes and the advent of sophisticated specific vaccine developmental technology and improved immunologic monitoring make the formulation of a safe and effective vaccine feasible. Small pox vaccine was the first vaccine to be used to treat herpes with no proven success (37). Although several vaccines have been available in Europe (9,10) and a subunit vaccine has been tested in the USA (32,33) the current double blind clinical studies in progress in the UK and USA with the Skinner subunit vaccine, appear to be the first major tests of a potentially effective vaccine (Table 3).

Kit and Kit (40), Black (7) and Meigner and Roizman (45) have recently reviewed the status and future of herpes vaccines. Table 3 is a modification of that from Kit and Kit, which summarizes their review. Dr. Roizman's review in this volume brings the reader up to date.

New data that may be of interest is an update on the Skinner vaccine data since Dr. Skinner's presentation at this symposium in 1985 (63). The formal data on 50 vaccinated normal, non-infected consorts of sexual partners with severe recurrent herpes has been completed. These consorts have been followed from 4-48 months representing a total of 694 patient months. Non of 49 subjects have contracted herpes genitalis. The one subject classified as infected, was a homosexual male diagnosed clinically by evaluation of two episodes of anal "fissuring" or "cracking" following frequent of anal intercourse with multiple partners. Cultures from the involved areas were negative during both episodes.

There have been no significant side effects of the vaccine. None of the subjects tested have shown any evidence of immunological reactivity to host cell or calf serum antigens.

The follow-up data available on patients with primary and severe recurrent genital herpes "treated" with the Skinner vaccine (63,65,81) continue to support some

**TABLE 3.** Herpes Simplex Virus Vaccines

| | |
|---|---|
| Inactivated Virus (19,52) | Formalin-treated extracts of HSV-2 infected rabbit kidney cells. Used in Bulgaria for recurrent herpes. Heat-inactivated HSV-2 derived from virus grown in chick cells (Lupidon G). Used in Germany, Austria, and France in treatment of recurrent genital herpes. |
| Subunit Vaccine (9) | Detergent (NP40) extract of HSV-2 infected chick embryo fibroblasts partially purified by centrifugation on sucrose gradients. Elicits antibodies and cellular immunity in human volunteers. |
| (62,63,65,81) | AcNFU$_1$(S-)MRC vaccine. Detergent (NP40) extract of HSV-1-infected human embryo lung cells purified by treatment with formaldehyde, ultracentrifugation to remove virus particles and precipitation of proteins with cold acetone. Administered to consorts of patients with genital herpes. |
| (32,33) | Glycoprotein subunit vaccine prepared using chick embryo fibroblasts infected with HSV-2. Glycoproteins released by Triton X-100, digested with DNase to eliminate viral genetic material, and purified on lectin affinity column and chromatography on Sephadex. Treated with formalin and formulated in alum adjuvant. Protective in mice and immunogenic in Cebus monkeys and man. |
| (43) | Purified glycoprotein D from HSV-1 and HSV-2-infected KB cells. Antigen administered several times with adjuvant. Protects mice against lethal challenge with HSV-1 and HSV-2. |
| Biosynthetic Polypeptides (77) | Immunologically active fusion protein containing types 1 or 2 HSV glycoprotein D, plus bacteriophage lambda cro and E. coli -glactosidase. Immunogenic in mice. |
| (6) | HSV-1 glycoprotein D produced by Chinese hamster cell line stably transformed by a recombinant plasmid that expresses glycoprotein D. Immunogenic in mice. |

./.

./. **TABLE 3.**

| | |
|---|---|
| Recombinant Hybrid Virus (16,54) | Recombinant vaccinia virus containing an insert of the HSV-1 glycoprotein D gene. Hybrid virus produces HSV-1 gD in infected cells. Protection against HSV-1 and cross-protection against HSV-2 in mice. |
| Modified Live Virus (45,59) | Attenuation of HSV by: 1)intermixing of HSV-1 and HSV-2 genes by recombination and 2) altering regulation of viral genes by engineering specific deletions in immediate early genes non-essential for virus replication in tissue culture. Pathogenicity studied only in mice. |
| (68) | Attenuation by multiple passages in thymidine kinase-positive and mutant, thymidine kinase-negative tissue-culture cells in the presence of high concentrations of bromodeoxyuridine. Modified viruses have multiple mutations in viral genome. Herpes-encoded thymidine kinase gene nonfunctional. Protects guinea pigs infected intravaginally with virulent HSV-2. |
| Immunologically Related non Pathogenic Virus (64) | Bovine mammalites virus (BMV) has been shown to over react with HSV and will prevent or modify HSV infection in animals. BMV is not known to infect humans and does not infect human cells in vitro. This virus is a possible source of vaccine antigens. |

effect in reducing frequency and severity of recurrences similar to that previously reported (Skinner, personal communication). Double blind placebo controlled clinical trials are underway in Chicago, Los Angeles, and London, utilizing the Skinner vaccine in patients with primary and recurrent herpes. The studies began in early 1987 and no data are available as yet.

Skinner et al. (64) proposed new approach to herpes vaccine development in a recent report in which he suggested the possibility of utilizing bovine mamillitis virus (BMV), which cross-reacts with the cross herpes simplex virus, as an alternative source of vaccine antigens. Since one of the problems of using the herpes simplex virus as the source of the vaccine antigens is the potential (though highly unlikely) of causing active disease or other serious side effects such as carcinogenesis with the vaccine, the use of a virus that is not pathogenic in humans would be of benefit. Skinner was unable to find evidence of human infection by BMV by search of the literature or field inquiry. BMV specific antibody was not detected in 21 control human sera or in 4 sera from personnel engaged in laboratory research with BMV. There was no replication or antigen synthesis by BMV in explant tissues or cell lines of human origin. This is an intriguing possibility to be considered with other methods of genetically engineered vaccines.

The only other point to make regarding vaccines, would be to consider a combination of vaccine and other modalities of treatment. Kit and Kit (40) suggested vaccine and chemotherapeutic agents. Vaccines and other BRM's might also be considered. Perhaps by the time of the next symposium more definitive answers will be available.

## CONCLUSIONS

Great strides have been made in the understanding of the agent and pathophysiology of genital herpes in recent years, however, prevention and cure remain elusive. Perhaps the crude vaccine currently being tested, if effective, will direct synthetic production of a more effective vaccine. The third generation antiviral compounds may lead to a non-toxic agent that eliminates the latent virus. With better understanding of the immune mechanisms involved in control of viral infection, replication and latency, perhaps a simple biologic modification of host immune mechanisms may be able to cure the disease or assist in effective vaccine or drug treatment.

## REFERENCES

1. Baggish, M.S. (1982): J. Reprod. Med., 27: 737-742.
2. Baker, D.A., and Milch, P.O. (1986): J. Reprod. Med., 31(S): 433-438.
3. Baker, D.A., Thomas, J., Epstein, J., Possilico, D., and Stone, M.L. (1982): Am. J. Obstet. Gynecol., 144: 346-349.
4. Barton, S.E., Munday, P.E., Kinghorn, G.R., van der Meijden, W.I., Stolz, E., Notowicz, A., Rashid, S., Schuller, J.L., Essex-Cater, A.J., Kuijpers, M.H.M., and Chanas, A.C. (1986): Genitourin. Med., 62: 247-250.
5. Becker, T.M., and Nahmias, A.J. (1985): Ann. Rev. Med., 36: 185-193.
6. Berman, P.W., Dowbenko, D., Lasky, L.A., Simonsen, C.C. (1983): Science, 222: 524-527.
7. Black, F.L. (1985): In: Herpes Viruses and Virus Chemotherapy, edited by R. Kuono, pp. 355-358, Elsevier Science Publishers.
8. Brown, A.Z., Berry, S., and Vontver, L.A. (1986): J. Reprod. Med., 31: 420-425.
9. Cappel, R., Sprecher, S., DeCuyper, F., and De

Braekeleer, J. (1985): J. Med. Virol., 16: 137–145.

10. Cappel, R., Sprecher, S., Rickaert, F., and DeCuyper, F. (1982): Arch. Virol., 73: 61–68.

11. Chanas, A.C. (1986): Genitourin. Med., 62: 247–250.

12. Chang, T. (1980): J. Infect., 2: 374–375.

13. Chen, M.H., Zhou, Z., Hartley, C.E., Cowan, M., and Skinner, G.R.B. (1986): Vaccine, 4: 249–252.

14. Corey, L., Benedetti, J.D., Critchlow, C.W., et al. (1982): Am. J. Med., 73(1A): 326–334.

15. Corey, L., and Spear, P.G. (1986): N. Engl. J. Med., 314: 749–757.

16. Cremer, K.J., Mackett, M., Wohlenberg, C., Notkins, A.L., and Moss, B. (1985): Science, 228: 737–739.

17. De Clerq, E., and Cassiman, J.J. (1986): In: Life Sciences, Vol. 38, pp. 281–289, Pergamon Press, USA.

18. Douglas, J.M., Jr, Judson, F.N., Levin, M.J., Bosso, J.A., Spruance, S.L., Johnston, J.M., Corey, L., McMillan, J.A., Weiner, L.B., and Frank, J.A., Jr. (1986): Antimicrob. Agents Chemother., 29: 464–467.

19. Dundarov, S., Andonov, P., Bakalov, B., Nechev, K., and Tomov, C. (1982): Dev. Biol. Stand., 52: 351–358.

20. Eby, G.A. (1985): Med. Hypotheses, 17: 157–165.

21. Eron, L.J., Toy, C., and Santomauro, D. (1985): In: Herpes Viruses and Virus Chemotherapy, edited by R. Kono, pp. 277–278, Elsevier Science Publishers.

22. Friedrich, E.G. (1973): Obstet. Gynecol., 43: 304–310.

23. Friedrich, E.G., and Masukawa, T. (1975): Obstet. Gynecol., 45: 337–339.

24. Freeman, D.J., Wenerstrom, R.N., and Spruance, S.L. (1985): Clin. Pharmacol. Ther., 38: 56–59.

25. Gibbs, R.S. (1986): J. Reprod. Med., 31: 395–397.

26. Goldenberg, R.L., and Nelson, K. (1975): Obstet. Gynecol., 46: 359–360.

27. Grossman, J.H., and Thornard-Neumann, E. (1985): J. Reprod. Med., 30: 675–676.

28. Grover, L., Kane, J., Kravitz, J., and Cruz, A. (1985): Obstet. Gynecol., 65: 284–287.

29. Growdon, W.A., Apocada, L., Cragun, J., Peterson, E.M., and de la Maza, L.M. (1987): JAMA, 257: 508–512.

30. Guinan, M.E., MacCalman, J., Kern, E.R., Overall, J.C., and Spruance, S.L. (1980): JAMA, 243: 1059–1061.

31. Halsos, A.M., Salo, O.P., Lassus, A., Tjotta, A.L., Hovi, K., Gabrielsen, B.O., and Fiddian, A.P. (1985): Acta Derm. Venereol., 65: 59–63.

32. Hilleman, M.R. (1984): Am. Intern. Med., 101:

852–858.

33. Hilleman, M.R., Larson, V.M., Lehman, E.D., Salerno, R.A., Conard, P.G., and McLean, A.A. (1981): In: The human herpes viruses: an interdisciplinary perspective, edited by A.J. Nahmias, W.R. Dowdle, and R.F. Schinazi, pp. 503–509, Elsevier, New York.

34. Hirsch, M.S., and Kaplan, J.C. (1987): Scientific American, 256: 76–85.

35. Kaufman, R.H., Gardner, H.L., Brown, D., Wallis, C., Rawls, W.E., and Melnick, J.L. (1973): Am. J. Obstet. Gynecol., 117: 1144–1146.

36. Kawana, T. (1985): In: Herpes Viruses and Virus Chemotherapy, edited by R. Kono, pp. 271–272, Elsevier Science Publishers.

37. Kern, A.B., and Schiff, B.L. (1959): J. Invest. Dermatol., 33: 99–102.

38. Kinghorn, G.R., Abeywickreme, I., Jeavons, M., Barton, I., Potter, C.W., Jones, D., and Hickmott, E. (1986): Genitourin. Med., 62: 186–188.

39. Kingsley, S.R., and Fiddian, A.P. (1985): In: Herpes Viruses and Virus Chemotherapy, edited by R. Kono, pp. 133–137. Elsevier Science Publishers.

40. Kit, S., and Kit, M. (1985): Clin. Obstet. Gynaecol., 28: 164–177.

41. Kuhls, T.L. (1986): J. Infect. Dis., 154: 437–442.

42. Li, J.H., Jerkovsky, M.A., and Rapp, F. (1975): Int. J. Cancer, 15: 190–202.

43. Long, D., Madara, T.J., Ponce de Leon, M., Cohen, G.H., Montgomery, P.C., and Eisenberg, R.J. (1984): Infect. Immun., 43: 761–764.

44. McLaren, C., Chen, M.S., Ghazzouli, I., Saral, R., and Burns, W.H. (1985): Antimicrob. Agents Chemother., 28: 740–744.

45. Meigner, B., and Roizman, B. (1985): Antiviral Research Suppl. 1: 259–265.

46. Mendelson, J., Clecner, B., and Eiley, S. (1986): Genitourin. Med., 62: 97–101.

47. Milch, P.O., Monheit, A.G., Burton, L., Rochelson, M.D., Metz, G., and Baker, D.A. (1986): Am. J. Obstet. Gynecol., 155: 399–400.

48. Mindel, A., Weller, I.V.D., Fajerty, A., Sutherland, S., Fiddian, A.P., and Adler, M.W. (1986): Genitourin. Med., 62: 28–32.

49. Monif, G.R.G., Kellner, K.R., and Donnelly, W.H. (1985): Am. J. Obstet. Gynecol., 152: 1000–1002.

50. Movshovitz, M., Schewach-Millet, M., Kriss-Leventon, S., Shoman, K., Doerner, T., and Revel, M. (1985): In: Herpes Viruses and Virus Chemotherapy, edited by R. Kono, pp. 285–292, Elsevier Science Publishers.

51. Nahmias, A.J., Keyserling, H.L., and Whitley, R. (1985): In: Herpes Viruses and Virus Chemotherapy, edited by R. Kono, pp. 145-147. Elsevier Science Publishers.
52. Nasemann, T., and Wassilew, S.W. (1979): Br. J. Vener. Dis., 55: 121-128.
53. Overall, J.C. (1982): In: The Human Herpes Virus, edited by A.J. Nahmias, W.R., Dowdle, R.F., Schinaz, pp. 447-462. Elsevier, New York.
54. Paoletti, E., Lipinskas, B.R., Samsonoff, C., Mercer, S., and Panicali, D. (1984): Proc. Natl. Acad. Sci. USA, 81: 193-197.
55. Peacock, J.E., and Sarubbi, F.A. (1983): Obstet. Gynecol., 61: 13S-18S.
56. Prusoff, W.H. (1959): Biochem. Biophys. Acta, 32: 395-396.
57. Rapp, F., Li, J.H., and Jerkofskyu, M. (1973): Virology, 55: 339-346.
58. Reichman, R.C. (1985): In: Herpes Viruses and Virus Chemotherapy, edited by R. Kono, pp. 149-154. Elsevier Science Publishers.
59. Roizman, B., Warren, J., Thuning, C.A., Fanshaw, M.S., Norrild, B., and Meignier, B. (1982): Dev. Biol. Stand., 52: 287-304.
60. Scott, T.F.M. (1986): Int. J. Dermatol., 25: 63-70.
61. Scott, T.F.M. (1986): Int. J. Dermatol., 25: 127-134.
62. Skinner, G.R.B., Woodman, C.B.J., Hartley, C.E., Buchan, A., Fuller, A., Durham, J., Synnot, M., Clay, J.C., Melling, J., Wiblin, C., and Wilkins, J. (1982): Br. J. Vener. Dis., 58: 381-386.
63. Skinner, G.R.B., Buchan, A., Durham, J., Cowan, M., Davies, J., Brookes, K., and Castrucci, G. (1987): Vaccine, 5: 55-59.
64. Skinner, G.R.B., Buchan, A., Fuller, A., Hartley, C.E., Hallworth, J.A., Muniu, E., and Holmes, P. (1986): In: Herpes and Papilloma Viruses, edited by G. De Palo, F. Rilke, and H. zur Hausen, pp. 354-365, Raven Press, New York.
65. Skinner, G.R.B., Fink, C.G., Cowan, M., Buchan, A., Fuller, A., Hartley, C.E., Durham, J., Wiblin, C., and Melling, J. (1987): Med. Microbiol. Immunol. (in press).
66. Spruance, S.L., and Freeman, D.J. (1985): In: Herpes Viruses and Virus Chemotherapy, edited by R. Kono, pp. 125-128, Elsevier Science Publishers.
67. Spruance, S.L., McKeough, M.B., and Cardinal, J.R. (1984): Antimicrob. Agents Chemother., 25: 10-15.
68. Standberry, L.R., and Kit, S. (1984): J. Cell. Biochem. (Suppl.), 8B: 208-215.
69. Straus, S.E. (1985): Ann. Intern. Med., 103: 404-419.

70. Straus, S.E., Seidlin, M., Takiff, H.E., Rooney, J.F., Lehrman, S.N., Bachrach, S., Felser, J.M., Di Giovanna, J.J., Grimes, G.J., Krakauer, H., Hallahan, C., and Alling, D. (1986): Antiviral Res., 6: 151–159.

71. Svennerholm, B., Vahlne, A., Lowhagen, G.B., Widell, A., and Lycke, E. (1985): Scand. J. Infect. Dis. (Suppl.), 47: 149–154.

72. Taylor, C.A., Hendley, J.O., Greer, K.E., and Swaltney, J.M. (1977): Arch. Dermatol., 113: 1550–1552.

73. Vontver, L.A., Reeves, W.C., Rattray, M., Corey, L., Remington, M.A., Tolentino, E., Schweid, A., and Holmes, K.K. (1979): Am. J. Obstet. Gynecol., 133: 548–554.

74. Wallin, J., Lernestedt, J.O., Ogenstad, S., and Lycke, E. (1985): Scand. J. Infect. Dis., 17: 165–172.

75. Wallis, C., and Melnick, J.L. (1965): Photochem. Photobiol., 4: 159–165.

76. Weinberg, A., Rasmussen, L., and Merigan, T.C. (1986): Infect. Dis., 154: 134–140.

77. Weis, J.H., Enquist, L.W., Salstrom, J.S., Watson, R.J. (1983): Nature, 302: 72–73.

78. Werner, G.H., and Zerial, A. (1985): In: The Herpesvirus, edited by B. Roizman, and C. Lopez, Vol. 4, pp. 395–416, Plenum Press, New York.

79. Wichmann, K., Vaheri, A., and Luukkainen, T. (1982): Am. J. Obstet. Gynecol., 142: 593–594.

80. Whitley, R.J. (1985): In: The Herpesvirus, edited by B. Roizman, and C. Lopez, Vol. 4, pp. 339–369, Plenum Press, New York.

81. Woodman, C.B.J., Buchan, A., and Fuller, A. (1983): Br. J. Vener. Dis., 59: 311–319.

# Topical Interferon-Beta Reduces Frequency of Recurrences in Labial and Genital Herpes: Double-Blind Placebo-Controlled and Phase IV Trials

M. Glezerman[1], M. Movshovitz[2], T. Doerner[3], J. Shoham[2] and M. Revel[4]

[1]Soroka Medical Center, Beer-Sheva,
[2]Sheba Medical Center, Tel-Aviv,
[3]InterYeda Ltd, Ness-Ziona,
[4]Department of Virology, Weizmann Institute of Science, Rehovot, Israel

The treatment of Herpes Simplex Virus (HSV) dermal infections is complicated by the recurrent nature of the disease (8). The basis for the latency state of the virus in sensory nervous ganglia afferent to the facial and genital areas is poorly understood, and so is the trigger which reactivates virus replication in the skin areas innervated by these ganglia (19). One hypothesis is that patients with recurrent herpes outbreaks about every month, have some impairment in cellular immunity which allows periodic virus reactivation (30,34). Indeed, HSV is wide spread in the human population: a 1973 USA survey showed HSV-1 in 45% of unselected trigeminal ganglia taken at autopsies (5), HSV-2 being found in 10% of sacral ganglia (4). The high incidence of periodic labial herpes (11), the increasing number of new cases of genital herpes (8), the severe objective and subjective discomfort caused by the recurrent eruptions, the danger of infection spreading to sexual partners and to newborns, and the associated cancer risk factor (3) emphasize the need for an efficient but also convenient treatment.

The antiviral nucleoside Acyclovir appears highly effective in reducing the risks of recurrence but only if taken systemically (e.g. orally), at high doses, and continuously (10,23,32,33). If treatment is not taken daily, recurrences remain frequent (33). In addition, if applied topically, acyclovir is not efficient against recurrences although it reduces virus proliferation and may fasten healing (6,9,18,28,29). On the other hand, in a preliminary trial, topical applications of human fibroblast interferon (IFN-β) had shown a prophylactic effect on recurrences of herpes labialis in addition to a notable reduction in the symptomatology, severity and duration of herpetic outbreaks (17). Since a treatment by local applications to the herpetic lesions would have advantages over systemic treatment, we carried out three trials of IFN-β ointment in labial and genital herpes, including a double-blind placebo-controlled trial and a phase IV study on 160 patients. The results of these studies and long-term follow-up on the rate of recurrences, done in several medical centers in Israel and in different groups of patients, are analyzed here. Topical applications of IFN-β during eruptions appears to provide a convenient and efficient means to reduce recurrences of herpes labial and genital infections to levels comparable to those achieved with continuous oral acyclovir.

## METHODS

### Interferon Ointment

Human IFN-β (FRONE$^R$, InterYeda, Ltd, Israel) was prepared from (rI)(rC)-superinduced foreskin fibroblasts and purified to > $10^7$ units/mg protein, the preparation containing essentially the IFN-$\beta_1$ subspecies (20). The IFN titers were determined by inhibition of the cytopathic effect (CPE) of vesicular stomatitis virus on human diploid fibroblasts FS11 cells (27) in comparison with the IFN-β international reference standard G-023-901-527 from NIH. The IFN-β cream was prepared with $10^5$ units IFN per gram in a polyethylene-glycol base, and presented in tubes of 5 g. The IFN-β gel contained $10^5$ units IFN per gram in a carboxymethyl cellulose base. Identical tubes of placebo gel were manufactured containing the same carrier gel without IFN. Storage of the cream and gel was at 4°C with a stability of one year.

### Open Trials

Patients with recurrent genital (13 men, 6 women) and facial herpes (2 men, 10 women) with mean age (± S.E.) of 31.3 years (± 1.8) and 28.6 years (± 1.9) were treated at the out-patient dermatology clinic of the Sheba Medical Center, Tel-Aviv. Recurrences every 0.5 - 3 months had been recorded during prolonged follow-up prior to treatment of 18 months (± 3.5) for genital herpes and 105 (± 18) for facial herpes (range 1-18 years). Virus was isolated as below, from each patient prior to IFN treatment. HSV-1 was found in all facial herpes cases and in one case with sacral localization.

HSV-2 was found in all other genital herpes. Details on individual patient were reported (25). Treatment protocol: at the time papules, vesicles or crusts were present, FRONE-cream was applied to the affected skin area 4 - 6 times daily (about $2x10^4$ units IFN-β). After visible lesions had disappeared, patients were instructed to apply the IFN-β cream twice a day also during remission and 6 times daily if prodromal symptoms of itching, burning or numbness appeared. Parameters recorded were 1) dates of recurrences, increased intervals between eruptions or prevention of eruptions, 2) improvement in symptoms of itching, burning, pain and fever in eventual recurrence, 3) reduction in duration of eruptions, 4) decrease in size or number of lesions in eventual recurrences, 5) side effects. Follow-up after initiation of treatment was on the average (+ S.E.) of 15 months (+ 1.3).

### Double-Blind Trial

The study was carried out in the Division of Obstetrics and Gynecology, Soroka Medical Center, Beer-Sheva. Patients with documented recurrent genital (6 men, 5 women) and facial herpes (2 men, 12 women), mean age 35 years (median 33.5, range 15-59) who had been followed for 1-27 years (mean 9.7, median 6), were enrolled when physical examination indicated acute herpetic infection. Confirmation of HSV infection was based on virus isolation and serological evidence of an HSV neutralizing titer exceeding 20. At this first visit blood tests were performed with the intent of eliminating from the study patients with liver, kidney or blood diseases. Pregnant woman were also excluded. When laboratory test had confirmed the herpes infection and when no other treatment had been used for at least 3 months, patients were instructed to apply the provided gel 4 times daily on the affected skin areas starting from the next subsequent attack. Identical coded tubes containing either 5g of IFN-β gel or only the carrier placebo gel were provided by InterYeda, Ltd. Neither patients nor medical team were aware of the tube contents. Gel was applied from the first sensation of impending outbreak of herpes dermal infection and until disappearance of visible lesions. In addition, patients applied 6 times daily a 3% chloramphenicol ointment. Patients were asked to maintain a log-sheet identified by the coded number of the tube used, to record occurrence of eruptions, duration, severity, symptoms (graded subjectively from 1 to 3), intercurrent diseases and frequency of drug administration. Follow-up visits were scheduled every 3 months or at onset of any subsequent attack. Patients who did not report back were not included. Code was

broken two years after enrollment of first patients,
every patient having been followed for at least one
year. Statistical analysis was done by two-tailed
Students T-test.

## Phase IV Study

Physicians prescribing FRONE[R] cream in 6 daily
applications during eruptions of HSV dermal infections
evaluated 151 patients with recurrent herpes and 16
primary cases for a minimum of one year. Virus isolation showed HSV-2 in genital herpes and HSV-1 in facial
and lower-back lesions.

## Virus Isolation

Samples were obtained prior to IFN treatment by
means of Virocult swabs from vesicular lesions unroofed
with a sterile needle. Cultures of African Green Monkey
Vero cells or Human embryo fibroblasts in M199 medium
with 500 U/ml penicillin, 500 $\mu$g/ml streptomycin and 50
U/ml mycostatin were infected and incubated 2-10 days
at 37°C until CPE appeared. Virus stocks were stored at
-70°C. HSV was identified by the indirect immunoperoxidase assay using HSV-positive and adenovirus-negative
sera.

## RESULTS

## Open Trial

The usefulness of topical applications of IFN-$\beta$
(FRONE[R]) cream in recurrent HSV dermal infections was
first analyzed in an open trial on 19 patients with
genital herpes and 12 patients with facial herpes, both
groups with a long history of recurrent eruptions.
After virus isolation, treatment was initiated at the
next eruption. IFN-$\beta$ ($10^5$ U/g) was applied 4-6 times
daily to the affected skin area, corresponding to about
$2 \times 10^4$ units of IFN. In preliminary experiments, this
dose of IFN-$\beta$ was found to reduce the titer of HSV-1 in
skin vesicles by more than two logs within 12-24 hours,
while placebo cream had no effect (25). This treatment
was continued during the period where papules, vesicu-
les or crusts were present. During remission, patients
were instructed to apply IFN-$\beta$ cream twice daily or, in
later cases, to suspend treatment. If prodromal symptoms of itching, burning or numbness appeared, treatment was resumed with 6 daily cream applications. The
therapy was continued for an average of 15 months and
patients were followed up to two years.
The main results of this study are summarized in
Table 1. During the observation period before treat-

ment, the average frequency of recurrence was one every 35 days for genital herpes and one every 40 days for labial herpes. With topical application of the IFN-β cream, a significant prolongation of the average remission time was observed in both groups to respectively 151 and 239 days (Table 1). Calculating the change in

**TABLE 1.** Effect of IFN-β Cream on Genital and Facial Herpes Infections

|  | GENITAL | | FACIAL | |
|---|---|---|---|---|
|  | Before Treatment | IFN-β Cream | Before Treatment | IFN-β Cream |
| Mean Time to Recurrence (days): | 35 | 151 | 40 | 239 |
| (S.E.): | (5.2) | (25.8) | (9.9) | (67.3) |
|  |  | p<0.001 |  | p<0.008 |
| Mean Frequency Decrease (fold): |  | 5.2 |  | 6.2 |
| (S.E.): |  | (0.89) |  | (1.77) |
| Mean Duration of Eruption (days): | 13.5 | 5.5 | 14.8 | 6.9 |
| (S.E.): | (1.51) | (0.49) | (1.13) | (0.69) |
|  |  | p<0.001 |  | p<0.001 |
| Response Rate (Per cent patients) |  |  |  |  |
| Reduced Pain, Itching |  | 100% |  | 90% |
| Reduced Severity |  | 89% |  | 80% |
| Prevention of Eruption |  | 42% |  | 50% |
| ≥ 5 X decreased frequency |  | 47% |  | 75% |
| ≥ 2 X decreased frequency |  | 73% |  | 83% |
| ≥ 2 X decreased duration |  | 76% |  | 70% |

frequency for each patient gives a 5-6 fold mean decrease in the rate of recurrence by topical IFB-β treatment. The individual data for the 31 patients reported before (25), revealed that two patients had no recurrence during the study and four others had less than one eruption per year. IFN treatment also reduced significantly the duration of eventual eruptions during the study from about 14 days to 5-7 days (Table 1). Taken together with the decrease in frequency, these data indicate that use of IFN-β cream reduced the number of days with herpes infection from about 100 to

10-12 days per year.

The percentage of patients responding to IFN-β topical applications was calculated for a number of parameters (Table 1). Alleviation of symptoms such as pain, feeling of itching and burning, was observed in over 90% of the cases. The number and size of lesions in eventual recurrences (severity) was reduced at least twofold in over 80% of the patients. Interestingly, application of IFN-β cream during the prodromal period could prevent eruption in almost half the patients. The ability of IFN to prevent an eruption is of significant importance for the patients and laboratory analyses showed some correlation to the sensitivity of the HSV strain isolated from the patients, to inhibition by IFN in vitro (25). The reduction in frequency of recurrence by a factor of 5 or more was observed more often in facial herpes than in genital herpes. However, we have noticed that 83% of the women with genital herpes achieved a 5-fold frequency reduction for only 30% of the men (25). Nevertheless, a 2-fold decrease in frequency was achieved in the vast majority of the patients in the two groups and of both sexes (Table 1). The reduction in lenght of the eruptions was also observed in over 70% of the patients.

### Double-Blind Placebo-Controlled Trial

Because placebo effects may not be negligible in herpes dermal infections, we carried out a two-year long double blind trial on a group of 25 patients with recurrent herpes simplex dermal infections. Patients were enrolled in this study during acute genital or facial herpetic infections, when positive HSV cultures were obtained. Most patients had a prolonged history of recurrent infections with an average of 9.2 years (range 1-27 years). Treatment with coded tubes of an IFN-β gel ($10^5$ U/g) or of placebo carrier gel was instituted in a double-blind protocol at the subsequent attack. Patients were instructed to apply the gel 4 times daily on the affected area starting with the first sensation of impending outbreak of Herpes infection and until the complete disappearance of visible lesions. Patients from both placebo or IFN-β gel groups also applied 3 times daily a 3% chloramphenicol ointment. Coded follow-up was at least a year and up to two years after beginning of treatment. At the end of the trial, 7 labial and 6 genital herpes patients had received placebo while 7 labial and 5 genital herpes patients had received IFN-β gel.

The effect of IFN-β and placebo on the rate of recurrence was studied by recording the number of herpetic eruptions per year (Table 2). Placebo produced no significant change in the number of recurrences,

**TABLE 2.** Double-Blind Placebo Control Trial with IFN-β Gel in Herpes

| | PLACEBO GROUP | | IFN-β GROUP | |
| --- | --- | --- | --- | --- |
| | Before Treatment | With Placebo | Before Treatment | With IFN-β Gel |
| Mean Eruptions per year (number): | 6.9 | 6.7 | 6.6 | 1.6 |
| (S.E.): | (1.58) | (1.35) | (1.6) | (0.18) |
| | | P>0.9 | | p<0.007 |
| Mean Frequency Decrease (fold): | | 1.09 | | 3.8 |
| (S.E.): | | (0.1) | | (0.79) |
| Mean Duration of Eruption (days): | 8.3 | 7.4 | 7 | 4.5 |
| (S.E.): | (0.82) | (0.76) | (0.79) | (0.63) |
| | | p=0.45 | | p<0.007 |
| Response Rate (Per cent patients): | | | | |
| Reduced Pain, Itching, Severity: | | 8% | | 92% |
| ≥ 3 X decreased frequency | | 0% | | 55% |
| ≥ 2 X decreased frequency | | 0% | | 64% |
| ≥ 2 X decreased duration | | 8% | | 50% |

which averaged 6.8 attacks per year. The application of IFN-β during the eruptions, produced a very significant reduction in the rate of recurrence to 1.6 attacks per year. When calculated for each patient individually, the mean decrease in frequency was 3.8 fold in the IFN-β group, no decrease being observed in the placebo group (Table 2). Both labial and genital herpes responded similarly. In the IFN-β group, 3/12 patients had one or less recurrence per year, 7/12 having two outbreaks per year. No patient treated with placebo achieved such results and the recurrences ranged from 4 to 20 per year.

IFN-β gel significantly reduced the duration of eventual eruptions (Table 2). Placebo had a slight effect on the duration of eruptions, but which was not significant. A small proportion of patients treated with placebo reported an improvement in the symptoms and duration of eruptions. However, the response rate in the IFN-β-treated group was much higher for all

parameters (Table 2). Most important, over half of the
patients receiving topical applications of IFN-β in
this double-blind protocol achieved a 3-fold decrease
in the rate of recurrence.

A cross-over arm was added to the trial, and all
patients in the placebo group received a 6 month treatment with IFN in a single blind protocol. A clear
reduction in symptoms was seen in 83% of the cases, the
duration of eruptions was reduced from 7.4 to 4.9 days
and frequency of attacks from 6.9 to 4 per year during
this short treatment (not shown). These results establish the efficacy of topical IFN treatment of herpetic
lesions on the rate of recurrence and symptomatology.
They further suggest that results are better after
several consecutive eruptions have been treated, which
may take more than 6 months.

### Phase IV Study

A total of 160 patients to whom FRONE[R]-cream had
been prescribed for treatment of herpetic dermal infections were followed by three physicians for a minimum
of one year. Patients applied the IFN-β cream six times
daily during eruptions until complete re-epithelisa-
tion. We analysed the follow-up sheets submitted by the
physicians, for 120 patients with genital herpes at
various locations, 10 with facial herpes and 30 with
labial herpes (Table 3). Besides 16 primary herpes
cases, patients had prolonged history of recurrent
disease which allowed to calculate the reduction in
disease frequency. The results varied slightly according to the site of eruption but 1/2 - 2/3 of the
patients achieved a 3-fold reduction in the rate of
recurrence, a higher proportion achieving at least a
two-fold reduction (Table 3). On third of the patients
had no recorded recurrence, the proportion being lowest
when the lesion were on the penis or vulva. The lenght
of eruptions and the number of visible lesions was
reduced in 70-80% of all patients. Symptoms of pain,
itching, burning were alleviated in the vast majority
of patients and were absent in more than half (Table
3). These response rates are satisfactory considering
the problems of compliance to treatment in such field
trials.

For about 80 patients of this phase IV trial, enough
data were available to evaluate more quantitatively the
effect of IFN-β cream applications. Table 4 shows that
the mean time to recurrence increased very significantly during the treatment period as compared to the
recorded data prior to IFN treatment. The mean frequency decrease was 5-fold for genital herpes at 4.4
fold for facial herpes, very comparable to what was
obtained in the first open trial (see Table 1). A

**TABLE 3.** Phase IV Study of IFN-β Cream on Recurrent Herpes

| Localization | Whole Genital Area | Penis | Vulva Vagina | Buttocks Crural Lowback | Labial Facial |
|---|---|---|---|---|---|
| Number of Cases | 24 | 61 | 24 | 11 | 40 |
| Lenght of Disease before Treatment (years): | 4.2 | 3.5 | 3 | 3.2 | 8.5 |
| Response Rate upon Treatment (% patients): | | | | | |
| Reduced Pain, Itching: | 80% | 79% | 77% | 91% | 86% |
| No Symptoms: | 59% | 40% | 47% | 49% | 58% |
| ≥ 2 X decreased frequency | 71% | 75% | 88% | 82% | 80% |
| ≥ 3 X decreased frequency | 59% | 62% | 63% | 73% | 52% |
| No Recurrence for 1 year | 35% | 25% | 12.5% | 46% | 32% |
| ≥ 2 X shorter eruptions | 78% | 69% | 84% | 77% | 68% |
| ≥ 2 X less lesions | 100% | 65% | 83% | 88% | 78% |

breakdown of the genital herpes cases, reveals that the decrease in frequency of eruptions was much higher in patients who prior to treatment had frequent recurrence occurring within less than two months. Patients with rare recurrences showed a smaller decrease (Table 4). A slightly higher reduction in frequency was obtained in women than in men. The mean duration of eventual eruptions during treatment was significantly reduced, as found in the other trials. Finally, treatment during the prodromal period could partially prevent eruptions in 39% of all patients, 13% showing no eruption at all (not shown). Side effects were minor: in the 160 patients enrolled, only two complained of a mild rash upon topical application of the IFN-β cream.

## DISCUSSION

The principal aim of treatment in herpetic cutaneous infections should be the reduction in frequency of recurrences and eventually their complete elimination. This ideally should be achieved through a simple and time-limited treatment which should also have the minimum risk and inconvenience for the daily life of the large numbers of patients to be treated. In several

**TABLE 4.** Phase IV Study of Genital and Facial Recurrent Herpes

| | GENITAL | | FACIAL | |
| | Before Treatment | IFN-β Cream | Before Treatment | IFN-β Cream |
|---|---|---|---|---|
| Mean Time to Recurrence (days): | 42 | 160 | 43 | 151 |
| (S.E.): | (4) | (15.9) | (5.2) | (23.9) |
| | | p<0.001 | | p<0.001 |
| Mean Frequency Decrease (fold): | | | | |
| All Patients: | | 5 | | 4.4 |
| (S.E.): | | (0.57) | | (0.67) |
| Patients with Frequent Recurrences (≤ 2 months): | | 5.5 | | |
| (S.E.) | | (0.65) | | |
| Patients with Rare Recurrences (≥ 2 months): | | 2.2 | | |
| (S.E.): | | (0.46) | | |
| Mean Duration of Eruptions (days): | 11 | 4.4 | 11.7 | 6 |
| (S.E.): | (0.63) | (0.45) | (0.7) | (0.8) |
| | | p<0.001 | | p<0.001 |

recent trials, the use of oral acyclovir at doses of 0.8 g per day was shown to reduce the rate of genital herpes recurrences from 8.6 to 0.6 per year in one study (23) or from 12 to 1.7 and 1.4 in another study for respectively 0.4 and 1.0 g acyclovir per day (10). However, the antiviral nucleoside acyclovir does not cure the disease since when therapy is terminated, the recurrence rate rebounds rapidly to its high level as before treatment (10,23,32). In addition, the suppressive effect of acyclovir is observed only if the drug is ingested at the high doses prophylactically every day but not if given a few days a week only (33). Topical applications of acyclovir to the lesions, although it reduces virus shedding and fastens somewhat healing (9,18), has no significant clinical benefit on the evolution and frequency of the recurrences. (6,9, 28). The continuous systemic prophylactic administration of a drug like acyclovir, besides problems of compliance, carries the risk of long-term toxicity, and also has the inherent danger of favoring emergence of drug-resistant HSV strains. Therefore, a time-limited

topical treatment, applied locally to the affected skin
area, would have – if proven effective on the rate of
recurrences – a very significant advantage for the
facial or genital herpes patient. Encouraged by early
results on the use of human interferon in topical
application as a cream or gel in labial and genital
herpes (16,17,24), we have carried out three clinical
trials to test more rigorously the effect of IFN-β on
the evolution of the disease and recurrence rate. Data
are reported here on 59 patients with facial herpes and
133 with genital herpes who received IFN-β topically
either in the hydrophobic cream or in the hydrophylic
gel.

In the first open trial, where each patient was
compared to its own past herpetic history, IFN-β cream
was applied several times a day during eruptions and
prophylactically twice a day during remissions. A 5-6
fold decrease in the frequency of recurrences measured
over a year of treatment was observed on the average in
the treated population. In total, 58% of the patients
achieved this mean reduction or a higher one (6 patients out of 31 having no recurrence during one year),
the results being best in facial herpes (75%) and in
women with genital herpes (75%) as detailed elsewhere
(25). In addition, the duration of an eventual recurrence was reduced twofold. During this study, we observed that IFN-β cream administration was not essential. On the other hand, in patients with prodrome, the
application of IFN-β cream 6 times daily as soon as the
first sensations appeared could prevent eruption alto-
gether in 45% of the cases.

In the second trial, carried out as a double-blind
placebo-controlled study, treatment was restricted to
the times when symptoms of eruption were apparent and
discontinued after the visible lesions had disappeared.
The results of this trial demonstrate that the topical
application of IFN-β reduces the number of recurrences
to an average of 1.6 per year while with placebo-gel it
remained at its pre-treatment level of 6.7 eruptions
per year. This effect of topical IFN-β (about 20,000
units daily) is comparable to what was reported for a
continuous daily dose of 400 mg oral acyclovir (1.7
eruptions/year), although with placebo the frequency of
recurrence was 9.7 on a yearly basis in that study
(10). As in the open trial, IFN-β gel in the double-
blind study, shortened the duration of eventual recurrences while placebo did not. Symptoms were alleviated
in 92% of the patients on IFN-β gel, for only 8% in
placebo. The somewhat smaller reduction in recurrence
frequency than in the open trial (3.8 fold versus 5-6
fold) may reflect the absence of psychological moti-
vation in the double-blind setting, or a higher efficacy of the hydrophobic cream over the hydrophilic gel.

Nevertheless, 4 patients out of the 11 treated with IFN-β gel, had 5-9 fold decreases in the frequency of recurrences. This double-blind placebo-controlled trial establishes that topical application of IFN-β on the herpetic labial and genital lesions is an effective means to suppress recurrences as well as to reduce severity and duration of outbreaks, and to alleviate symptoms.

The third tiral was a phase IV protocol involving 40 facial herpes. and 120 genital herpes patients. This study was carried out with IFN-β (FRONE[R])-cream given only during eventual eruptions. The results collected from this relatively large population indicate a good response for alleviation of symptoms, decrease in number and duration of lesions, and reduction in frequency of recurrences. About one third of all patients reported no recurrence for one year after the first episode treated. Women with vulval or vaginal herpes had a worse result than other genital or facial herpes patients. The mean decrease of frequency in genital and facial herpes was similar to that in the first open trial. Interestingly, the frequency decrease was greater in patients with frequent recurrences than in patients with more spaced episodes. This trial also included 14 patients with primary herpes, 2 facial and 12 genital: twelve of these had no recurrence during the year following the treatment of the first episode (2 genital herpes patients having recurrences at 30 and 240 days). In comparison, treatment of the first episode by oral acyclovir had no effect on the rate of subsequent recurrences or on the time to first recurrence (22). Topical acyclovir is not considered today as an efficient treatment to suppress herpes simplex recurrences (28,29) and Iododeoxyuridine cream also had no effect on time to healing and recurrence rate (28). Thus IFN-β seems to be at present the only agent effective topically on recurrent herpes simplex cutaneous infections.

In topical use, IFN-β cream or gel was practically devoid of side effects. The local application of IFN is not only convenient but may be a condition for efficacy of IFN therapy of recurrent herpes. Indeed, Eron et al. (12) reported that $3 \times 10^7$ units of recombinant IFN-α2b given systemically by subcutaneous injections had no effect on frequency or duration of recurrences in genital herpes. One possible explanation is that even at these high doses of IFN injected systemically, the serum levels are only about 100 U/ml after 4-6 hours (15). With topical IFN, doses of $10^4$ units can be achieved with 0.1 g of ointment applied directly on the lesions several times a day. The non-intact skin probably facilitates contact of the protein with the target cells. Others also recently reported beneficial

effects of topical IFN  on herpetic skin lesions  (14).
We know very little about the mechanism by which  IFN-β
acts on the herpes simplex recurrent infections. It  is
likely that in addition to the antiviral effect on  HSV
replication seen in cultured cells and in the  herpetic
vesicles (2,25),  effects on  the  immune response  are
involved which may include increase in HLA on the  cell
surface, enhanced antigen  presentation and more  efficient killing  of  virus infected  cells  by  activated
killer  lymphocytes  and  monocytes  (26,31).  Cellular
immunity appears  important in  recurrent herpes  cutaneous infections  (30,34). The  antiviral effect  could
help reducing recurrences by a reduction in the  amount
of virus  which  replicates  in the  skin  lesions  and
thereafter a  reduced reinfection  of  neurones by  the
ascending route  (19). In  mice, it  has been  observed
that after HSV inoculation, virus can be isolated  from
contralateral ganglions and also in lymphnodes  serving
the inoculation site; a diffusion of virus through  the
lymphatic system has been  considered to explain  these
experimental results (19). This may explain why topical
IFN-β treatment is better than systemic IFN injections,
since topical treatment could prevent dissemination  in
lymphnodes (19) and uptake of IFN-β through the  lymphatic system has been observed in rabbits (7). The  fact
that a potent inhibitor of HSV replication as acyclovir
is not effective topically further supports the  notion
that a combined immune  and antiviral effect is at  the
base of topical IFN-β efficacy on herpes recurrences.
     Our study shows that about one third of the patients
in the double-blind  trial and in  the phase IV  study,
had no recurrence for  at least a  year after a  single
course of  topical  IFN-β applications  of  10-15  days
during an eruption.  Although this is  a far from  complete cure, it suggests  that higher doses of IFN-β  or
combinations with  other biological  modifiers such  as
IFN-γ and TFN-α or  β, which have been shown to help the
immune system  to  kill virus-infected  cells  (1),  in
particular HSV-infected cells (21), should be tried  to
further improve  the  fraction of  recurrence-free  patients. Combinations  of IFN cream  with acyclovir  may
also be of interest as the two compounds show synergism
(13). The  first  results of  a  double-blind  placebo-
controlled and phase IV  trials presented here  already
warrant to consider the use of IFN-β cream as a simple,
convenient and effective way of treatment for  recurrent
facial and genital herpes.

## REFERENCES

1. Aderka, D.,  Novick, D., Hahn,  T., Fischer,  D.G.,
   and  Wallach, D.  (1985):  Cell.  Immunol.,  92:
   218-225.

2. Armstrong, J.A., Skicki-Mullen, M.B., Breinig, M.K., and Ho, M. (1983): Antimicrob. Agents Chemother., 24: 137-139.
3. Aurelian, L. (1986): In: Herpes and Papilloma Viruses, edited by G. De Palo, F. Rilke, and H. zur Hausen, pp. 63-82, Raven Press, New York.
4. Baringer, J.R. (1974): N. Engl. J. Med., 291: 828-830.
5. Baringer, J.R., and Swolevand, P. (1973): N. Engl. J. Med., 288: 648-650.
6. Barton, I.G., Kinghorn, G.R., Rowland, M., Jeavons, M., Al-Omer, L.S., and Potter, C.W. (1984): Antiviral Res., 4: 293-300.
7. Bocci, V. (1985): Immunol. Today, 6: 7-9.
8. Corey, L., Adams, H.G., Baron, Z.A., and Holmes, K.K. (1983): Ann. Intern. Med., 98: 958-972.
9. Corey, L., Benedetti, J.K., Critchlow, C.W., et al. (1982): Am. J. Med., 73: 326-334.
10. Douglas, J.M., Critchlow, C., Benedetti, J., Mertz, G.J., Connor, J.D., Hintz, M.A., Fahnlander, A., Remington, M., Winter, C., and Corey, L. (1984): N. Engl. J. Med., 310: 1551-1556.
11. Embil, J.A., Stephens, R.G., and Manuel, F.R. (1975): Can. Med. Assoc. J., 113: 627-635.
12. Eron, L.J., Harvey, L., Toy, C., and Santomauro, D. (1986): Antimicrob. Agents Chemother., 30: 608-610.
13. Fraser-Smith, E.B., Eppstein, D.A., Marsh, Y.V., and Matthews, T.R. (1984): Antimicrob. Agents Chemother., 25: 563-565.
14. Friedman-Kien, A.E., Klein, R.J., Glaser, R.D., and Czelusniak, S.M. (1986): J. Am. Acad. Dermatol., 15: 989-995.
15. Gutterman, J.U., Fine, S., Quesada, J., Horning, S., Levine, J.F., Alexanian, R., Bernhardt, L., Kramer, M., Spiegel, H., Colburn, W., Trown, P., Merigan, T., and Dziewanowski, Z. (1982): Ann. Intern. Med., 96: 549-556.
16. Ikic, P., Smerdel, S., Rajninger-Miholic, M., Soos, E., and Jusic, D. (1975): In: Symposium on Clinical Use of Interferon. Proc. Yugoslav Acad. Sci. and Arts, pp. 195-202.
17. Isacsohn, M., Berson, B., Sternberg, I., and Morag, A. (1983): Isr. J. Med. Sci., 19: 959-962.
18. Kinghorn, G.R., Turner, E.B., Barton, I.G., Potter, C.W., Burke, C.A., and Fiddian, A.P. (1983): Antiviral Res., 3: 291-301.
19. Klein, R.J. (1985): Antiviral Res. Suppl., 1: 111-120.
20. Knight, E., and Fahey, D. (1981): J. Biol. Chem., 256: 3609-3611.
21. Koff, W.C., and Fann, A.V. (1986): Lymphokine Res., 5: 215-222.

22. Mertz, G.J., Critchlow, C.W., Benedetti, J., Reichman, R.C., Dolin, R., Connor, J., Redfield, D.C., Savoia, M.C., Richman, D.D., Tyrrel, D.L., Miedzinski, L., Portnoy, J., Keeney, R.E., and Corey, L. (1984): JAMA, 252: 1147-1151.
23. Mindel, A., Faherty, A., Hindley, D., Weller, I.V.D., Sutherland, S., Fiddian, A.P., and Adler, M.W. (1984): Lancet, ii: 57-59.
24. Moller, B., and Berg, K. (1983): 2nd International TNO Meeting on the Biology of the Interferon System. Abstracts P10b.
25. Movshovitz, M., Schewach-Millet, M., Kriss-Leventon, S., Shoham, J., Doerner, T., and Revel, M. (1985): In: Herpes Viruses Chemotherapy, edited by R. Kono, pp. 285-292. Elsevier Science Publishers, Amsterdam.
26. Munoz, A., Carrasco, L., and Fresno, M. (1983): J. Immunol. 131: 783-787.
27. Novick, D., Eshhar, Z., Gigi, O., Marks, Z., Revel, M., and Rubinstein, M. (1983): J. Gen. Virol., 64: 905-910.
28. Reichman, R.C. (1985): In: Herpes Viruses Chemotherapy, edited by R. Kono, pp. 149-154, Elsevier Science Publishers, Amsterdam.
29. Shaw, M., King, M., Best, J.M., Banatvala, A.A., Gibson, J.R., and Klaber, M.R. (1985): Br. Med. J., 291: 7-9.
30. Sheridan, J.F., Beck, M., Aurelian, L., and Radowsky, M. (1985): J. Infect. DIs., 152: 449-456.
31. Stanwick, T.L., Campbell, D.E., and Nahmias, A.J. (1982): Cell. Immunol., 70: 132-140.
32. Strauss, S.E., Takiff, H.E., Seidlin, M., Bachrach, S., Lininger, L., DiGiovanna, J.J., Western, K.A., Smith, H.A., Lehrman, S.N., Creagh-Kirk, T., and Alling, D.W. (1984): N. Engl. J. Med., 310: 1545-1550.
33. Strauss, S.E., Seidlin, M., Takiff, H.E., Rooney, J.F., Lehrman, S.N., Bachrach, S., Felser, J.M., DiGiovanna, J.J., Grimes, G.J., Krakauer, H., Hallaha, C., and Alling, D. (1986): Antiviral Res., 6: 151-159.
34. Torseth, J.W., and Merigan, T.C. (1986): J. Infect. Dis., 153: 979-984.

# Interferon Therapy in Laryngeal Papillomatosis

## A. Bomholt

*ENT Department, Roskilde Hospital, Roskilde, Denmark*

Many forms of therapy have been advocated for laryngeal papillomatosis. The most important of these has been, and appears to remain, surgery. The most dramatic symptom in laryngeal papillomatosis is upper airway obstruction and the only way to achieve immediate relief is by surgical removal of the papillomas. Until 30–40 years ago this was done without general anaesthesia. The technique used in direct laryngoscopy was at that time not as refined as today and the light in the laryngoscope was of poor quality. Consequently, it was difficult to identify the fine structures of the larynx and to perform a precise removal of the papillomas. Inadequate removal of papillomas and scarring of the larynx explain very well why direct laryngoscopy was often combined with tracheotomy, especially in children.

A breakthrough in surgery was achieved in the 1960's with the introduction of the binocular operating microscope. Prior to this introduction, the attitude in favour of general anaesthesia gained ground, and the situation was thereby considerably improved for the patient.

The most recent surgical advance has been the introduction of the $CO_2$ laser. This technique is undoubtedly superior in some respects to microsurgical removal. Thus, the laser makes it possible to perform precise evaporization of papillomas with minimal or no bleeding, and the risk of scarring or damaging the fine structures of the larynx is thereby minimized. In addition, it produces little adjacent tissue reaction, for which reason immediate postoperative complications, especially airway obstruction, are rare. The laser technique cannot be considered a curative treatment and a positive effect on the recurrence rate has as yet not been demonstrated (7).

Irradiation was introduced in the 1920's and was hoped to be effective in cases of papillomas showing an unusual tendency to recur rapidly. Treatment was given in a dosage almost as great as that which was used for carcinoma (9). Several years later, malignant degeneration of papillomas was noted in patients having received irradiation to the neck (12). In other patients, the growth of the larynx was arrested and, consequently, the larynx became stenotic. Fortunately, this treatment was abandoned in the 1950's.

The introduction of several topical and systemic medications emphasizes the demand for an adjuvant to surgical management. The various agents include steroid hormones, antibiotics, antimetabolites, bleomycin, podophyllum and various types of vaccine. None of these agents have gained ground in the daily clinic.

Interferons are proteins produced and secreted from certain cells which have been exposed to viruses, double stranded RNA, mitogens or small molecular weight agents (14). Interferon was first described in 1957 by Isaacs and Lindenmann (8).

Interferons possess a wide range of biological properties, including antiviral activity, antiproliferative effects, alterations of cell membrane receptors and antigens, and variety of profound effects on the immune system (13).

The first clinical study on interferon therapy for juvenile laryngeal papillomatosis was reported in 1981 by Haglund et al. (6). The original idea of treating laryngeal papillomas was based on an observation made in 1971. In a patient suffering from cervical carcinoma in situ, it was noted that plantar warts disappeared during interferon treatment. Because of the supposed common viral etiology of plantar warts and juvenile laryngeal papillomas, a pilot study was started in 1976. The study comprised 7 patients, most of whom were infants with an aggressive tumour growth requiring numerous endoscopic removals of papillomas. Some of the patients were tracheotomized. The initial dose of interferon was 3 mill. IU given by IM injections 3 times weekly. In the first two cases, tumour tissue was not removed before interferon treatment was initiated and a dramatic reduction of tumour massess was noted. The remaining patients underwent endoscopic removal of as much of the papillomatous tumour masses as possible before interferon treatment was initiated. During treatment, lasting from 12 to 21 months, tumour control was achieved in all 7 cases. The Swedish group concluded from the study that tumour growth could be controlled, that regrowth occurred when interferon was decreased or discontinued, that papillomas regressed when interferon was increased or reinitiated, and that the papillomas showed degeneration in response to interferon treatment. It remained, however, to be determined what doses and which time schedules should be used in order to achieve optimal results.

This study was soon after followed by two American studies, the findings of which confirmed those of the Swedish study (5,11). As a result of the early positive results in children, a study on treatment of adult patients was conducted in Denmark (1). Eight patients were treated for three weeks with a low dose of interferon prior to surgery. The results showed reduced tumour size in 5 cases. Following surgery, the interferon dose was increased and during the postsurgical treatment lasting 5 months, small papillomas were noted in only 1 patient. However, follow-up evaluations 7-11 months after treatment showed recurrence in 4 patients.

Because of the study design with interferon treatment prior to surgery, histological and ultrastructural studies were performed (3,4). The principal light microscopical findings in the interferon treated papillomas comprised: increased atypia, change in intraepithelial differentiation, sclerosis of the underlying stroma and infiltration of plasma cells, in particular. Compared with untreated papillomas, no difference in ultrastructure was found by transmission electron microscopy. By scanning electron microscopy significant alterations, comprising a smooth and oedematous surface with a uniform microvilli pattern of the superficial cells, were observed after interferon therapy.

These 4 pilot studies have been followed by other uncontrolled studies. It is noteworthy, however, that treatment of less than 100 patients has been reported from 1981 to 1985. In September 1986, an open-labelled, randomized, cross-over study, comprising 66 patients, was reported at a meeting in Finland and showed a statistically proven effectiveness of interferon (10).

It has often been reported that patients treated with interferon will experience side effects. Few hours after systemic administration the body temperature will rise and the patient will experience influenza-like symptoms. The attack normally lasts a few hours and in the course of treatment this reaction will subside. A decrease in WBC is often noted, but it returns to normal values if the dose is reduced or treatment discontinued. Similar observations have been made with respect to liver toxicity. Mild erythema may occur but serious allergic reactions to treatment have not been reported. Apart from the initial rise in temperature, fatique seems to be the most troublesome reaction. However, patients with a good response to treatment will often experience a greater degree of well-being because of the improvement of voice and sustained free airways. Only few patients have not been able to tolerate or accept interferon treatment and fatal complications have not been reported.

## CONCLUSION

Papilloma growth can in most cases be controlled by interferon, but recurrence will often occur when treatment is discontinued. Interferon therapy can only be considered an adjuvant to surgical management. The optimal dose-time schedules have still to be determined. The treatment is safe and well-tolerated in most cases.

The good prognosis of most cases of laryngeal papillomatosis should be taken into consideration when selecting patients for treatment (2). Interferon adjuvant therapy seems particularly justified in patients with long-lasting and aggressive tumour growth or when the disease cannot be controlled by surgery alone.

## REFERENCES

1. Bomholt, A. (1983): Arch. Otolaryngol., 109: 550–552.
2. Bomholt, A. (1987): Laryngeal papillomatosis. Raven Press (this volume).
3. Bomholt, A., and Horn, T.(1985): Acta Otolaryngol., 100: 304–308.
4. Bomholt, A., Ostergaard, B., and Horn, T. (1986): Acta Otolaryngol., 102: 131–135.
5. Goepfert, H., Sessions, R.B., Gutterman, J.U., Cangir, A., Dichtel, W.J., and Sulek, M. (1982): Ann. Otol. Rhinol. Laryngol., 91: 431–436.
6. Haglund, S., Lundquist, P.G., Cantell, K., and Strander, H. (1981): Arch. Otolaryngol., 107: 327–332.
7. Irwin, B.C., Hendrickse, W.A., Pincott, J.R., Bailey, C.M., and Evans, J.N. (1986): J. Laryngol. Otol., 100: 435–445.
8. Isaac, A., and Lindenmann, J. (1957): Proc. R. Soc. Lond., 147: 258.
9. Jackson, C., and Jackson, C. (1945): Diseases of the Nose, Throat and Ear. W.B. Saunders Co., Philadelphia.
10. Kashima, H.K., Leventhal, B., Whisnant, J.K., and Weck, P.K. (1986): The 1986 ISIR-TNO Meeting of the Interferon System. J. Interferon Research 6, suppl. 1.
11. McCabe, B.F., and Clark, K.F. (1983): Ann. Otol. Rhinol. Laryngol., 92: 2–7.
12. Rabbet, W.F. (1965): Ann. Otol., 74: 1149–1163.
13. Stewart, W.E. (1981): The interferon system. Springer Verlag, New York.
14. Torrence, P.F., and De Clercq, E. (1977): Pharmacol. Ther., 2: 1–7.

# Subject Index